FMGEMS
COMPREHENSIVE
EXAMINATION
REVIEW

FMGEMS

COMPREHENSIVE

EXAMINATION

REVIEW

1458 MULTIPLE-CHOICE QUESTIONS AND
REFERENCED, EXPLANATORY ANSWERS

SIXTH
EDITION

Prepared by a Board of 51
Distinguished Physicians and Educators

MEDICAL EXAMINATION PUBLISHING COMPANY

Medical Examination Publishing Company
A Division of Elsevier Science Publishing Company, Inc.
52 Vanderbilt Avenue, New York, New York 10017

© 1986 by Elsevier Science Publishing Company, Inc.

This book has been registered with the Copyright Clearance Center, Inc. For further information, please contact the Copyright Clearance Center, Salem, Massachusetts.

Library of Congress Cataloging in Publication Data

ECFMG/FMG examination review.
   FMGEMS comprehensive examination review.

   1. Medicine—Examinations, questions, etc.
I. Title. [DNLM: 1. Foreign Medical Graduates.
2. Medicine—examination questions.   W 18 E17]
R834.5.E25   1986   610.76   86-13542
ISBN 0-444-01050-5

Current printing (last digit)
10 9 8 7 6 5 4 3

Manufactured in the United States of America

Contents

About the Authors

Part 1

Michael A. Baker, M.D., F.R.C.P.(C), F.A.C.P., *Professor of Medicine*, University of Toronto, *Director of Oncology and Hematology*, Toronto General Hospital, Toronto, Ontario, Canada

Sidney A. Cohn, Ph.D., *Professor Emeritus*, Department of Anatomy, The University of Tennessee Center for the Health Sciences, Memphis, Tennessee

Ivan Damjanov, M.D., *Professor of Pathology*, Hahnemann University School of Medicine, Philadelphia, Pennsylvania

Louis E. Grenzer, M.D., P.A., *Instructor*, Department of Medicine, Mercy Hospital, Saint Joseph Hospital, and University of Maryland Medical School, Baltimore, Maryland

Charles W. Kim, M.S.P.H., Ph.D., *Assistant Professor of Medicine and Microbiology*, School of Medicine, Health Sciences Center, State University of New York at Stony Brook, Stony Brook, New York

Leonard J. Kryston, M.D., *Assistant Cinical Professor of Medicine*, University of Pennsylvania School of Medicine, *Head*, Endocrine Section, Division of Medicine, Pennsylvania Hospital, Philadelphia, Pennsylvania

N. LeRoy Lapp, M.D., *Professor of Medicine*, Pulmonary Disease Section, Department of Medicine, West Virginia University Medical Center, Morgantown, West Virginia

John R. McCullough, Ph.D., *Senior Scientist*, Inflammation/ Atherosclerosis Research, Pharmaceuticals Division, Ciba-Geigy Corporation, Summit, New Jersey

Alvin E. Parrish, M.D., F.A.C.P., *Professor of Medicine*, The George Washington University Medical Center, Washington, D.C.

Edward L. Petsonk, M.D., *Assistant Professor of Medicine*, Pulmonary Disease Section, Department of Medicine, West Virginia University Medical Center, Morgantown, West Virginia

James L. Poland, Ph.D., *Associate Professor*, Department of Physiology and Biophysics, Medical College of Virginia, Health Sciences Division, Virginia Commonwealth University, Richmond, Virginia

William Pryse-Phillips, M.D., F.R.C.P., F.R.C.P.(C), *Professor of Medicine (Neurology)*, Memorial University of Newfoundland, St. John's, Newfoundland, Canada

Martin J. Raff, M.D., *Professor of Medicine, Assistant Professor of Microbiology, Chief*, Section of Infectious Diseases, Department of Medicine, University of Louisville School of Medicine, Louisville, Kentucky

Joseph Renn, M.D., *Clinical Associate Professor of Medicine*, Pulmonary Disease Section, Department of Medicine, West Virginia University Medical Center, Morgantown, West Virginia

Sanford Simon, Ph.D., *Associate Professor of Biochemistry*, Department of Biochemistry, School of Medicine, Health Sciences Center, State University of New York at Stony Brook, Stony Brook, New York

William A. Sodeman, Jr., M.D., *Deputy Dean for Academic Affairs, Professor and Chairman*, Department of Comprehensive Medicine, University of South Florida College of Medicine, Tampa, Florida

Peter C. Ungaro, M.D., *Professor of Medicine*, Divisions of Hematology and Oncology, University of North Carolina School of Medicine; *Associate Chief*, University Medical Service, New Hanover Memorial Hospital, Wilmington, North Carolina

Steven J. Wees, M.D., F.A.C.P., *Assistant Clinical Professor of Internal Medicine*, University of Nebraska College of Medicine, Omaha, Nebraska

Part 2

Barbara Ann Allen, M.S.W., Ph.D., *Clinical Associate Professor*, Department of Psychiatry and Behavioral Sciences, University of Oklahoma, Tulsa Medical College, Tulsa, Oklahoma

James R. Allen, M.D., F.R.C.P.(C), *Professor and Chairman*, Department of Psychiatry and Behavioral Sciences, University of Oklahoma, Tulsa Medical College; Chief of Staff, Children's Medical Center, Tulsa, Oklahoma

Lawrence W. Brown, M.D., *Associate Professor of Pediatrics and Neurology*, The Medical College of Pennsylvania, Philadelphia, Pennsylvania

Cheng T. Cho, M.D., Ph.D., *Professor*, Department of Pediatrics, Infectious Diseases, The University of Kansas College of Health Sciences and Hospital, Kansas City, Kansas

William P. Coleman III, M.D., *Associate Clinical Professor of Dermatology*, Tulane University School of Medicine, New Orleans, Louisiana

John W. Downing, Jr., M.D., F.A.C.C., *Professor of Pediatrics*, Howard University College of Medicine, Washington, D.C.

Ralph W. Hale, M.D., *Professor and Chairman*, Department of Obstetrics and Gynecology, University of Hawaii at Manoa, John

A. Burns School of Medicine, Kapiolani—Children's Medical Center, Honolulu, Hawaii

Aram S. Hanissian, M.D., *Pediatric Rheumatologist*, Baptist Memorial Hospital East, Memphis, Tennessee

Charles E. Hollerman, M.D., *Chairman*, Department of Pediatrics, Mercy Hospital, Pittsburgh, Pennsylvania

Wellington Hung, M.D., Ph.D., *Professor of Child Health and Development*, George Washington University School of Medicine and Health Sciences; *Chairman*, Department of Endocrinology and Metabolism, Children's Hospital National Medical Center, Washington, D.C.

Leslie Iffy, M.D., *Professor of Obstetrics and Gynecology*, University of Medicine and Dentistry of New Jersey, New Jersey Medical School; *Director*, Division of Maternal-Fetal Medicine, Newark, New Jersey

Stephen A. Koff, M.D., *Associate Professor and Chief*, Pediatric Urology, The Ohio State University Children's Hospital, Columbus, Ohio

Frederick M. Karrer, M.D., *Instructor in Surgery*, Pediatric Surgery Research Fellow, University of Colorado School of Medicine, Denver, Colorado

Michael I. Kulick, D.D.S., M.D., Plastic and Reconstructive Surgery, San Francisco, California

Albin B. Leong, M.D., *Clinical Assistant Professor*, Department of Pediatrics, University of California, Davis, School of Medicine, Davis; *Pediatric Pulmonologist/Allergist*, Kaiser Permanente Medical Center, Sacramento, California

William M. Liebman, M.D., *Director*, Pediatric Gastroenterology, Children's Hospital Medical Center of Northern California (Oakland) and of San Francisco, California

John R. Lilly, M.D., *Professor of Surgery,* University of Colorado School of Medicine; *Chief,* Pediatric Surgery, University Hospital, Denver, Colorado

Kimball I. Maull, M.D., *Professor and Chairman,* Department of Surgery, University of Tennessee Memorial Research Center and Hospital, Knoxville, Tennessee

W. Frederick McGuirt, M.D., *Associate Professor of Otolaryngology,* The Bowman Gray School of Medicine of Wake Forest University, North Carolina Baptist Hospital, Winston-Salem, North Carolina

James G. McMurtry III, M.D., *Associate Professor of Clinical Neurological Surgery,* Columbia University; *Associate Attending Physician of Clinical Neurological Surgery,* Neurological Institute, Columbia Presbyterian Medical Center; *Chief,* Neurological Surgery, Lenox Hill Hospital, New York, New York

Henry S. Metz M.D., *Professor and Chairman,* Department of Ophthalmology, University of Rochester School of Medicine and Dentistry, Rochester, New York

Thomas D. Miale, M.D., *Chief,* Pediatric Hematology-Oncology, Department of Pediatrics, Southern Illinois University School of Medicine, Springfield, Illinois

J. David Moorehead, M.D., *Assistant Professor of Urology,* Loma Linda University School of Medicine, *Pediatric Urologist,* Loma Linda University Medical Center, Loma Linda, California

Alan E. Oestreich, M.D., Division of Radiology, Children's Hospital Medical Center, Cincinnati, Ohio

Shirley K. Osterhout, M.D., *Assistant Professor,* Department of Pediatrics, Duke University School of Medicine; *Director,* Duke Poison Control Center; *Assistant Dean for Student Affairs,* Duke University School of Medicine, Durham, North Carolina

M. D. Ram, B.Sc., M.D., M.S. (Surg.), Ph.D., F.R.C.S. (Eng.), F.R.C.S. (Ed.), F.R.C.S. (Can.), F.A.C.S., *Professor of Surgery and Surgeon,* Albert B. Chandler Medical Center, University of Kentucky College of Medicine; *Chief,* Surgical Service, Veterans Administration Medical Center, Lexington, Kentucky

Raymond M. Russo, M.D., F.A.A.P., *Professor of Pediatrics,* University of Medicine and Dentistry of New Jersey, Rutgers Medical School, Piscataway; *Chief,* Ambulatory Services, Robert Wood Johnson-University Hospital, New Brunswick, New Jersey

James R. Ryan, M.D., *Associate Professor,* Department of Orthopedic Surgery, Wayne State University School of Medicine, Detroit, Michigan

R. Michael Sly, M.D., *Professor of Child Health and Development,* George Washington University School of Medicine and Health Sciences; *Director of Allergy and Immunology,* Children's Hospital National Medical Center, Washington, D.C.

Richard J. Thurer, M.D., *Professor of Surgery, Thoracic and Cardiovascular Surgery,* University of Miami School of Medicine, Miami, Florida

Jorge E. Uceda, M.D., *Assistant Clinical Professor of Surgery,* The University of Texas Health Science Center at Dallas, Southwestern Medical School, Dallas, Texas

John E. Williams, M.D., *Clinical Assistant Professor of Pediatrics,* University of Medicine and Dentistry of New Jersey, New Jersey Medical School; *Associate Director and Chief,* Section of Developmental and Behavioral Pediatrics, Institute for Child Development, Hackensack Medical Center, Newark, New Jersey

Raymond O. West, M.D., M.P.H., *Adjunct Professor of Epidemiology,* Loma Linda University School of Health, Loma Linda, California

Preface

FMGEMS Comprehensive Examination Review is designed as a study aid for candidates preparing to take the Foreign Medical Graduate Examination in the Medical Sciences.

The examination is administered semiannually in centers throughout the world. It is a comprehensive exam whose purpose is to both test and develop the candidate's acumen in the principal fields of medicine. The examination comprises several question types: one best response, matching, modified matching, multiple true-false, and situation. Because the *FMGEMS Comprehensive Examination Review* closely simulates the exam in both content and format, the reader can become familar and comfortable with the actual test experience. In this sense, both Parts 1 and 2 of the *FMGEMS Comprehensive Examination Review* are an invaluable aid.

Part 1 covers in 718 questions the basic sciences of anatomy, biochemistry, microbiology, pathology, pharmacology, and physiology, as well as the specialties of internal medicine, cardiology, endocrinology, gastroenterology, hematology, infectious diseases, nephrology, neurology, oncology, pulmonary medicine, and rheumatology. Part 2 covers in 740 questions the specialties of pediatrics, obstetrics and gynecology, surgery, psychiatry, and public health and community medicine. Each answer is fully explained and referenced to current major works in the field. Candidates are urged to pursue these sources for further concentrated study.

Acknowledgments

I would like to take this opportunity to thank all of the Contributing Authors for taking time out of their busy schedules to prepare this review book. You have touched my life, and I know your efforts will be appreciated by those who use this book in preparing for their exam.

Thank you,

Lisa M. Teitz
Former Associate Editor, MEPC

Disclaimer

The authors have made every effort to thoroughly verify the answers to the questions which appear on the following pages. However, as in any text, some inaccuracies and ambiguities may occur; therefore, if in doubt, please consult your references.

The Publisher

FMGEMS
COMPREHENSIVE
EXAMINATION
REVIEW

BASIC
SCIENCES

1
Anatomy
Sidney A. Cohn, Ph.D.

DIRECTIONS: Each of the questions or incomplete statements below is followed by five suggested answers or completions. Select the **one** that is best in each case.

1.1. Each of the following muscles plays an important role in flexion of the humerus EXCEPT the
  A. coracobrachialis
  B. subscapularis
  C. deltoid
  D. pectoralis major
  E. biceps brachii

1.2. The important sinoatrial nodal artery of the heart is usually a branch of the
  A. left coronary
  B. circumflex
  C. right coronary
  D. anterior interventricular
  E. posterior interventricular

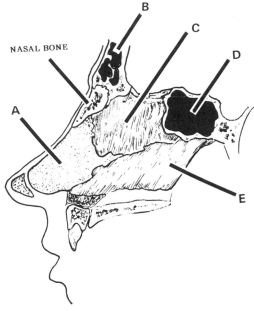

Figure 1

1.3. Each of the lettered structures in Figure 1 forms a major portion of the nasal septum EXCEPT the
 A. septal cartilage
 B. frontal bone
 C. ethmoid bone
 D. sphenoid bone
 E. vomer bone

1.4. Each of the following structures is located in both the superior and posterior mediastina EXCEPT the
 A. vagus nerve
 B. phrenic nerve
 C. thoracic duct
 D. esophagus
 E. azygos vein

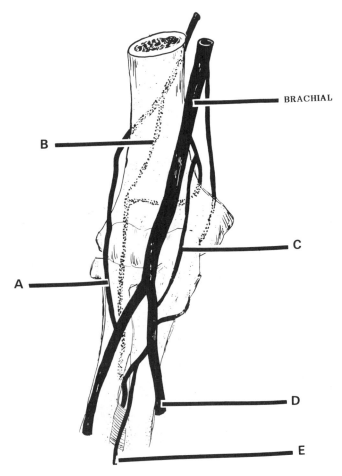

BRACHIAL

B

C

A

D

E

Figure 2

1.5. Each of the lettered arteries in Figure 2 is correctly identified
below EXCEPT the
   A. radial collateral
   B. middle collateral
   C. posterior ulnar collateral
   D. ulnar
   E. anterior interosseous

1.6. The greater petrosal nerve, a branch of the facial nerve, supplies parasympathetic innervation to glands in each of the following regions EXCEPT the
   A. soft palate
   B. lacrimal gland
   C. nasal mucosa
   D. hard palate
   E. parotid gland

1.7. The muscles of the anterior compartment of the leg consist of all of the following EXCEPT the
   A. peroneus tertius
   B. extensor hallucis longus
   C. extensor digitorum longus
   D. peroneus longus
   E. tibialis anterior

1.8. One of the most frequent types of epithelial attachments is known as the
   A. desmosome
   B. lysosome
   C. ribosome
   D. centrosome
   E. peroxisome

1.9. Which of the following hormones produced by the anterior hypophysis stimulates body growth?
   A. Lactogenic hormone
   B. Luteinizing hormone
   C. Adrenocorticotrophic hormone
   D. Somatotrophic hormone
   E. Thyrotrophic

1.10. Each of the following organs is lined by stratified squamous epithelium EXCEPT the
   A. ureter
   B. pharynx
   C. vagina
   D. hard palate
   E. esophagus

1.11. The adult red bone marrow gives rise to each of the following cells of the blood EXCEPT the
  A. erythrocyte
  B. monocyte
  C. neutrophil
  D. basophil
  E. eosinophil

1.12. The cerebellar cortex contains each of the following nerve cell types EXCEPT the
  A. purkinje
  B. stellate
  C. basket
  D. satellite
  E. granule

1.13. The carotid sinus, a baroreceptor that responds to changes in blood pressure, is associated with the
  A. facial nerve
  B. vagus nerve
  C. glossopharyngeal nerve
  D. trigeminal nerve
  E. accessory nerve

1.14. Lesions of the spinal trigeminal tract would probably result in loss of
  A. two-point discrimination
  B. pain sense
  C. taste
  D. pressure sense
  E. kinesthesis

1.15. Which of the following is the most common type of anorectal malformation?
  A. Anal agenesis
  B. Membranous atresia
  C. Anorectal agenesis
  D. Rectal atresia
  E. Anal stenosis

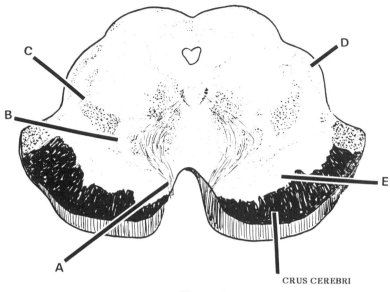

Figure 3

1.16. Each of the lettered structures in Figure 3 is correctly identified below EXCEPT the
   A. abducens nerve
   B. red nucleus
   C. medial meniscus
   D. brachium of inferior colliculus
   E. substantia nigra

DIRECTIONS: The group of questions below consists of five lettered headings followed by a list of numbered words or statements. For each numbered word or statement, select the **one** lettered heading that is most closely associated with it. Each lettered heading may be selected once, more than once, or not at all.

Match each muscle with the type of action it produces at the hip joint.
   A. Abduction
   B. Flexion
   C. Medial rotation
   D. Lateral rotation
   E. Adduction

1.17. Gracilis

1.18. Iliopsoas

1.19. Quadratus femoris

1.20. Rectus femoris

1.21. Biceps femoris

DIRECTIONS: The set of lettered headings below is followed by a list of numbered words or phrases. For each numbered word or phrase select
   (A) if the item is associated with A only
   (B) if the item is associated with B only
   (C) if the item is associated with both A and B
   (D) if the item is associated with neither A nor B

   A. The functional component for taste (SVA) is associated with this cranial nerve
   B. The functional component for branchial arch musculature (SVE) is associated with this cranial nerve
   C. Both
   D. Neither

1.22. Facial

1.23. Trigeminal

1.24. Vagus

1.25. Oculomotor

1.26. Accessory

DIRECTIONS: For each of the questions or incomplete statements below, **one or more** of the answers or completions given is correct. Select
- **(A)** if only 1, 2, and 3 are correct
- **(B)** if only 1 and 3 are correct
- **(C)** if only 2 and 4 are correct
- **(D)** if only 4 is correct
- **(E)** if all are correct.

1.27. The organelles that are found in the cytoplasm include
1. ribosomes
2. endoplasmic reticulum
3. Golgi apparatus
4. secretory granules

1.28. Cells associated with the gastric glands of the stomach are the
1. parietal cells
2. goblet cells
3. chief cells
4. paneth cells

1.29. Syndactyly, a condition in which the digits are webbed or fused, is
1. most commonly seen between the third and fourth fingers
2. seen more often in the foot than in the hand
3. the most common limb malformation
4. due to hereditary factors

1.30. Muscles innervated by the ulnar nerve include the
1. pronator teres
2. supinator
3. extensor carpi ulnaris
4. adductor pollicis

1.31. The hypothalamus has afferent connections with the
1. anterior thalamic nucleus
2. stria terminalis
3. medial forebrain bundle
4. fornix

DIRECTIONS: This section of the test consists of a situation followed by a series of questions. Study the situation and select the **one** best answer to each question following it.

Questions 1.32–1.36: A young man was driving into town with his 22-year-old date. As he entered an intersection, a car in the opposing traffic lane ran a red light and hit the passenger side of his car broadside. His date was severely injured. Upon radiologic examination at the hospital, her right humerus showed an oblique fracture through the middle of the shaft. Neurologic examination revealed a loss of ability to extend the forearm and wrist drop. There was a cutaneous loss over the dorsum of the thumb, index, and middle fingers. The resident in the emergency room removed a tourniquet that had been applied to her arm at the scene of the accident, and noted blood spurting from a laceration in the region of the anatomic snuffbox.

1.32. Fractures through the middle of the humeral shaft would probably involve which of the following bony landmarks?
A. Deltoid tuberosity
B. Surgical neck
C. Radial groove
D. Medial epicondyle
E. Olecranon

1.33. The artery, which appears to be lacerated in the anatomic snuffbox, is the
A. radial
B. ulnar
C. brachial
D. superficial radial nerve
E. middle collateral

1.34. The cutaneous loss over the dorsum of the hand is probably due to a loss of the
  A. dorsal cutaneous branch of the ulnar nerve
  B. digital branches of the median nerve
  C. posterior antebrachial cutaneous nerve
  D. superficial radial nerve
  E. digital branches of the ulnar nerve

1.35. Inability to extend the forearm would most likely indicate paralysis of the
  A. coracobrachialis muscle
  B. brachialis muscle
  C. triceps brachii muscle
  D. extensor carpi radialis muscle
  E. extensor digitorum muscle

1.36. Injury to which of the following nerves is most likely to result in wrist drop?
  A. Musculocutaneous
  B. Ulnar
  C. Median
  D. Radial
  E. Axillary

Answers and Comments

1.1. **(B)** Flexion of the humerus takes place through the actions of the anterior fibers of the deltoid, the clavicular fibers of the pectoralis major, the biceps brachii, and the coracobrachialis muscles. The subscapularis is involved in extension, adduction, and medial rotation of the humerus (Ref. 2, p. 132).

1.2. **(C)** The sinoatrial nodal artery, which supplies the specialized myocardium, the sinoatrial node, the structure responsible for initiation of the heart beat, is usually a branch of the right coronary artery (Ref. 2, p. 337).

1.3. **(B)** The major portion of the nasal septum is formed by the septal cartilage and by contributions from the ethmoid, vomer, sphenoid, maxilla, and palatine bones. The frontal bone has only a minor contribution to the septum (Ref. 1, pp. 173–174).

1.4. (B) The phrenic nerve descends from the neck into the superior mediastinum by passing superficially to the subclavian artery. It then enters the middle mediastinum by passing anteriorly to the root of the lung (Ref. 2, pp. 321, 334−335).

1.5. (C) The collateral circulation around the elbow involves anastomoses between branches of the deep brachial arteries with branches of the ulnar and radial arteries. The artery wrongly identified in Figure 2 is the anterior ulnar recurrent (Ref. 1, p. 718).

1.6. (E) The parotid gland receives its parasympathetic innervation from the lesser petrosal nerve, a branch of the glossopharyngeal nerve. The other regions listed, as well as a part of the nasal pharynx and paranasal sinuses, are innervated by the greater petrosal nerve (Ref. 2, pp. 196, 243).

1.7. (D) The muscles found in the anterior compartment of the leg are the tibialis anterior, extensor hallucis longus, extensor digitorum longus, and peroneus tertius. The peroneus longus is found in the lateral compartment of the leg (Ref. 2, pp. 559−560).

1.8. (A) The desmosome is the most frequent type of epithelial attachment. It is also one of the earliest known types. Desmosomes were recognized in light microscopy as "intercellular bridges" (Ref. 3, pp. 119−122).

1.9. (D) Each of the hormones listed is produced by the anterior hypophysis. It is the somatotrophic hormone (STH) that stimulates body growth, especially the development of long bones by increasing the activity of cartilage cells in the epiphyses (Ref. 3, pp. 787−788).

1.10. (A) The ureter is lined for its entire length by transitional epithelium. This type of epithelium is characteristic of most of the urinary system (Ref. 3, p. 677).

1.11. (B) In the normal adult the development of erythrocytes and granular leukocytes is generally limited to the bone marrow. Monocytes and lymphocytes develop in the lymphoid organs although it has been shown that numerous lymphocytes and monocytes are also produced in the bone marrow (Ref. 3, pp. 427−437).

1.12. **(D)** The cerebellar cortex contains five different types of nerve cells: basket cell, stellate cell, purkinje cell, granule cell, and Golgi type II cell. Satellite cells form a capsule around the bodies of the spinal ganglion cells (Ref. 4, pp. 181, 456−461).

1.13. **(C)** The carotid sinus is a baroreceptor located at the bifurcation of the common carotid artery. It responds to changes in blood pressure and these impulses are conveyed centrally by way of the glossopharyngeal nerve (Ref. 4, p. 352).

1.14. **(B)** Lesions of the spinal trigeminal tract could probably result in the loss of thermal, pain, and tactile senses in the regions innervated by the trigeminal nerve (Ref. 4, pp. 324, 398).

1.15. **(C)** Low defects of the anorectal region include: anal agenesis, anal stenosis, membranous atresia, rectal atresia, and anorectal agenesis. Anorectal agenesis is the most common type of anorectal malformation (Ref. 5, p. 250).

1.16. **(A)** The oculomotor nerve can be visualized in a transverse section through the upper portion of the midbrain. Fibers of the abducens nerve pass through the pontine tegmentum and lateral to the corticospinal tract and emerge from the brainstem at the caudal border of the pons (Ref. 4, p. 421).

1.17. **(E)** The gracilis muscle is an important adductor of the thigh and it also assists in flexing the leg at the knee (Ref. 1, p. 563).

1.18. **(B)** The iliopsoas muscle is often thought of as two muscles, the psoas major and iliacus. The primary action of the iliopsoas muscle is to flex the thigh. It also flexes the pelvis (Ref. 1, p. 557).

1.19. **(D)** The quadratus femoris muscle has its origin from the tuberosity of the ischium and inserts into the linea quadrata. It is a lateral rotator of the thigh (Ref. 1, p. 570).

1.20. **(B)** The quadriceps femoris muscle consists of four parts: the vastus lateralis, vastus medialis, vastus intermedius, and the rectus femoris. The rectus femoris is a flexor of the thigh. The entire quadriceps is an extensor of the leg (Ref. 1, pp. 562−563).

1.21. (D) The biceps femoris muscle has two heads, a long and a short head. Its primary action is to flex the leg. The long head also extends the thigh and rotates it laterally (Ref. 1, pp. 571–572).

1.22. (C) The facial nerve supplies taste fibers (SVA) to the anterior two-thirds of the tongue. It also innervates (SVE) all branchial arch muscles derived from the second arch (Ref. 4, p. 385).

1.23. (B) The muscles derived from the first branchial arch are innervated (SVE) by the trigeminal nerve (Ref. 4, p. 393).

1.24. (C) The vagus nerve conveys sensory fibers for taste (SVA) from the root of the tongue and epiglottis. It also innervates (SVE) the branchial muscles derived from the fourth arch (Ref. 4, p. 342).

1.25. (D) The oculomotor nerve conveys nerve fibers (GSE) to ocular muscles and parasympathetic fibers (GVE) to the constrictor pupillae and the ciliary muscle of accommodation (Ref. 4, p. 426).

1.26. (B) The accessory nerve innervates (SVE) the sternocleido-mastoid and trapezius muscles which are thought to be derived from branchial arches in conjunction with the vagus nerve (Ref. 4, p. 341).

1.27. (A) Secretory granules are considered cytoplasmic inclusions rather than organelles. Such inclusions are products of cellular activity and include pigment, lipid droplets, and glycogen. Cytoplasmic organelles are essential for cellular activity (Ref. 3, pp. 30–63).

1.28. (B) The cells found in the mucosa of the stomach are parietal, chief, mucous neck, and enteroendocrine (Ref. 3, pp. 532–542).

1.29. (E) Syndactyly is the most common limb malformation. It is seen more frequently in the foot than in the hand and most often occurs between the third and fourth fingers and second and third toes. Hereditary factors are implicated (Ref. 5, pp. 370–372).

1.30. (D) The muscles innervated by the ulnar nerve include the medial half of the flexor digitorum profundus, flexor carpi ulnaris, abductor digiti minimi, flexor digiti minimi brevis, opponens digiti minimi, adductor pollicis, all interossei, the two medial lumbricals, and the palmaris brevis (Ref. 1, pp. 1217−1219).

1.31. **(E)** The hypothalamus has afferent connections with the stria terminalis, medial forebrain bundle, fornix, anterior thalamic nucleus, hippocampohypothalamic fibers, and ventral amygdalofugal pathway (Ref. 4, pp. 560−564).

1.32. **(C)** The radial groove begins on the posterior aspect of the humerus and runs obliquely downward and forward. Within this groove will be found the radial nerve and deep brachial artery. Thus, fractures in the middle of the humeral shaft will involve this groove (Ref. 2, p. 88).

1.33. **(A)** The radial artery in its descent on the forearm moves from the ventral aspect of the radius to the dorsum of the hand, where it passes deeply between the first and second metacarpal bones. In this latter part of its course it lies in the anatomic snuffbox, a triangular depression formed by the extensor pollicis longus and extensor pollicis brevis muscles (Ref. 2, pp. 99, 112).

1.34. **(D)** The superficial radial nerve, a totally cutaneous nerve, arises in the cubital fossa and descends in the forearm under the brachioradialis muscle to reach and supply the dorsum of the thumb, the index, and the middle fingers (Ref. 2, 62−63).

1.35. **(C)** Inability to extend the forearm indicates paralysis of the triceps brachii, a muscle innervated by the radial nerve (Ref. 2, pp. 85−86).

1.36. **(D)** Injury to the radial nerve, which supplies all of the extensors of the hand, would result in wrist drop. This nerve is more frequently paralyzed than any other branch of the brachial plexus (Ref. 2, pp. 90−91, 142).

References

1. Clemente, C.D.: *Gray's Anatomy of the Human Body*, 30th Ed., Lea and Febiger, Philadelphia, 1985.

2. Woodburne, R.T.: *Essentials of Human Anatomy*, 7th Ed., Oxford Press, London and Toronto, 1983.

3. Kelley, D.E., Wood, R.L., and Enders, A.C.: *Bailey's Textbook of Histology*, 18th Ed., Williams and Wilkins, Baltimore, 1984.

4. Carpenter, M.B.: *Human Neuroanatomy*, 8th Ed., Williams and Wilkins, Baltimore, 1983.

5. Moore, K.L.: *The Developing Human*, 3rd Ed., W.B. Saunders, Philadelphia, 1982.

2

Biochemistry
Sanford Simon, Ph.D.

DIRECTIONS: Each of the questions or incomplete statements below is followed by five suggested answers or completions. Select the **one** that is best in each case.

2.1. A disease which has its basis in the failure to carry out the normal repair process following exposure of DNA to UV light is
   A. scleroderma
   B. lupus erythematosus
   C. xeroderma pigmentosum
   D. Kleinfelter's syndrome
   E. Burkitt's lymphoma

2.2. Which of the following agents would NOT introduce a base-pair *substitution* into DNA?
   A. Nitrous acid
   B. 5-Bromodeoxyuridine
   C. Ethylmethane sulfonate
   D. Acridine orange
   E. Nitrogen mustard

2.3. Polypeptides which are secreted by cells are
  A. synthesized in the cisternae of the endoplasmic reticulum
  B. synthesized with a so-called signal peptide sequence attached to the C-terminal end of the nascent chain
  C. generally processed posttranslationally by a peptidase in the extracytoplasmic side of the endoplasmic reticulum
  D. generally synthesized off a polycistronic mRNA and then cleaved into individual subunits posttranslationally
  E. none of the above

2.4. To detect a particular gene in a mixture of restriction endonuclease fragments from a digest of DNA,
  A. the mRNA for the gene product should be used with reverse transcriptase to make a cDNA
  B. the restriction endonuclease fragments should be reacted with antibodies to the gene product
  C. the restriction endonuclease fragments should be annealed to see which fragments hybridize with each other
  D. the restriction endonuclease fragments should be used as templates to make a number of cDNA copies
  E. the restriction endonuclease fragments should be hybridized to the intact DNA

2.5. In the metabolism of arachidonic acid
  A. thromboxane A_2 may be formed via the cyclooxygenase pathway
  B. prostacyclin I_2 may be formed via the lipoxygenase pathway
  C. prostaglandin E_2 is formed via the cyclooxygenase pathway whereas prostaglandin F_{2a} is formed via the lipoxygenase pathway
  D. HETE may be formed via the cyclooxygenase pathway
  E. the active metabolites may persist for several days, especially in the presence of antiinflammatory drugs

2.6. In the ischemic heart muscle, a drop in pH can result in inhibition of glycolysis because
  A. the affinity of phosphohexoisomerase for AMP as a negative effector is increased
  B. the affinity of aldolase for ATP as a negative effector is increased
  C. the affinity of phosphofructokinase for ATP as a negative effector is increased
  D. the affinity of hexokinase for glucose as a positive effector is decreased.
  E. the affinity of pyruvate kinase for cAMP as a positive effector is decreased

2.7. The mechanism of catalysis invoked for the enzyme lysozyme makes use of
  A. cooperative interactions among subunits
  B. half-of-the-sites reactivity
  C. distortion and strain of the substrate
  D. isozyme interactions
  E. an acyl enzyme intermediate

2.8. Two substrates, A and A′, are bound to the same active site of an enzyme with equal affinity, but the catalytic constant for A′ is four orders of magnitude smaller than that for A. Which of the following statements is true?
  A. In the presence of a fixed amount of A′, the conversion of A to product will occur at a significantly reduced rate, regardless of how much A is added to the enzyme
  B. A′ may be considered as a competitive inhibitor of A, with a K_I for A′ approximately equal to the K_M for A
  C. A′ may be considered as a noncompetitive inhibitor of A
  D. If an amount of A equal to the K_M for A is added to the enzyme, then the observed velocity of the reaction will be independent of the amount of A′ added
  E. The K_I for A′ is four orders of magnitude smaller than the K_M for A

2.9. Two isozymes of an enzyme, E_H and E_M, have been isolated: the turnover number for E_H is twice as big as that for E_M. Which of the following statements is true?

A. The K_M of E_H for a substrate would be twice as large as the K_M of E_M for the same substrate

B. The specific activity of E_H was two orders of magnitude greater than that of E_M

C. The V_M for a substrate with E_H was twice the value of V_M for the same substrate with E_M

D. The molecular weight of E_H was half that of E_M

E. The Q_{10} of E_H would be twice as large as that of E_M

2.10. An enzyme preparation has been purified to high constant specific activity and is submitted to starch gel electrophoresis under nondenaturing conditions. When the gel is stained for protein or for enzymatic activity, five bands can be visualized. The same enzyme preparation is also submitted to starch gel electrophoresis in the presence of 8 M urea and stained for protein; under these conditions only two bands can be visualized. A simple explanation for this is that the enzyme is

A. a tetramer composed of two different types of subunits

B. a pentamer of five different types of subunits

C. a pentamer under nondenaturing conditions and a dimer in the presence of 8 M urea

D. a urease

E. most likely creatine phosphokinase

2.11. The role of cAMP-dependent protein kinase in the metabolism of glycogen is

A. to activate phosphorylase kinase by catalyzing its phosphorylation and to inhibit glycogen synthetase by catalyzing its dephosphorylation

B. to activate both phosphorylase kinase and glycogen synthetase by catalyzing their phosphorylation

C. to inhibit both phosphorylase kinase and glycogen synthetase by catalyzing their phosphorylation

D. to activate phosphorylase kinase and to inhibit glycogen synthetase by catalyzing their phosphorylation

E. to activate phosphorylase kinase by catalyzing its phosphorylation; the enzyme is without effect on glycogen synthetase

2.12. Calcium can serve as an activator of glycogenolysis if it is bound to

    A. calcitonin
    B. calciferol
    C. kallekrein
    D. cap binding protein
    E. calmodulin

2.13. Allysine residues are condensed into desmosine in

    A. collagen
    B. keratin
    C. elastin
    D. tropomyosin
    E. fibroin

2.14. The enzyme argininosuccinate synthetase provides

    A. the carbonyl group of urea by catalyzing the condensation of ornithine and glutamic acid
    B. one of the two nitrogens of urea by catalyzing the condensation of citrulline and aspartic acid
    C. the carbonyl group and one nitrogen of urea by catalyzing the condensation of arginine and succinic acid
    D. the carbonyl group and one nitrogen of urea by catalyzing the condensation of carbamoyl phosphate and citrulline
    E. the carbonyl group of urea by catalyzing the condensation of citrulline and fumarate

2.15. The effect of allopurinol on xanthine oxidase results in

    A. increased levels of hypoxanthine and decreased levels of xanthine and uric acid
    B. decreased levels of xanthine and hypoxanthine and increased levels of uric acid
    C. increased levels of xanthine and hypoxanthine and decreased levels of uric acid
    D. increased levels of xanthine, hypoxanthine, and uric acid
    E. decreased levels of xanthine, hypoxanthine, and uric acid

2.16. In the metabolism of bile salts
- **A.** cholic acid is converted into deoxycholic acid in the liver
- **B.** cholic acid is converted into lithocholic acid in the colon
- **C.** deoxycholic acid is converted into chenodeoxycholic acid in the colon
- **D.** chenodeoxycholic acid is converted into lithocholic acid in the colon
- **E.** chenodeoxycholic acid is converted into taurocholic acid in the colon

---

DIRECTIONS: Each group of questions below consists of five lettered headings or a diagram with lettered components followed by a list of numbered words or statements. For each numbered word or statement, select the **one** lettered heading that is most closely associated with it. Each lettered heading may be selected once, more than once, or not at all.

- **A.** Oxytocin
- **B.** Insulin
- **C.** Thyroxin
- **D.** Corticotropin-releasing factor
- **E.** Thyrotropin-releasing factor

2.17. A nine amino acid peptide with a single internal disulfide bridge

2.18. A tripeptide with blocked amino and carboxyl termini

2.19. A mono-amino-mono-carboxy-amino acid

- **A.** Hexosaminidase A deficiency
- **B.** Sphingomyelinase deficiency
- **C.** Arylsulfatase deficiency
- **D.** Iduronidase deficiency
- **E.** Iduronate sulfatase deficiency

2.20. Results in dysostosis multiplex, mental retardation; is sex linked

2.21. Results in mental retardation, cherry red spot on macula; has high incidence in Ashkenazic Jews

2.22. Results in metachromatic leukodystrophy

For Questions 2.23−2.25, refer to Figure 4

2.23. Sulfonamides interfere with incorporation of this moiety in bacteria which synthesize E

2.24. Methotrexate is a competitive inhibitor of the enzyme which catalyzes the reduction of this moiety

2.25. Jejunal conjugases recognize this moiety

For Questions 2.26−2.28, refer to Figure 5

2.26. This curve is most likely to fit the V vs. S dependence of a monomeric enzyme

2.27. If curve B describes the substrate dependence of the velocity of a reaction catalyzed by an enzyme in the absence of effectors, this curve would describe the effect of addition of an effector which stabilizes the T state in the model of Monod, Wyman, and Changeux.

Figure 4

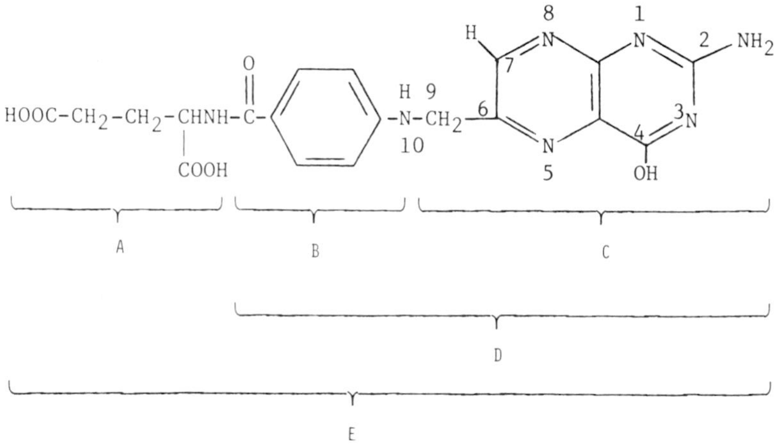

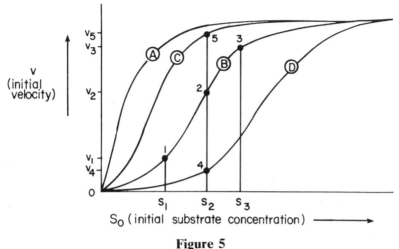

Figure 5

2.28. This curve would also describe the binding of oxygen to hemoglobin Kempsey, a mutant which is permanently locked into the R conformation, according to the model of Monod, Wyman, and Changeux.

For Questions 2.29 and 2.30, refer to Figure 6

2.29. A defect in this enzyme gives rise to Cori type V (McArdle's) storage disorder

2.30. A defect in this enzyme gives rise to type III (Cori's) limit dextrinosis

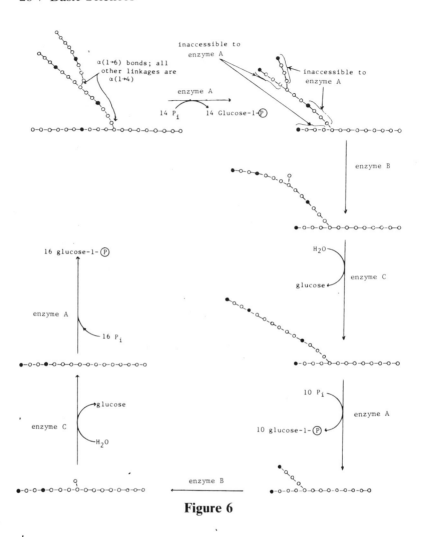

Figure 6

DIRECTIONS: Each set of lettered headings below is followed by a list of numbered words or phrases. For each numbered word or phrase select

(A) if the item is associated with A only
(B) if the item is associated with B only
(C) if the item is associated with both A and B
(D) if the item is associated with neither A nor B

A. Palmitate biosynthesis
B. Palmitate β oxidation
C. Both
D. Neither

2.31. Uses NADP≦NADPH as the redox coenzyme

2.32. Uses dolichol phosphate as a carrier

2.33. Occurs primarily in the mitochondria

2.34. Involves a β-hydroxy intermediate in the pathway

A. Tetrahydrofolate
B. S-adenosylmethionine
C. Both
D. Neither

2.35. Deficiency state may result in urinary excretion of formaminoglutamic acid (FIGlu)

2.36. Deficiency state presents with megaloblastosis complicated by neurologic involvement

2.37. Required for conversion of phosphatidylethanolamine to phosphatidylcholine

2.38. Required for donation of one carbon fragment in purine biosynthesis

DIRECTIONS: For each of the questions or incomplete statements below, **one or more** of the answers or completions given is correct. Select

(A) if only 1, 2, and 3 are correct
(B) if only 1 and 3 are correct
(C) if only 2 and 4 are correct
(D) if only 4 is correct
(E) if all are correct

2.39. In the control of oxygen affinity of hemoglobin
1. removal of the C-terminal amino acid of the α and β chain decreases oxygen affinity
2. binding of CO to two subunits of a hemoglobin molecule increases the affinity of the remaining two subunits for oxygen
3. human fetal hemoglobin (hemoglobin F) has a lower oxygen affinity than adult hemoglobin (hemoglobin A) in the presence of physiologic concentrations of 2,3-diphosphoglyceric acid
4. lowering the pH of a hemoglobin solution decreases oxygen affinity

2.40. In the regulations of glycolysis
1. a high AMP/ATP ratio has a positive effector action on phosphofructokinase and a negative effector action on fructose-1,6-diphosphatase
2. glucose-6-phosphate feedback inhibits hexokinase whereas fructose-1,6-diphosphate feedforward activates pyruvate kinase
3. the Pasteur effect is the inhibition of glucose utilization observed when oxygen consumption is initiated
4. accumulation of citrate can activate phosphofructokinase, the rate limiting enzyme of glycolysis

2.41. Diseases associated with defects in amino acid metabolism include

1. Hartnup disease, a defect in tryptophan absorption, which may present with symptoms of niacin deficiency
2. alcaptonuria, a defect in tyrosine catabolism, which may present with ochronosis
3. phenylketonuria, a defect in conversion of phenylalanine to tyrosine, which may present with mental retardation
4. Refsum's disease, a defect in the oxidative decarboxylation of leucine, isoleucine, and valine, which may present with neurologic complications

2.42. In establishing the molecular basis of thalassemias

1. fragments released by restriction endonuclease digestion of DNA of patients with βδ-thalassemia are reduced in size, indicating that deletion of part of the genes for the globin chains has occurred
2. most of the cases of β-thalassemia are associated with point mutations that lead to rapid denaturation of the nascent chains
3. C_0t curves of cDNA made from the reticulocyte mRNA of patients with Cooley's anemia show that reduced levels of β globin gene mRNA must have been present
4. the α-thalassemias are more common than the β-thalassemias because the hemoglobin which is present in the α-thalassemic patients has normal oxygen affinity whereas that which is present in β-thalassemic patients has abnormally high oxygen affinity

2.43. In the biosynthesis of the adrenocorticosteroids

1. the zona glomerulosa is especially rich in 18-hydroxylase and 18-dehydrogenase activity but not in 17α-hydroxylase activity
2. the absence of 11β-hydroxylase may lead to an accumulation of 11-deoxycorticosterone, an intermediate with significant mineralocorticoid activity
3. the intermediate, dehydroepiandrosterone (DHEA), accumulates in cases of 3β-dehydrogenase deficiency, leading to a virilizing syndrome
4. glucocorticoids, mineralocorticoids, androgens, and estrogens are all synthesized from the common intermediate, pregnenolone

DIRECTIONS: This section of the test consists of situations, each followed by a series of questions. Study each situation and select the **one** best answer to each question following it.

Questions 2.44 – 2.45: A woman has brought her 1-year-old baby to a clinic for a routine examination. You discover that the baby has a hemoglobin level of 11 g/dl. The mother has brought the child, who is fretfully sucking his milk bottle, to your office. You have already established that the child did not recently suffer any abnormal blood loss. A Coombs' test has proved negative.

2.44. If you discovered on interview that the child's sister suffered from dactylitis and recurrent *H. influenzae* infections with the first manifestations of painful swelling of the fingers starting at about 6 months of age, you might
  A. order a restriction endonuclease map to test for β-thalassemia
  B. order a p_{50} determination to test for a hemoglobin with abnormal oxygen affinity
  C. order a hemoglobin electrophoresis and solubility test to detect a hemoglobin that polymerizes in the deoxygenated state
  D. order a platelet count to test for idiopathic thrombocytopenic purpura
  E. order an enzyme screen for glucose-6-phosphate dehydrogenase deficiency

2.45. If you discovered instead that the child's major source of nutrition for the first year had been cow's milk, with no supplementation, you might
  A. order a lactose tolerance test for lactase insufficiency
  B. order a serum iron to test for iron deficiency
  C. order a Schilling test for vitamin B_{12} deficiency
  D. order a serum folate for confirmation of megaloblastosis
  E. see whether the hemoglobin level rises after administration of vitamin K

Questions 2.46 – 2.48: A 30-year-old patient with extensive athero-sclerosis is being investigated for a possible biochemical basis for his vascular disease. Fibroblasts from the patient have been obtained and grown in tissue culture for biochemical assays. Results obtained so far show that the function of the low density lipoprotein (LDL) receptors on the patient's fibroblasts is defective. The patient's serum lipoprotein profile has been determined and been found to be distinctly abnormal. A program of therapy based on the use of the compounds mevinolin and compactin has been proposed.

2.46. The use of mevinolin and compactin is intended to
  A. activate synthesis of HDL
  B. inhibit the activity of β-hydroxy-β-methylglutaryl CoA reductase
  C. inhibit the conversion of VLDL to LDL
  D. provide substitutes for the missing LDL receptors
  E. inhibit hepatic synthesis of VLDL

2.47. A defect or abnormality in which of the following proteins might account for the abnormal function of the LDL receptors?
  A. lipoprotein lipase
  B. vinculin
  C. lecithin – cholesterol acyl transferase
  D. clatherin
  E. apoprotein A

2.48. The fact that the patient has experienced premature athero-sclerosis indicates that
  A. the defect in LDL receptors is probably confined to cells of the vasculature and does not involve the liver.
  B. the HDL/LDL ratio in the patient's circulation has been chronically elevated above normal
  C. too much cholesterol has been esterified with fatty acids rather than being employed for cell membrane synthesis.
  D. cells in the intimal layer of the vasculature have accumu-lated deposits of crystalline LDL
  E. the patient has not been able to synthesize HDL and LDL in his vasculature

Answers and Comments

2.1. **(C)** The diseases xeroderma pigmentosum, Fanconi's anemia, Bloom's syndrome, and ataxia telangiectasia are all associated with defects in DNA repair (Ref. 1, pp. 392–393).

2.2. **(D)** Acridine dyes are intercalating agents which introduce an extra base-pair insertion into DNA. The other mutagens listed all produce base-pair substitutions (Refs. 1, pp. 418–419; 2, pp. 636–637).

2.3. **(C)** Secretory proteins are synthesized on endoplasmic reticulum-bound ribosomes with a signal peptide sequence of amino acids attached at the amino terminal end. This signal peptide sequence is cleaved by a peptidase in the luminal side of the endoplasmic reticulum (Ref. 2, pp. 713–714).

2.4. **(A)** The technique of restriction endonuclease mapping to isolate a desired gene is generally carried out by hybridizing a cDNA probe, synthesized from the mRNA for the gene product, to the electrophoretically separated fragments of genomic DNA which has been digested with restriction endonucleases (Ref. 2, pp. 732–733, 765).

2.5. **(A)** The cyclooxygenase pathway is responsible for the biosynthesis of prostaglandins (including those of the E and F series), prostacyclin, and thromboxanes. The lipoxygenase pathway is responsible for synthesis of HETE. Aspirin and other nonsteroidal antiinflammatory agents inhibit the cyclooxygenase pathway (Ref. 1, pp. 821–834).

2.6. **(C)** Phosphofructokinase is the rate limiting enzyme in the glycolytic pathway. It is subject to allosteric regulation, with AMP as a positive effector and ATP as a negative effector. The affinity of the enzyme for ATP is increased as the pH is lowered (Refs. 1, pp. 190–191; 2, pp. 542–543; 3, pp. 353–358).

2.7. **(C)** The fourth sugar in the hexasaccharide binding site of lysozyme is distorted into a "half-chair" configuration, favoring formation of the carbonium ion intermediate (Ref. 2, pp. 135–148).

2.8. (B) Competitive inhibitors are frequently substrate analogues which can bind in the same site as the substrate but which undergo reaction only very slowly or not at all (Ref. 1, pp. 109−112, 119−121).

2.9. (C) The maximum velocity, V_M, may be related to the turnover number if the total concentration of enzyme sites $[E]_o$, is known. $V_M = k_3[E]_o$, where k_3 is the turnover number (Ref. 2, p. 114).

2.10. (A) Lactic dehydrogenase exemplifies a group of isozymes consisting of tetrameric proteins composed of two subunits. The two subunits are electrophoretically separable under denaturing conditions, e.g., 8 M urea, but when they combine randomly to form tetramers, five different tetrameric isozymes may be separated (Ref. 1, pp. 134, 200−204).

2.11. (D) In the liver, cAMP stimulates glycogenolysis and inhibits glycogenesis by activating protein kinase to phosphorylate both glycogen synthetase and phosphorylase kinase (Ref. 1, pp. 268−269, 280−281).

2.12. (E) Calmodulin is a calcium-dependent regulatory protein which activates a number of enzymes, including phosphorylase kinase, cAMP phosphodiesterase, and kinases involved in non-muscle contractile processes in cells (Ref. 3, pp. 208−210).

2.13. (C) Desmosine and isodesmosine are cyclic products of aldol condensation and Schiff-base reactions of allysine and lysine residues; they are found uniquely in elastin (Ref. 1, pp. 462−464).

2.14. (B) Argininosuccinate synthetase catalyzes the condensation of citrulline and aspartic acid to form argininosuccinate, which is then cleaved with argininosuccinate lyase to form fumarate and arginine. The aspartic acid α-amino group appears in urea, along with the second amino group and carbonyl derived from carbamoyl phosphate (Ref. 1, pp. 590−593).

2.15. (C) Allopurinol inhibits both the conversion of hypoxanthine to xanthine and the conversion of xanthine to uric acid, two reactions catalyzed by xanthine oxidase. The resultant reduction in uric acid levels, associated with buildup of the more soluble precursors, forms an important therapeutic modality for treatment of gout (Ref. 1, pp. 520−522).

2.16. **(D)** The primary bile acids, cholate and chenodeoxycholate, are synthesized and conjugated with glycine or taurine in the liver, and are then converted to their corresponding secondary bile acid forms, deoxycholate and lithocholate, in the colon via the action of the bacterial flora (Ref. 1, pp. 923−931).

2.17. **(A)** Oxytocin and vasopressin are nonapeptides released from larger precursor proteins in neurons arising in the supraoptic and parventricular nuclei of the hypothalamus. The two hormones accumulate at the endings of these neurons in the posterior pituitary (Ref. 1, pp. 1218−1220).

2.18. **(E)** Thyrotropin-releasing hormone is a tripeptide, pyroglutamylhistidylprolinamide (Ref. 1, p. 662).

2.19. **(C)** Thyroxin is an α-amino acid synthesized by condensation of tyrosine residues on thyroglobulin (Ref. 1, pp. 650−654).

2.20. **(E)** Hunter's syndrome is a sex-linked deficiency of iduronate sulfatase, leading to accumulation of dermatan sulfate and heparan sulfate (Ref. 3, p. 427).

2.21. **(A)** Tay-Sachs disease is a deficiency of hexosaminidase A, leading to accumulation of ganglioside G_{M2} (Ref. 3, p. 530).

2.22. **(C)** Metachromatic leukodystrophy is a sphingolipid storage disease associated with mental retardation and a characteristic staining pattern of neurons due to accumulation of sulfatides. It is a deficiency of a sulfatase known by its assay procedure as arylsulfatase A (Ref. 3, p. 528).

2.23. **(B)**
2.24. **(C)**
2.25. **(A)** The illustration shows the structure of folic acid, a complex molecule composed of glutamic acid, p-aminobenzoic acid, and a pteridine ring system. Folic acid synthesis in bacteria is

antagonized by p-aminobenzoate analogs such as sulfonamides and isoniazid. Folic acid is stored in foodstuffs as polyglutamate precursors, but all except one glutamic acid residue are removed by intestinal conjugases. Reduction of the pteridine ring system yields dihydrofolate, and then, via dihydrofolate reductase, an enzyme that is competitively inhibited by methotrexate, the biologically active form, tetrahydrofolic acid (Ref. 1, pp. 485−489, 1063).

2.26. (A)
2.27. (D)
2.28. (A) Monomeric enzymes rarely display cooperative sigmoidal kinetics, but rather display hyperboic Michaelis−Menten kinetics. Stabilization of the low affinity or T structure of an allosteric enzyme, according to the model of Monod, Wyman, and Changeux, shifts the V vs. S curve to the right, indicating increasing substrate concentrations required to achieve half-maximal velocity. Hemoglobin Kempsey, a mutant locked in the high affinity R conformation, binds oxygen in a noncooperative fashion with a myoglobinlike curve, even though it retains its tetrameric structure (Ref. 1, pp. 124−128, 743).

2.29. (A)
2.30. (C) Glycogenolysis is accomplished via the sequential action of three enzymes: phosphorylase, glucosyl transferase, and debranching enzyme [amylo-(1-6) glucosidase]. Defects in phosphorylase and in debranching enzyme lead to accumulation of glycogen in glycogen storage diseases. Types V and VI glycogen storage diseases (McArdle's and Hers'), due to phosphorylase deficiency, are associated with accumulation of glycogen of normal structure, whereas type III glycogen storage disease (Cori's) is associated with accumulation of limit dextrins (Ref. 1, pp. 277−279, 285).

2.31. (A)
2.32. (D)
2.33. (B)
2.34. (C) β-Oxidation of fatty acids makes use of NAD, whereas synthesis makes use of NADP. These reactions are compartmentalized, with synthesis taking place in the cytoplasm and degradation in the mitochondria. Both synthesis and degradation involve β-hydroxy intermediates, attached to acyl carrier protein in the cytoplasm and to coenzyme A in the mitochondria. Dolichol phos-

phates, polyprenol derivatives, are used in the synthesis of glyco-proteins (Refs. 1, pp. 892–907; 2, pp. 714–717).

2.35. (A)
2.36. (D)
2.37. (B)
2.38. (A) Folate deficiency may present with megaloblastic anemia accompanied by excretion of FIGlu and AICA. Megaloblastic anemia with neurologic involvement and methylmalonic aciduria is due to vitamin B_{12} deficiency. S-adenosyl methionine is used in methylation of phosphatidylethanolamine, norepinephrine, and DNA and RNA, but not in purine or pyrimidine synthesis (Ref. 1, pp. 620, 1062–1072).

2.39. (C) Stabilization of the C-terminal ends of hemoglobin in salt bridges lowers the oxygen affinity; removal of the C-terminal residues destabilizes the low affinity conformation. Binding of any gaseous ligand to some of the subunits of hemoglobin increases the affinity of the remaining subunits for any other gaseous ligand. The organic phosphate binding site in human fetal hemoglobin lacks positive charges and thus 2,3-diphosphoglycerate is bound less strongly. The Bohr effect is the lowering of oxygen affinity of hemoglobin by protons (Ref. 1, pp. 700–728).

2.40. (A) ATP is a negative effector of phosphofructokinase and a positive effector of fructose-1,6-diphosphatase. Glucose-6-phosphate acts as a product inhibitor of hexokinase, whereas fructose-1,6-diphosphate is a positive effector of pyruvate kinase. Citrate is another negative effector of phosphofructokinase. The Pasteur effect is the depression of the rate of glycolysis by oxygen, thought to be due to a combination of factors, including high ATP levels generated by oxidative phosphorylation and the depletion of ADP and inorganic phosphate from the cytoplasm by the mitochondria (Ref. 1, pp. 205–206, 230–232).

2.41. (A) Defective catabolism of the branched chain amino acids, leucine, isoleucine, and valine is associated with the inborn error of metabolism called maple syrup urine disease. Refsum's disease is an abnormality in the catabolism of odd numbered fatty acids (Ref. 1, pp. 617, 628–629, 632, 638, 673, 887–888).

2.42. **(B)** Most thalassemias are due to defects in mRNA production from one of the globin genes. Except for a few α-chain termination mutations that produce elongated α chains, the globin chains synthesized in the thalassemias are normal in amino acid sequence. Gene deletions have been demonstrated for the βδ thalassemias, although not for most of the β thalassemias (Ref. 1, pp. 729−739).

2.43. **(E)** The adrenal cortex is divided into the zona fasciculata, where the glucocorticoids are synthesized; the zona glomerulosa, where the mineralocorticoids are synthesized; and the zona reticularis, where the androgens and estrogens are synthesized. Several forms of congenital adrenal hyperplasias have been described, in which deficiency of one of the enzymes along the pathway from pregnenolone to the gluco- and mineralocorticoids and sex hormones has been identified (Ref. 1, pp. 1225−1235).

2.44. **(C)** Sickle cell disease, in which the patient is homozygous for hemoglobin S, is associated with characteristic infarctions leading to painful crises and to loss of splenic function, resulting in a high incidence of infections. The constellation of symptoms associated with the disease can be traced to aggregation of the deoxyhemoglobin S molecules into fiberlike polymers (Ref. 1, pp. 747−751).

2.45. **(B)** Iron deficiency anemia is a common complication of a highly restricted dietary intake confined to milk in the first few years of life. It generally responds readily to oral iron supplements (Ref. 1, pp. 688−695; 3, pp. 1230−1233).

2.46. **(B)** Mevinolin and compactin are inhibitors of β-hydroxy-β-glutaryl CoA reductase. By inhibiting the endogenous synthesis of cholesterol, they reduce total body cholesterol levels (Refs. 1, pp. 931−969; 3, pp. 512−514).

2.47. **(D)** LDL bound to specific receptors on the plasma membrane is internalized by formation of clatherin-coated pits. In the absence of clatherin, the receptors do not cluster and bind LDL effectively (Refs. 1, pp. 931−969; 3, pp. 512−514).

2.48. **(C)** The biochemical basis of the atherosclerotic plaque is the formation of inclusions of cholesterol esters. The cholesterol that is esterified in the cells of the vasculature arises from intracellular degradation of excessively high levels of LDL. Such LDL would normally be cleared efficiently from the circulation by the liver (Refs. 1, pp. 931–969; 3, pp. 512–514).

References

1. Bhagavan, N.V.: *Biochemistry*, Lippincott, Philadelphia, 1978.

2. Stryer, L.: *Biochemistry*, W.H. Freeman, San Francisco, 1981.

3. Devlin, T.M.: *Textbook of Biochemistry*, J. Wiley, New York, 1982.

3

Microbiology
Charles W. Kim, M.S.P.H., Ph.D.

DIRECTIONS Each of the questions or incomplete statements below is followed by five suggested answers or completions. Select the **one** that is best in each case.

3.1. As compared to the primary antibody response, the secondary antibody response is characterized by
   A. longer lag period between encounter with antigen and appearance of antibodies
   B. antibody production at a slower rate
   C. higher antibody titers at peak of response
   D. lower antibody titers at peak of response
   E. antibodies with lower affinity for antigen

3.2. All of the following diseases are prevented by immunogens that are infectious (attenuated) viruses EXCEPT
   A. measles
   B. influenza
   C. mumps
   D. rubella
   E. yellow fever

3.3. Which one of the extracellular products of β-streptococci is responsible for surface colony hemolysis on a blood plate?
A. Streptolysin O
B. Streptolysin S
C. Streptokinase A
D. Streptokinase B
E. Erythrogenic toxin

3.4. All of the following features describe tuberculin hypersensitivity EXCEPT
A. in the U.S., 0.1 ml of standardized PPD is injected intradermally
B. reactions of less than 10 mm in diameter at 48 hr are recorded as doubtful
C. intense reactions can cause necrosis
D. severe reactions can cause scarring
E. OT is still the preferred tuberculin for skin testing in the U.S.

3.5. When viruses of more than one type infect the same cell, in certain cases, multiplication of one type of virus may be inhibited by the other. This phenomenon is known as
A. complementation
B. genetic recombination
C. viral interference
D. abortive infection
E. none of the above

3.6. Concerning cryptococcosis:
A. chronic meningitis is a frequent manifestation
B. *Cryptococcus neoformans* appears as a thin-walled organism in the spinal fluid
C. the organism develops arthrospores at room temperature
D. the organism has multiple buds in tissue
E. none of the above

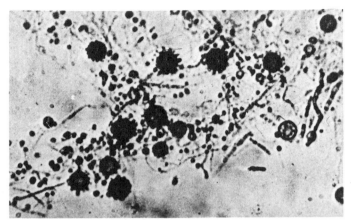

Figure 7

3.7. Which stage of *Plasmodium falciparum* is generally NOT seen in peripheral blood?
   A. Young trophozoite
   B. Older trophozoite
   C. Microgametocyte
   D. Macrogametocyte
   E. Schizont

3.8. Large round to pyriform tuberculate macroconidia on Sabouraud's glucose agar at room temperature are shown in Figure 7. They are
   A. *Cryptococcus neoformans*
   B. *Histoplasma capsulatum*
   C. *Blastomyces dermatitidis*
   D. *Candida albicans*
   E. *Aspergillus fumigatus*

3.9. *Chlamydia psittaci*
   A. causes disease only in psittacine birds
   B. causes psittacosis in humans via discharges of infected birds
   C. contains only RNA
   D. has cell walls that are related to gram-positive bacteria
   E. is still considered to be a virus

3.10. Legionnaires' disease
   A. is caused by a gram-positive bacillus
   B. has an incubation period of more than one month
   C. is caused by *Legionella pneumophila*, which can survive in water
   D. is limited to the continental U.S.
   E. occurs only sporadically

3.11. The microfilaria shown in Figure 8 is sheathed and appears in largest numbers at night. It is
   A. *Wuchereria bancrofti*
   B. *Mansonella ozzardi*
   C. *Onchocerca volvulus*
   D. *Dipetalonema perstans*
   E. *Dipetalonema streptocerca*

3.12. All of the following statements characterize genital herpes simplex EXCEPT
   A. primary genital herpes is a venereally transmitted exogenous infection
   B. it is generally caused by HSV type 2 (HSV-2)
   C. skin and mucous membrane lesions of HSV-1 and HSV-2 are easily distinguishable
   D. the sexual partner may have symptomatic or asymptomatic genital infection
   E. the virus replicates in cells of the stratum spinosum

3.13. The most frequent cause of purulent meningitis in infants is
   A. *Streptococcus pneumoniae*
   B. *Haemophilus influenzae*
   C. *Neisseria meningitidis*
   D. *Listeria monocytogenes*
   E. none of the above

3.14. The helminth egg shown in Figure 9 measures $114-180$ μm $\times$ $45-73$ μm and is found in stool or can be recovered by rectal biopsy. It is
   A. *Schistosoma mansoni*
   B. *Schistosoma haematobium*
   C. *Schistosoma japonicum*
   D. *Paragonimus westermani*
   E. *Fasciola hepatica*

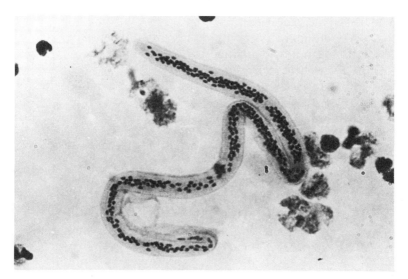

Figure 8

Figure 9

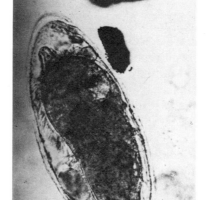

3.15. Bacterial exotoxins
  A. are found only within the parent organism
  B. cannot be detoxified by formaldehyde
  C. are heat stable
  D. are produced by gram-positive and gram-negative organisms
  E. are less toxic than strychnine

3.16. Regarding human T cell leukemia virus (HTLV):
  A. it is a human retrovirus
  B. it is closely related to other retroviruses
  C. its major core protein, p24, is identical to p24 of bovine leukemia virus
  D. it is not present in peripheral blood T lymphocytes
  E. there is only one type

3.17. Lyme disease
  A. was named after the founder of the disease
  B. is characterized by a particular skin eruption
  C. is prevalent during the winter months
  D. is transmitted by the soft tick
  E. is geographically distributed primarily in the South

3.18. The following statements describe babesiosis EXCEPT
  A. the etiologic agent infects the red blood cells
  B. it has been reported in humans and animals
  C. it is transmitted by various species of ticks
  D. the organisms appear as ring-like structures in the red blood cell
  E. it has been reported only in splenectomized persons

3.19. Regarding *Campylobacter*:
  A. it is gram-positive
  B. it is curved
  C. it is nonmotile
  D. it has only one species: *C. fetus*
  E. it does not cause fatal infections

3.20. The following statements describe cryptosporidiosis EX-CEPT
  A. it is caused by the coccidian, *Cryptosporidium*
  B. it has been reported in immunosuppressed and immunocompetent individuals
  C. the organism is generally found on the mucosal surface of the intestine
  D. the organism is spherical measuring approximately 4 μm
  E. it is found only in humans

3.21. Concerning cephalosporins:
  A. cephalosporin C resembles penicillin in structure but not its mode of action
  B. cephalosporin C possesses a β-lactam ring that is fused with a six-member dihydrothiazine ring like penicillins
  C. they are active against most organisms susceptible to the penicillins
  D. the first generation cephalosporins are effective even against indol-positive *Proteus* strains and *Pseudomonas* species
  E. the newer second and third generation cephalosporins are less resistant to the action of cephalosporinases produced by gram-negative organisms

---

DIRECTIONS: The set of lettered headings below is followed by a list of numbered words or phrases. For each numbered word or phrase select
  (A) if the item is associated with A only
  (B) if the item is associated with B only
  (C) if the item is associated with both A and B
  (D) if the item is associated with neither A nor B

  A. RNA genome
  B. Membranous envelope
  C. Both
  D. Neither

3.22. Orthomyxoviruses

3.23. Adenoviruses

3.24. Paramyxoviruses

3.25. Picornaviruses

3.26. Herpesviruses

DIRECTIONS: For each of the questions or incomplete statements below, **one or more** of the answers or completions given is correct. Select
   (A) if only 1, 2, and 3 are correct
   (B) if only 1 and 3 are correct
   (C) if only 2 and 4 are correct
   (D) if only 4 is correct
   (E) if all are correct

3.27. In the Arthus reaction
   1. immune aggregates that fix C must be formed in tissues
   2. polymorphonuclear leukocytes are attracted
   3. reactions are not limited to the skin
   4. there is no tissue damage

3.28. Phenotypic mechanisms of drug resistance include
   1. increased destruction of the drug
   2. increased activation of the drug
   3. formation of an altered receptor
   4. increased permeability

3.29. Interferons are
   1. virus-specific
   2. cell-specific
   3. produced by a limited number of animal viruses
   4. produced only in small amounts

3.30. Concerning *Blastomyces dermatitidis*:
  1. large, spherical, thick-walled budding forms are found from lesions
  2. it grows as a yeastlike organism at 37°C
  3. it grows as a filamentous moldlike organism at room temperature
  4. it produces a single bud during yeast phase

3.31. Regarding IgM class of immunoglobulins:
  1. human IgM molecule is a pentamer made up of five four-chain subunits
  2. in humans, IgM accounts for about 5−10% of the serum immunoglobulins
  3. they are formed early in an immune response
  4. they were also known as 19S antibodies

DIRECTIONS: This section of the test consists of a situation followed by a series of questions. Study the situation and select the **one** best answer to each question following it.

Questions 3.32.−3.36: A 6-year-old boy was admitted to a university hospital because of a severe cough and vomiting of 7-day duration. Two weeks prior to admission to the hospital, he had developed signs of upper respiratory infection with rhinitis, fever, and a hacking cough. The cough became severe, paroxysmal, and ended with an inspiratory crowing sound. He vomited at the end of paroxysm. History indicated that he had not been immunized during infancy. The total white cell count was 50,000/mm^3 with predominance of small mature lymphocytes.

3.32. Based on the history and findings, the most likely diagnosis is
  A. croup
  B. diphtheria
  C. measles
  D. pertussis
  E. common cold

3.33. If this is pertussis
   A. infants under 6 months always develop typical paroxysms
   B. the patient is never cyanotic
   C. the period of highest communicability is during catarrhal and early paroxysmal stages
   D. immunity is not developed after one attack
   E. hyperleukocytosis is characteristic of infants under 6 months of age

3.34. The etiologic agent of pertussis is
   A. a coccobacillus of 0.5 μm in length
   B. motile
   C. not encapsulated
   D. identical to *H. influenzae*
   E. never pleomorphic

3.35. All of the following statements refer to the standard active immunization used against pertussis EXCEPT
   A. utilizes DPT
   B. primary injection series is given at 2–3 months of age
   C. series is completed by 4–5 months of age
   D. a booster is given at 1 year of age
   E. a booster is neither given nor necessary before school age

3.36. The choice culture medium for the isolation of *Bordetella pertussis* is
   A. EMB plate
   B. B-G plate
   C. S-S plate
   D. Sabouraud's agar
   E. corn meal agar

Answers and Comments

3.1. (**C**) In the secondary response, higher antibody titers are seen as a consequence of a shorter lag period and a more persistent antibody production at a higher rate (Ref. 3, p. 420).

3.2. (B) Inactivated influenza virus is used as the immunogen in the prevention of influenza (Ref. 3, p. 448).

3.3. (B) Streptolysin S is oxygen-stable and is responsible for surface colony hemolysis in which no red cells are visible on microscopic examination (Ref. 3, p. 608).

3.4. (E) Old tuberculin was originally described by Koch. However, a more refined tuberculin, purified protein derivative (PPD), is now used as the tuberculin for the Mantoux test (Ref. 3, p. 733).

3.5. (C) When influenza A virus, as interfering virus, is inoculated into the allantoic cavity followed 24 hr later by influenza B virus as challenge virus, the multiplication of the second inoculum is partially or totally inhibited. Interference depends on timing and on viral concentrations (Ref. 3, pp. 1002–1003).

3.6. (A) Chronic meningitis is the most frequent pattern in the chronic, disseminated form of cryptococcosis (Ref. 3, p. 834).

3.7. (E) Schizogony does not usually take place in the peripheral blood in falciparum malaria. Hence, schizonts are not ordinarily seen, except in moribund patients (Ref. 4, p. 80).

3.8. (B) In fact, mycologic diagnosis of histoplasmosis can be established on the basis of the characteristic large round to pyriform tuberculate macroconidia (8–16 μm in diameter) (Ref. 2, p. 1144).

3.9. (B) Chlamydiae are shed in secretions from eyes, nostrils, and feces of infected birds. The organism remains viable in dried feces, and can be cultured from feathers and dust in the vicinity of infected birds (Ref. 1, p. 808).

3.10. (C) *L. pneumophila* can survive for months in distilled water and for over a year in tap water (Ref. 1, p. 836).

3.11. (A) The microfilariae of *W. bancrofti* are sheathed. They are found at their greatest density at night, generally between 10:00 PM and 2:00–4:00 AM. The microfilariae of other filariae listed are not sheathed and do not show periodicity (Ref. 4, p. 234).

3.12. (C) The pathology and pathogenesis of genital herpes simplex appear to be analogous to those of oropharyngeal infections caused by HSV-1. The skin and mucous membrane lesions of both HSV-1 and HSV-2 are indistinguishable (Ref. 1, p. 1041–1042).

3.13. (B) Although over 80% of the cases of purulent meningitis are caused by *H. influenzae, N. meningitidis,* and *S. pneumoniae,* the most frequent cause is *H. influenzae* and it is highest among infants during the second six months of life (Ref. 1, p. 1060).

3.14. (A) The egg of *S. mansoni* possesses a characteristic lateral spine, which projects from the side of the egg near one pole (Ref. 4, p. 159).

3.15. (D) Gram-positive organisms (e.g., *B. anthracis, Clostridium,* and *C. diphtheria*) as well as gram-negative organisms (e.g., *E. coli, Shigella, V. cholerae*) produce exotoxins (Ref. 1, pp. 42, 43).

3.16. (A) HTLV is a human retrovirus, which has been isolated from peripheral blood T lymphocytes. Recent evidence suggests that there is more than one type. HTLV is not closely related to any known retrovirus, but its major core protein, p24, displays some relatedness to the p24 of bovine leukemia virus (Ref. 2, p. 951).

3.17. (B) Lyme disease is characterized by a particular skin eruption, erythema chronicum migrans. Approximately 85% of recognized cases of Lyme disease have the rash, which frequently begins at the site of a tickbite and slowly expands to an annular, erythematous single lesion (Ref. 2, p. 737).

3.18. (E) Human cases of babesiosis have been reported in splenectomized persons as well as in patients with intact spleens (Ref. 4, p. 136).

3.19. (B) *Campylobacter* is derived from the Greek word *campylo* meaning "curved." The organism is curved and measures 1.5 to 5 μm in length (Ref. 2, p. 742).

3.20. (E) Cryptosporidiosis was known as a parasite of the intestinal tracts of many different vertebrates until 1976 when it was reported in an immunocompetent child and also in an immunosuppressed adult male (Ref. 4, p. 70).

3.21. **(C)** The cephalosporins are widely used antibiotics and are active against most organisms susceptible to the penicillins. They have been useful alternatives in patients who are allergic to penicillin (Ref. 2, p. 197).

3.22. **(C)** Orthomyxoviruses have RNA genome and are enveloped (Ref. 3, pp. 855, 1121).

3.23. **(D)** Adenoviruses contain double-stranded DNA molecules with no envelope (Ref. 3, pp. 855, 1049).

3.24. **(C)** Paramyxoviruses have RNA genome and are enveloped (Ref. 3, pp. 855, 1140).

3.25. **(A)** Picornaviruses contain RNA but do not possess a lipid envelope (Ref. 3, pp. 855, 1097).

3.26. **(B)** Herpesviruses contain double-stranded DNA and an encompassing envelope (Ref. 3, pp. 855, 1062).

3.27. **(A)** The principal requirement for Arthus reaction is the formation in tissues of immune aggregates that fix C; the resulting C fragments attract the neutrophils. Their released lysosomal enzymes cause tissue damage. The reaction can occur when antigen is injected almost anywhere, i.e., it is not limited to the skin (Ref. 3, p. 485).

3.28. **(B)** Increased destruction of the drug is the usual mechanism of plasmid-borne resistance. The formation of an altered receptor is an important mechanism, e.g., the alteration in specific ribosomal proteins by one-step mutations increases many times the level of resistance (Ref. 3, pp. 123–124).

3.29. **(C)** Interferons are cell-specific in both their production and their effects. A given interferon inhibits viral multiplication most effectively in cells of the species in which it was produced. Although interferons are produced in small amounts, they can be obtained in highly pure form because they are very stable and can be specifically adsorbed (Ref. 3, pp. 1003–1004).

3.30. **(E)** Direct microscopic examination of material from lesions show several large, spherical, thick-walled budding forms. When cultured, it develops as a yeastlike organism at 37°C or as a filamentous moldlike organism at room temperature. In the yeastlike phase it produces a single bud attached by a wide septum to the parent cell (Ref. 2, pp. 1146, 1149).

3.31. **(E)** 19S antibodies, assigned to the IgM class, are formed early in antibody response. In humans and other mammals, IgM accounts for about 5–10% of the serum Igs. The pentamer is made up of five four-chain subunits each with a pair of H (μ) chains and a pair of κ or λ L chains (Ref. 3, p. 349).

3.32. **(D)** Clinical manifestations of pertussis are those of any early respiratory infection with a hacking cough and fever. The disease, particularly in older children, is marked by crescendo development of inexorable paroxysmal coughing, the end of which may be marked by a massive single inspiratory stroke causing the whoop. Vomiting occurs frequently at the end of a paroxysm. In a majority of cases, estimated to be 80% in unimmunized infants and children, hyperleukocytosis and lymphocytosis develop during the paroxysmal stage. The WBC may rise to greater than 100,000/mm^3 with a predominance of small mature lymphocytes, which appear in circulation as a result of discharge of the marginal pool under the influence of the lymphocyte-promoting factor of *B. pertussis* (Ref. 1, pp. 788–789).

3.33. **(C)** Bacilli are recovered from the nasopharynx most frequently during the catarrhal (preparoxysmal) and early paroxysmal stages. This correlates with the period of highest communicability (Ref. 1, p. 788).

3.34. **(A)** In optimal liquid or semisolid medium, *B. pertussis* is a highly uniform, minute coccobacillus measuring approximately 0.5 μm in length (Ref. 1, p. 787).

3.35. **(E)** Booster is repeated one or two times before school age (Ref. 1, p. 791).

3.36. **(B)** The B-G culture medium originally described by Bordet and Gengou, with minor modifications, is still the preferred medium for the isolation of *B. pertussis* (Ref. 1, p. 789).

References

1. Braude, A.L.: *Infectious Diseases and Medical Microbiology*, 2nd Ed., W.B. Saunders, Philadelphia, 1986.

2. Joklik, W.K., Willett, H.P., and Amos, D.B.: *Zinsser Microbiology*, 18th Ed., Appleton-Century-Crofts, Norwalk, CT, 1984.

3. Davis, B.D., Dulbecco, R., Eisen, H.N., and Ginsberg, H.S.: *Microbiology*, 3rd Ed., Harper & Row, Hagerstown, MD, 1980.

4. Markell, E.K. and Voge, M.: *Medical Parasitology*, 5th Ed., W.B. Saunders, Philadelphia, 1981.

4

Pathology
Ivan Damjanov, M.D.

DIRECTIONS Each of the questions or incomplete statements below is followed by five suggested answers or completions. Select the **one** that is best in each case.

4.1. Enlargement of an organ due to an increased number of normal constituent cells is called
  A. hypertrophy
  B. hyperplasia
  C. metaplasia
  D. anaplasia
  E. dysplasia

4.2. Fatty liver may be caused by all of the following EXCEPT
  A. excessive entry of free fatty acids into the liver
  B. interference with conversion of fatty acids to phospholipids in the liver
  C. impaired lipoprotein secretion from the liver
  D. decreased apoprotein synthesis in the liver
  E. decreased esterification of fatty acids to triglycerides in the liver

4.3. Which of the following clotting factors has a central role and initiates clotting, fibrinolytic, and kinin systems?
  A. Prothrombin
  B. Fibrinogen
  C. Antihemophilic factor VIII
  D. Hageman factor (XII)
  E. Stewart factor

4.4. Hyperacute rejection of renal allograft occurs due to
  A. preformed circulating antibodies in the recipient
  B. antigen antibody complexes present in the recipient
  C. suppressor T cell activation
  D. cytotoxic T cell activation
  E. natural killer cell activation

4.5. Which of the following conditions is considered to be a primary immunodeficiency?
  A. DiGeorge's syndrome
  B. Alport's syndrome
  C. Fanconi's syndrome
  D. Potter's syndrome
  E. Down's syndrome

4.6. Most malignant tumors of the urinary bladder are histologically classified as
  A. squamous cell carcinoma
  B. adenocarcinoma
  C. fibrosarcoma
  D. transitional cell carcinoma
  E. none of the above

4.7. Clear cell adenocarcinoma of the vagina and vaginal adenosis appear to be more common in the following groups than in the general population?
  A. Prostitutes
  B. Nuns
  C. Women on oral contraceptives
  D. Women exposed prenatally to diethylstilbestrol
  E. Women infected with herpes simplex type II

4.8. Which of the following is a thyroid malignant tumor with the best long-term prognosis?
- **A.** Papillary adenocarcinoma
- **B.** Follicular carcinoma
- **C.** Medullary carcinoma
- **D.** Small-cell undifferentiated carcinoma
- **E.** Epidermoid carcinoma

4.9. Staphylococcal food poisoning occurs due to
- **A.** entry of virulent staphylococci into the stomach
- **B.** entry of virulent staphylococci into the blood circulation from the intestine
- **C.** entry of nonvirulent staphylococci into the small intestine, whose content is normally sterile
- **D.** entry of virulent staphylococci into the large intestine following broad spectrum antibiotic therapy and the elimination of normal intestinal flora
- **E.** ingestion of preformed enterotoxin formed by staphylococci in the contaminated food

4.10. Aschoff bodies in the myocardium are the hallmark of carditis in
- **A.** systemic lupus erythematosus
- **B.** rheumatoid arthritis
- **C.** scleroderma
- **D.** polyarteritis nodosa
- **E.** rheumatic fever

4.11. Which of the following lymphoproliferative disorders represents a T-cell malignancy?
- **A.** Multiple myeloma
- **B.** Burkitt's lymphoma
- **C.** Sézary's syndrome-mycosis fungoides
- **D.** Hodgkin's disease
- **E.** Most chronic lymphocytic leukemias

4.12. The typical features of viral pneumonia are
   A. intraalveolar infiltrates composed of polymorpho-nuclear leukocytes
   B. interstitial infiltrates composed of mononuclear cells
   C. intrabronchial mucus plugs
   D. peripheral atelectasis
   E. subapical emphysema recognized easily on x-ray examination as patchy radiolucencies

4.13. Acidophilic or "Councilman-like" bodies found in a liver biopsy suggest the diagnosis of
   A. congestive hepatomegaly
   B. alcoholic cirrhosis
   C. viral hepatitis
   D. primary liver cell tumor
   E. extrahepatic biliary obstruction

4.14. Carcinoma of the gallbladder, which has not yet spread, is frequently (70%) associated with
   A. liver disease
   B. gallstones
   C. obstructive jaundice
   D. disorders of fat metabolism
   E. pancreatic disease

4.15. Most of the carcinomas of the pancreas are located in the
   A. head of the pancreas
   B. body of the pancreas
   C. tail of the pancreas
   D. islets of Langerhans
   E. aberrant pancreatic tissue

4.16. The tumor illustrated in Figure 10 is a(n)
   A. squamous cell carcinoma
   B. teratoma
   C. sarcoma
   D. papilloma
   E. adenoma

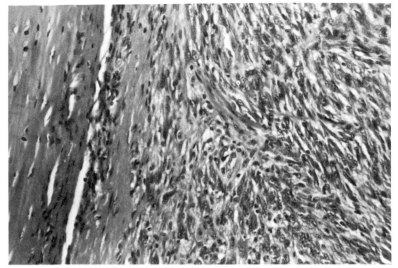

Figure 10

4.17. Most breast carcinomas present histologically as
   A. infiltrating duct carcinoma
   B. medullary carcinoma
   C. colloid carcinoma
   D. Paget's disease
   E. infiltrating lobular carcinoma

DIRECTIONS: Each group of questions below consists of five lettered headings followed by a list of numbered words or statements. For each numbered word or statement, select the **one** lettered heading that is most closely associated with it. Each lettered heading may be selected once, more than once, or not at all.

   A. Vitamin A deficiency
   B. Vitamin D deficiency
   C. Vitamin K deficiency
   D. Thiamine (vitamin B_1) deficiency
   E. Nicotinamide deficiency

4.18. Dementia, dermatitis, and diarrhea

4.19. Congestive heart disease

    A. Deficient synthesis of α and β globin chains of hemo-
        globin
    B. Low iron in serum
    C. Circulating autoantibodies
    D. Vitamin B_{12} deficiency
    E. Bone marrow aplasia

4.20. Megaloblastic anemia

4.21. Thalassemia

4.22. Hemolytic anemia of systemic lupus erythematosus

DIRECTIONS: The set of lettered headings below is followed by a list of numbered words or phrases. For each numbered word or phrase select
    (A) if the item is associated with A only
    (B) if the item is associated with B only
    (C) if the item is associated with both A and B
    (D) if the item is associated with neither A nor B

    A. Antibodies to glomerular basement membrane
    B. Circulating immune complexes
    C. Both
    D. Neither

4.23. Nephritis of systemic lupus erythematosus

4.24. IgA nephropathy (Berger's disease)

4.25. Goodpasture's syndrome

4.26. Lipoid nephrosis ("nil" disease)

4.27. Membranoproliferative glomerulonephritis, type I

DIRECTIONS: For each of the questions or incomplete statements below, **one or more** of the answers or completions given is correct. Select

    (A) if only 1, 2, and 3 are correct
    (B) if only 1 and 3 are correct
    (C) if only 2 and 4 are correct
    (D) if only 4 is correct
    (E) if all are correct

4.28. Numerical chromosomal abnormalities are found in
    1. phenylketonuria
    2. Down's syndrome
    3. Tay-Sachs disease
    4. Klinefelter's syndrome

4.29. Caseous necrosis
    1. is a combination of coagulative and liquefaction necrosis
    2. may be caused by casein released from tissues under the influence of strong acids
    3. is usually encountered in tuberculous infection
    4. is a hallmark of granulomas of sarcoidosis

4.30. Disorder(s) of skin pigmentation associated frequently with internal malignant tumors is (are)
    1. nevocellular nevus
    2. melasma
    3. lentigo
    4. acanthosis nigricans

4.31. Osteomalacia is characterized by
    1. inadequate production of osteoid matrix in the growing bones
    2. inadequate mineralization of newly formed osteoid matrix
    3. increased resorption of calcium from the bone trabeculae
    4. increased fragility of the bones

DIRECTIONS: This section of the test consists of situations, each followed by a series of questions. Study each situation and select the **one** best answer to each question following it.

Question 4.32: A 45-year-old man presented with intractable peptic ulcers, gastric hyperacidity, and diarrhea. These symptoms did not respond to intensive antipeptic ulcer therapy. Elevated levels of gastrin were demonstrated biochemically in the serum. The patient underwent exploratory laparotomy and a tumor was found.

4.32. Where was the tumor most likely located?
- **A.** Stomach
- **B.** Duodenum
- **C.** Pancreas
- **D.** Small intestine
- **E.** Liver

Question 4.33: Subsequent studies on the same patient revealed that he had evidence of a congenital familial disorder that was diagnosed as multiple endocrine adenomatosis type I.

4.33. A tumor was found in which of the following organs?
- **A.** Parathyroid, adrenal cortex, pituitary
- **B.** Pituitary, testis, adrenal cortex
- **C.** Pituitary, adrenal cortex, parathyroid
- **D.** Pituitary, thyroid, adrenal medulla
- **E.** Adrenal medulla

Questions 4.34 – 4.35: The pediatrician palpated an intraabdominal mass in a 6-month-old child. The mass had apparently replaced the left kidney. On x-ray examination a normal right kidney was demonstrated and the left kidney was surgically removed (Figure 11).

4.34. The most likely diagnosis is
- **A.** cystic renal dysplasia
- **B.** adult polycystic renal disease occurring in childhood
- **C.** infantile polycystic disease of the kidney
- **D.** fibrocystic disease
- **E.** cystinosis

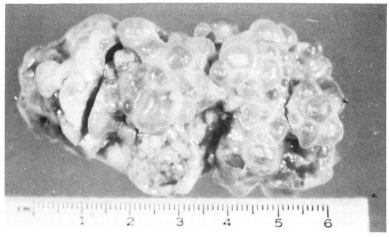

Figure 11

4.35. This disorder is
   A. inherited as autosomal dominant
   B. inherited as autosomal recessive
   C. inherited as sex-linked dominant
   D. inherited as sex-linked recessive
   E. sporadic without familial clustering

Question 4.36: A young man presented with fever, leukocytosis, and testicular pain and swelling. Clinical studies confirmed the diagnosis of infectious orchitis. At surgery the epididymis was swollen and contained pus. You are looking as the bisected testis (Figure 12).

4.36. The lesion most likely represents
   A. mumps orchitis
   B. syphilitic orchitis
   C. bacterial orchitis
   D. herpesvirus-induced orchitis
   E. mycoplasma-induced orchitis

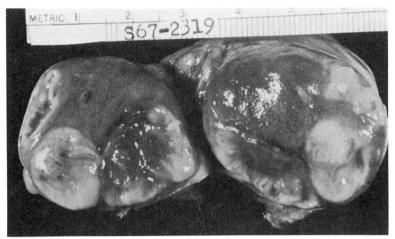

METRIC

S67-2319

Figure 12

Answers and Comments

4.1. (B) Hyperplasia is an enlargment of an organ due to the increased number of cells normally forming the tissues of that organ. Hypertrophy refers to an increase in size of cells, unaccompanied by proliferation of these cells. Metaplasia, anaplasia, and dysplasia refer to the changes in the biological character and the morphology of cells in a tissue (Ref. 1, pp. 31–34).

4.2. (E) Fatty change of liver cells may be due to excessive influx of fat, inadequate utilization and deficient export of fat in form of lipoproteins. Answers A–D all refer to these biochemical processes. Increased esterification of fatty acids would also cause fatty liver; however, the answer E alludes to decreased esterification, i.e., the opposite process, and is therefore not considered a cause of fatty change in the liver (Ref. 1, pp. 18–21).

4.3. (D) Cascade leading to the activation of these systems begins with the activation of Hageman factor (Ref. 1, pp. 53–54).

4.4. (A) Hyperacute rejection occurs within minutes after transplantation and is due to cytotoxic complement-dependent, preexisting antibodies in the host. Antibodies attack the vascular endothelium leading to fibrinoid degeneration of blood vessels and massive intravascular thrombosis (Ref. 1, p. 173).

4.5. (A) DiGeorge's syndrome comprises the congenital deficiency of thymus and parathyroid glands, which develop from the third and fourth pharyngeal pouches. These children have tetany and impaired cell-mediated (thymus-dependent) immunity (Ref. 1, p. 207).

4.6. (D) Transitional cell carcinoma is the most common malignant neoplasm of the urinary bladder. Most tumors of the urinary bladder are transitional cell neoplasm. These tumors are either flat or papillary and vary from well differentiated (grade I) to moderately well differentiated (grade II) to undifferentiated (grade III). Approximately 5% of urinary bladder tumors are classified as squamous cell carcinoma. Adenocarcinomas and various forms of sarcoma are very rare (Ref. 1, pp. 1071–1076).

4.7. (D) Prenatal exposure to diethylstilbestrol (DES) has been linked to an unusually high incidence of clear cell adenocarcinoma of the vagina. Most tumors have been diagnosed in postpubertal young women. In the general population this form of cancer is extremely rare. Vaginal adenosis is a benign condition also related to prenatal exposure to DES. It could represent a precursor of adenocarcinoma, but in most instances it heals spontaneously without serious consequences (Ref. 1, p. 447).

4.8. (A) Papillary carcinoma is the most common malignancy of the thyroid. It is also the malignant tumor with the best prognosis. The tumor has a tendency to metastasize to regional lymph nodes of the neck. Although metastases are found in local lymph nodes of 50% of the patients at the time of diagnosis, most patients (85%) will survive 15–20 years following the removal of the tumor and the involved lymph nodes (Ref. 1, pp. 1218–1224).

4.9. (E) Symptoms of food poisoning develop several hours following the ingestion of food that contains the preformed enterotoxins secreted by the staphylococci. Symptoms, such as diarrhea, nausea, abdominal cramps, and vomiting, are transient and the patient recovers as soon as the enterotoxins have been neutralized and metabolized, usually within 24 hours of poisoning (Ref. 1, p. 305).

4.10. (E) Fully developed Aschoff bodies are pathognomonic of rheumatic carditis. They consist of focal fibrinoid necrosis surrounded by mononuclear and multinucleated histiocytes. These bodies undergo healing through fibrosis. Approximately 50% of patients undergoing surgery for rheumatic valvular heart disease have Aschoff bodies in the myocardium (Ref. 1, p. 572).

4.11. (C) Sézary's syndrome and mycosis fungoides are typical T-cell lymphoproliferative disorders. Mycosis fungoides presents with skin lesions whereas the patients with Sézary's syndrome have not only skin infiltrates but also neoplastic cells in circulation. In later stages of the disease internal organs are also infiltrated by the neoplastic lymphocytes. The neoplastic cells have deeply indented nuclei (cerebriform nuclei) and have all the surface markers of T lymphocytes (Ref. 1, p. 665).

4.12. (A) In contrast to bacterial pneumonias, which cause massive exudation into the alveoli, viral pneumonitis is an interstitial disease with very little intraalveolar cellular exudation. Alveoli may contain fluid or fibrin. Viruses induce a response of lymphocytes and macrophages (Ref. 1, pp. 734–738).

4.13. (C) Acidophilic bodies represent liver cells that have undergone coagulation necrosis. These round eosinophilic (red) bodies usually do not have a visible nucleus and they appear extruded into the sinusoids. Typically such cell injury is induced by viral infections such as viral hepatitis or yellow fever. In the livers affected by yellow fever these bodies were originally described by Councilman (Ref. 1, p. 906).

4.14. (B) Gallstones are found in most patients with gallbladder tumors suggesting that there is a causal relationship between the two conditions. It is also possible that conditions predisposing to formation of gallstones predispose to gallbladder cancer (Ref. 1, pp. 953–954).

4.15. **(A)** Most carcinomas of the pancreas originate from the epithelial cells lining the ducts and are most often located in the head (60%). Approximately 20% are located in the body and 5–10% in the tail of the pancreas (Ref 1, p. 969).

4.16. **(C)** This tumor is composed of elongated cells forming intertwining bundles. Thus it is a mesenchymal malignant tumor, i.e., sarcoma (Ref. 1, p. 215).

4.17. **(A)** Most breast tumors originate in the ducts and have the histologic appearance of infiltrating duct carcinoma. Due to a pronounced desmoplastic reaction of the stroma these tumors are typically firm ("scirrhous") (Ref. 1, pp. 1180–1186).

4.18. **(E)** Deficiency of nicotinamide causes pellagra, a disease characterized by three Ds—dementia, dermatitis, and diarrhea. The disease is endemic in the poverty stricken parts of the world. Nicotinamide deficiency may develop in chronic alcoholics, and may accompany various gastrointestinal disorders or conditions characterized with increased demand for this vitamin, like pregnancy, lactation, infections, and hyperthyroidism (Ref. 1, pp. 415–416).

4.19. **(D)** Thiamine deficiency may cause cardiac beriberi presenting chiefly with congestive heart failure. The pathogenesis of heart failure is not fully understood. The pathologic changes in the heart are nonspecific and consist of dilation of the ventricles and atria and excessive flabbiness of the myocardium (Ref. 1, p. 413–414).

4.20. **(D)** Megaloblastic anemia is caused by a deficiency of either B_{12} or folic acid, although a small number of cases appear to have a disease that does not respond to either B_{12} or folic acid. Deficiency may be due to decreased intake or increased requirement (Ref. 1, pp. 630–635).

4.21. **(A)** There are several forms of thalassemia such as thalassemia major and thalassemia minor. Alpha thalassemia is characterized by deficient synthesis of α-chain hemoglobin and β thalassemia by a deficient synthesis of β chain (Ref. 1, pp. 622–627).

4.22. **(C)** In most patients suffering from systemic lupus erythematosus, there are autoantibodies to various cellular components. Some of these may cause hemolytic anemia (Ref. 1, p. 180–187).

4.23. **(B)** In systemic lupus erythematosus the glomerular lesions are induced by deposition of circulating DNA–antiDNA complexes (Ref. 1, pp. 1021–1022).

4.24. **(D)** IgA nephropathy (Berger's disease) is characterized by the deposition of IgA in the mesangium of the glomeruli usually with complement. The reasons for the deposition of IgA are not known. There is no evidence that IgA circulates in the form of immune complexes. Most likely the deposited IgA locally activates complement via the alternate pathway (Ref. 1, p. 1019).

4.25. **(A)** Goodpasture's syndrome is the prototype of a kidney disease caused by antibodies to glomerular basement membrane. Disruption of the basement membrane is accompanied by deposition of fibrin and formation of extracapillary crescents (Ref. 1, pp. 1010–1011).

4.26. **(D)** Lipoid nephrosis is a disease of unknown pathogenesis. There is no evidence of injury due to specific antiglomerular basement membrane antibodies or circulating immune complexes. Immunofluorescent microscopic examination of the kidney will usually yield negative results, i.e., no immunoglobulins or complement will be found in the glomeruli. By light microscopy the glomeruli appear normal. By electron microscopy one may usually find fusion of the foot processes of the epithelial cells in the glomeruli (Ref. 1, pp. 1014–1015).

4.27. **(B)** Most cases of membranoproliferative glomerulonephritis type I have circulating immune complexes in serum. By electron microscopy the deposits of immune complexes present as dense aggregates in the subendothelial location, but also in other locations (Ref. 1, pp. 1016–1018).

4.28. **(B)** Down's syndrome is in most instances characterized by trisomy of the chromosome 21 and Klinefelter's syndrome by more than one X chromosome. In both instances the karyotype of the affected individual contains an abnormal number of chromosomes. Phenylketonuria and Tay-Sachs disease are inborn errors of metabolism. Although in both diseases the enzyme defect has been identified, the chromosomal analysis will not show any structural or numerical chromosomal changes (Ref. 1, pp. 126–129).

4.29. (B) Caseous necrosis is usually found in the center of granulomas caused by *Mycobacterium tuberculosis*. It is a combination of coagulation and liquefaction necrosis. The name has been derived from the cheesy appearance of the lesions on gross examination. The caseous consistency has been attributed to the lipopolysaccharides released from the capsule of *M. tuberculosis*, but the exact pathogenesis of the lesion and the reasons for caseation are not known. Presence of caseous necrosis helps distinguish tuberculous granuloma from granulomas of sarcoidosis (Ref. 1, pp. 64, 341).

4.30. (D) Acanthosis nigricans is a clinically important paraneoplastic skin lesion. It occurs in middle-aged and older persons and presents as a hyperpigmented patch on the skin of the flexural areas (axillae, groins, anogenital area) and neck. In most instances the underlying malignancy is localized in the stomach (Ref. 1, p. 256).

4.31. (C) Osteomalacia has many causes which all lead to inadequate mineralization of bone matrix. It represents the adult counterpart of rickets. The production of osteoid matrix is not impaired. The bones contain increased amounts of osteoid which is not mineralized and thus lacks firmness. Fractures are therefore common (Ref. 1, pp. 1327–1329).

4.32. (C) The patient had a Zollinger-Ellison syndrome. The gastrin-producing tumors are most often localized in the pancreas, but 13% of gastrinomas are in the duodenum (Ref. 1, pp. 987–988).

4.33. (C) Multiple endocrine adenomatosis type I (MEA-I) presents with tumor or hyperplasia of the pituitary, parathyroid, adrenal cortex, and pancreas. This is in contrast with MEA-II which presents with medullary carcinoma of the thyroid and pheochromocytoma (Ref. 1, p. 988).

4.34. **(A)** Cystic renal dysplasia is the most common form of unilateral renal cystic disease and typically presents as an intraabdominal mass. The other kidney is usually normal. Bilateral disease is less common and those children develop renal insufficiency soon after birth (Ref. 1, p. 999).

4.35. **(E)** Cystic renal dysplasia occurs sporadically and is not considered a heredofamilial condition. This contrasts with the autosomal dominant inheritance of the adult form of polycystic renal disease and the autosomal recessive inheritance of the infantile form of renal polycystic disease (Ref. 1, p. 999).

4.36. **(C)** The photograph depicts abscesses of the testis. Viruses, spirochetes, and mycoplasma do not produce purulent lesions, i.e., abscesses. Thus the lesions represents a form of bacterial orchitis, most likely caused by pyogenic staphylococci or streptococci (Ref. 1, pp. 1088–1089).

Reference

1. Robbins, S.L., Cotran, R.S., and Kumar, V.: *Pathologic Basis of Disease, 3rd Ed.*, W.B. Saunders, Philadelphia, 1984.

5

Pharmacology
John R. McCullough, Ph.D.

DIRECTIONS: Each of the questions or incomplete statements below is followed by five suggested answers or completions. Select the **one** that is best in each case.

5.1. Cimetidine is

   A. a histamine analog which can be substituted for histamine as a test of gastric secretion

   B. a liberator of histamine from mast cells and basophils

   C. an H_1-receptor blocker which also inhibits gastric secretion

   D. a selective H_1-receptor blocker with much less sedating properties

   E. a selective H_2-receptor blocker which inhibits gastric secretion

5.2. The drug of choice in the initial treatment of status epilepticus is intravenous

   A. carbamazepine

   B. diazepam

   C. lidocaine

   D. meprobamate

   E. clonazepam

5.3. Figure 13 is a graph of the membrane responsiveness, relating the maximum rate of rise of phase zero of a cardiac action potential to the activation potential. Curve I is the normal relationship. One of the actions of antiarrhythmic agents, such as quinidine, is
  A. a shift in the responsiveness relationship along curve I to less negative potentials
  B. a shift in the responsiveness relationship from curve II to curve I to improve conduction
  C. a shift in the responsiveness relationship along curve II to more negative potentials
  D. a shift in the responsiveness relationship from curve I to curve II
  E. none of the above

Figure 13

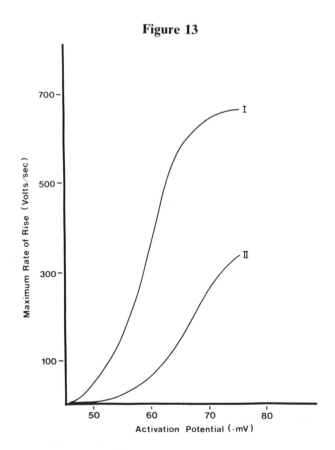

5.4. Which of the following is a potassium-sparing diuretic?
   A. Furosemide
   B. Ethacrynic acid
   C. Chlorothiazide
   D. Hydrochlorothiazide
   E. Triamterene

5.5. Cyclosporine A is
   A. a cytotoxic immunosuppressive agent affecting B lymphocytes
   B. a cytotoxic immunosuppressive agent affecting T lymphocytes
   C. an analog of cyclophosphamide useful in the treatment of severe rheumatoid arthritis
   D. an immunosuppressive agent inhibiting the expression of effector T lymphocytes
   E. an immunosuppressive agent affecting the generation of suppressor lymphocytes

5.6. Which of the following anesthetics has poor analgesic properties?
   A. Methoxyflurane
   B. Nitrous oxide
   C. Ketamine
   D. Thiopental
   E. Innovar (fentanyl + droperidol)

5.7. The drug of choice in the treatment of a suspected opiate overdose is
   A. oxymorphone
   B. levallorphan
   C. naloxone
   D. pentazocine
   E. nalbuphine

5.8. In a neurally stimulated skeletal muscle, an effective dose of d-tubocurarine would produce which of the following changes in the contractions?
  A. No change in frequency, but a reduction in amplitude
  B. An increase in frequency, but a reduction in amplitude
  C. An initial increase in frequency and amplitude followed by reduction
  D. An initial increase in frequency followed by a reduction in frequency
  E. None of the above

5.9. Plasma glucose levels are lowered by sulfonylureas by
  A. reducing oxidative phosphorylation and stimulating anaerobic glycolysis
  B. stimulating insulin release
  C. inhibiting the glycogenolytic actions of glucagon
  D. prolonging the half-life of circulating insulin by inhibiting its metabolism
  E. none of the above

5.10. Orthostatic hypotension following treatment with trimethapan is due to
  A. dilation of arterioles
  B. failure of the reflexes to bring about compensatory vasoconstriction
  C. dilation of veins
  D. inhibition of acetylcholine release from preganglionic nerve terminals
  E. none of the above

5.11. All the following statements concerning the mixed function oxygenases involved in drug metabolism are true EXCEPT
  A. treatment of a patient with certain drugs such as phenobarbital will induce the synthesis of additional oxygenase
  B. the oxygenase reactions include hydroxylations of aromatic rings and of alkyl side chains
  C. the activity of the oxygenases is lower in the neonate
  D. the hydroxylation or oxidation requires NADPH and oxygen
  E. the oxygenases are located in the mitochondria of liver cells

5.12. The main pharmacodynamic property of digitalis in congestive heart failure is
   A. to decrease venous pressure
   B. to alleviate edema by promoting diuresis
   C. to decrease diastolic size by increasing contractility
   D. to decrease blood volume
   E. none of the above

5.13. All of the following will increase the toxicity of digitoxin EXCEPT
   A. cholestyramine
   B. quinidine
   C. furosemide
   D. thioridazine
   E. isoproterenol

5.14. Local anesthetics act by
   A. forming areas of nerve block along a neuron
   B. binding to a chloride receptor on the nerve membrane
   C. blocking calcium channels of nerve membranes
   D. increasing the potassium conductance, making it harder to reach threshold for the action potential
   E. inhibiting the transient increase in sodium conductance underlying the action potential

5.15. Which of the following agents intercalates with DNA?
   A. Thioguanine
   B. Adriamycin
   C. Chlorambucil
   D. Vinblastine
   E. Bleomycin

5.16. A single 700-mg dose of a new drug was given to a 70-kg patient by intravenous bolus. Figure 14 plots the plasma concentration of the drug vs. time after administration. The apparent volume of distribution of the new drug in this patient is
   A. 700 L
   B. 70 L
   C. 7 L/kg
   D. 0.1 L/kg
   E. 0.7 L/kg

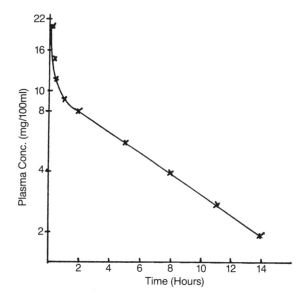

Figure 14

DIRECTIONS: Each group of questions below consists of five lettered headings followed by a list of numbered words or statements. For each numbered word or statement, select the **one** lettered heading that is most closely associated with it. Each lettered heading may be selected once, more than once, or not at all.

A. Phentolamine
B. Metoprolol
C. Pindolol
D. Labetalol
E. Propranolol

5.17. An antagonist of α- and β-adrenoceptors

5.18. A β-adrenoceptor antagonist with intrinsic sympathomimetic activity

A. Cephalosporins
B. Erythromycins
C. Polymyxins
D. Idoxuridine
E. Tetracyclines

5.19. Binds to the 50s subunit of the microbial ribosome interfering with protein synthesis

5.20. Interferes with cell-wall synthesis

5.21. Interferes with the synthesis of functional DNA

DIRECTIONS: Each set of lettered headings below is followed by a list of numbered words or phrases. For each numbered word or phrase select
(A) if the item is associated with A only
(B) if the item is associated with B only
(C) if the item is associated with both A and B
(D) if the item is associated with neither A nor B

A. Ephedrine
B. Methoxamine
C. Both
D. Neither

5.22. Most effects are due to norepinephrine release

5.23. Not deaminated by monoamine oxidase

A. Lithium carbonate
B. Chlorpromazine
C. Both
D. Neither

5.24. Useful in the treatment of severe violent mania

5.25. Useful in the treatment of schizophrenia

5.26. Useful in the treatment of anxiety

DIRECTIONS: For each of the questions or incomplete statements below, **one or more** of the answers or completions given is correct. Select
  (A) if only 1, 2, and 3 are correct
  (B) if only 1 and 3 are correct
  (C) if only 2 and 4 are correct
  (D) if only 4 is correct
  (E) if all are correct.

5.27. Figure 15 represents dose–response curves for several drugs. According to the receptor theory of drug action
  1. curves I and III could represent two agonists with equal efficacy, drug I being more potent than drug III
  2. curves I and III could represent the response to an agonist before (I) and after (III) treatment with a competitive antagonist
  3. curves I and II could represent two drugs with similiar potencies but drug I is a full agonist whereas II is a partial agonist
  4. curves I and II could represent the response to an agonist before (I) and after (II) treatment with a noncompetitive antagonist

5.28. The rationale(s) for the use of the fixed combination trimethoprim-sulfamethoxazole as an antimicrobial is (are)
  1. trimethoprim improves the solubility of sulfamethoxazole excreted in the urine
  2. sulfamethoxazole is a competitive antagonist of para-aminobenzoic acid, preventing its incorporation into folic acid
  3. trimethoprim and sulfamethoxazole together act non-competitively to inhibit tetrahydrofolate synthesis
  4. trimethoprim inhibits dihydrofolate reductases preventing the formation of tetrahydrofolate

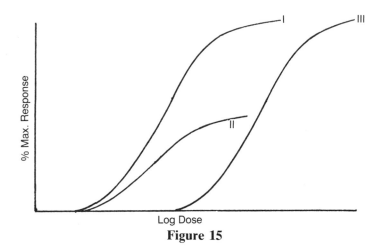

Figure 15

5.29. Cardiac glycosides increase the contractility of the cardiac muscle by
   1. slowing the rate, thus allowing the muscle time to relax
   2. increasing the ATPase activity of the contractile proteins
   3. increasing the activity of the sodium pump
   4. increasing the fraction of Ca^{2+} exchanged for Na^+

5.30. With respect to the treatment of epilepsies
   1. phenytoin, carbamazepine, and phenobarbital are used for tonic-clonic (grand mal) seizures
   2. primidone and phenobarbital are used for absence (petit mal) seizures
   3. clonazepam and ethosuximide are used for absence (petit mal) seizures
   4. mephobarbital is superior to phenobarbital and can be used in lower doses

5.31. Glucocorticoids
   1. interact with intracellular receptors in target cells
   2. promote disposition of glycogen in the liver
   3. suppress the inflammatory response as a result of hypersensitivity reactions
   4. exhibit relatively more potency for sodium retention than mineralocorticoids

DIRECTIONS: This section of the test consists of situations, each followed by a series of questions. Study each situation and select the **one** best answer to each question following it.

Questions 5.32—5.33: A 45-year-old male musician is brought from the concert hall to the emergency room suffering from shortness of breath. Upon examination the following symptoms are noted: hypotension, bradycardia, AV block, bronchial congestion, and diarrhea. The patient is depressed, but otherwise alert. An oral history reveals that the patient took several "migraine" tablets to calm his performance jitters.

5.32. The migraine pills were most likely
  A. diazepam
  B. amitriptylene
  C. propranolol
  D. methysergide
  E. diphenhydramine hydrochloride

5.33. The treatment for this drug overdose is
  A. atropine
  B. dopamine
  C. phenoxybenzamine
  D. hemodialysis
  E. none

Question 5.34: A 3-year-old child who has eaten some "wild berries" is rushed to the emergency room with dry mucous membranes, dilated unresponsive pupils, tachydardia, dry flush, rash, and fever.

5.34. The treatment of choice is
  A. small dose of acetycholine
  B. large dose of acetylcholine
  C. isoflurophate (diisopropyl phosphorofluoridate)
  D. neostigmine
  E. physostigmine

Questions 5.35–5.36: A 30-year-old male is seen exhibiting the following symptoms: hypertension, sweating, palpitations, tachycardia, headache, and weight loss. Hematology reveals increased fasting glucose levels. Analysis of urinary catecholamines indicates increased excretion. Cardiomyopathy was also found.

5.35. A pheochromocytoma is suspected and the pharmacologic diagnostic test(s) may include
  A. injection of a small dose of propranolol to prevent tachycardia
  B. injection of histamine or tyramine to stimulate catecholamine release
  C. injection of phenoxybenzamine to prevent blood pressure rise
  D. injection of a monoamine oxidase inhibitor to increase urinary catecholamine excretion
  E. none of the above

5.36. From the results of the diagnostic test(s) surgery is indicated. In preparation for the removal of the tumor, the patient's tachycardia and hypertension are treated with
  A. propranolol
  B. phenoxybenzamine then propranolol
  C. propranolol then phentolamine
  D. nitrites and digitalis
  E. digitalis alone

Answers and Comments

5.1. (E) Cimetidine is a selective competitive antagonist of H_2 receptors and has virtually no activity on H_1 receptors. It inhibits histamine-induced gastric acid release and is used in hypersecretory states. H_1-receptor blockers do not antagonize gastric acid secretion (Refs. 1, pp. 609–632; 2, pp. 183–193; 3, p. 437).

5.2. (B) Diazepam is the drug of choice, but phenytoin or a barbiturate (pentobarbital, phenobarbital, etc.) IV may also be given to control convulsions (Refs. 1, pp. 339–361, 470–471; 2, p. 317; 3, p. 907; 4, p. 302).

5.3. (D) Quinidine and quinidinelike antiarrhythmic agents, such as lidocaine, propranolol, and procainamide, reduce both the amplitude of the action potential and its rate of rise. Since the amplitude and rate of rise are dependent upon the membrane potential, at any given potential these agents reduce the response compared to control. This has the effect of reducing conduction velocity, thereby slowing arrhythmias. Note: these agents have other actions that add to their antiarrhythmic activity (Refs. 1, pp. 761–792; 3, pp. 225–258).

5.4. (E) Only triamterene (and spironolactone) of those diuretics listed are potassium-sparing (Refs. 1, pp. 908–909; 2, pp. 160–169).

5.5. (D) Cyclosporine A inhibits effector T lymphocytes without affecting suppressor or B lymphocytes. It is useful in preventing rejection of transplanted organs (Ref. 4, pp. 1433–1448).

5.6. (D) Thiopental and other ultrashort-acting barbiturates are very poor analgesics and may actually be antianalgesic at low blood concentrations. All the other agents provide profound analgesia although their anesthetic potencies vary (Ref. 1, pp. 286–297).

5.7. (C) Naloxone, a competitive opiate antagonist, is the drug of choice in a narcotic overdose because it lacks agonist activity and thus does not further depress respiration. Levallorphan also is a competitive antagonist, but possesses agonist activity that may intensify respiratory depression. Oxymorphone (a pure agonist), and nalbuphine, and pentazocine (mixed agonist-antagonists) are used for their agonist activities (Refs. 1, pp. 494–534; 2, pp. 264–279; 3, p. 1019; 4, pp. 67–86, 1871–1873).

5.8. (A) d-Tubocurarine is a competitive antagonist of acetylcholine (ACh) at the neuromuscular junction; therefore, only a reduction in contraction amplitude is seen. Depolarizing agents, such as succinylcholine, cause an initial period of rapid stimulation followed by a depolarizing block of ACh receptor (Refs. 1, pp. 220–232; 2, pp. 210–215).

5.9. (B) Sulfonylureas stimulate insulin release from the pancreas. They are useful in the treatment of maturity-onset diabetes (Refs. 1, pp. 1510–1514; 2, pp. 385–388; 3, pp. 530–533).

5.10. (B) Although ganglionic blocking agents, such as trimethaphan, dilate arterioles and veins, it is the blockade of the vasomotor reflexes that results in postural hypotension (Ref. 1, pp. 215–217).

5.11. (E) The liver microsound oxygenase system is located in the smooth endoplasmic reticulum of liver cells. These enzymes generally convert active lipid-soluble substances to inactive, more polar, water-soluble metabolites which are easier to excrete. The activity of this system is low at birth, leading to a longer half-life of a drug in an infant than in an adult (Refs. 1, pp. 13–19; 2, pp. 11–13; 3, pp. 146–147).

5.12. (C) The principal action of cardiac glycosides is their ability to increase the force of contraction. The other effects (i.e., increased cardiac output; reduced cardiac size, blood volume, and venous pressure; diuresis) beneficial to patients with congested heart failure are all a result of the positive inotropic action. Slowing of ventricular rate in atrial fibrillation or flutter is a second important action. Digitalis has other actions which may be explained on the basis of its actions on vascular smooth muscles and the autonomic nervous system (Refs. 1, pp. 729–756; 2, pp. 135–146).

5.13. (A) Cholestyramine can bind digitoxin, decreasing its reabsorption from the intestine. Quinidine can increase plasma concentrations, perhaps by displacing glycoside bound to tissues. Furosemide can lead to hypokalemia and digitalis toxicity. Thioridazine can have a quinidinelike action, and can lead to more sympathetic tone through its antimuscarinic action. Increased sympathetic tone and/or β-agonists, such as isoproterenol, increase the likelihood of arrhythmias in patients taking digitalis (Ref. 1, pp. 414, 729–756, 843).

5.14. (E) Local anesthetics block the increase in sodium conductance underlying the upstroke of the action potential. They apparently must react with sites on the internal surface of the membrane. These sites are believed to be the sodium channels, which must first be activated (or opened) before the local anesthetic can block them (Ref. 1, pp. 301–302).

5.15. (B) All of these agents are antineoplastic agents. Adriamycin intercalates with DNA inhibiting RNA synthesis. Chlorambucil is an alkylating agent which cross-links DNA strands. Bleomycin causes breaks in DNA and prevents repair. Thioguanine inhibits purine biosynthesis, and vinblastine binds to the mitotic spindle apparatus causing disruption of mitosis (Refs. 1, pp. 1252–1305; 2, pp. 477–499; 3, pp. 804–821).

5.16. (D) When a drug is administered as a single IV dose, initially the plasma concentration falls rapidly as the drug is distributed throughout the body. The second phase represents first-order elimination of the drug. This line is extrapolated to give a plasma concentration at zero time, namely 10 mg/100 ml

apparent volume of distribution

$$= \frac{\text{total amount in body}}{\text{plasma concentration}} = \frac{700 \text{ mg}/70 \text{ kg}}{10 \text{ mg}/100 \text{ ml}}$$
$$= \frac{10 \text{ mg/kg}}{100 \text{ mg/L}} = 0.1 \text{ L/kg}$$

or for the 70-kg patient 7L (Ref. 1, pp. 21–22).

5.17. (D)

5.18. (C) Labetalol competively antagonizes both α- and β-adrenoceptors and lacks selectivity for β-receptor subtypes. Pindolol is a nonselective β-blocker and possesses the ability to act as a partial agonist (intrinsic sympathomimetic activity). Phentolamine is a competitive α-antagonist. Propranolol is a nonselective β-antagonist whereas metroprolol is a cardioselective β-antagonist (Refs. 1, pp. 178–198; 4, pp. 655–662, 718–728).

5.19. (B)

5.20. (A)

5.21. (D) Erythromycins, lincomycins, and chloramphenicol bind to the 50s subunit of the microbial ribosome to inhibit protein synthesis. Both tetracyclines and aminoglycoside antibiotics bind to different receptors on the 30s subunit. Cephalosporins and penicillins inhibit the transpeptidation reaction which involves the terminal cross-linking of linear glycopeptides in bacterial cell-wall synthesis. Polymyxins bind to bacterial cell membranes rich in phosphatidylethanolamine, and disrupt transport mechanisms leading to cell lysis. Idoxuridine is an example of analogs of nucleic acid bases which are incorporated into the DNA of DNA viruses. They cause either an inhibition of DNA synthesis or a nonfunctional DNA structure (Refs. 1, pp. 1081, 1129−1130, 1164−1165, 1183, 1192, 1222−1223, 1229, 1240−1243; 2, pp. 530−533, 544, 549, 553, 556, 561, 576, 590−591; 3, pp. 743−776).

5.22. (A)

5.23. (C) Most of the effects of ephedrine are due to its ability to release norepinephrine. It does have some partial agonist activity for α-receptors as well as direct CNS stimulatory actions. Methoxamine is primarily a direct α-agonist with little β-activity. Both ephedrine and methoxamine have substituted α-carbons, protecting them from inactivation by monoamine oxidase thus prolonging their duration of action (Ref. 1, pp. 141−144, 163−166).

5.24. (C)

5.25. (B)

5.26. (D) Lithium carbonate is the drug of choice for mania. Since its onset of action is slow, an antipsychotic agent such as chlorpromazine, can be coadministered to control bizarre behavior at the beginning of therapy. Antipsychotic agents (phenothiazines, thioxanthenes, butyrophenones, etc.) are more effective for schizophrenia. Anxiety is best relieved with a long-acting sedative such as phenobarbital or a benzodiazepine (Refs. 1, pp. 339−354, 395−418, 430−434, 437−442; 2, pp. 226−238, 251−262; 3, pp. 842−848, 856−868).

5.27. (E) All the answers are correct. Curves I and III could represent two agonists with equal efficacy (since they both are able to produce the same maximal response) but differing potency (a higher concentration of III than of I is needed to produce the same response). Curves I and III could represent the effects of a competitive antagonist, namely a parallel shift in the dose response relationship without affecting the maximum response (i.e., a higher concentration of I is needed in the presence of the competitive antagonist). Curves I and II could represent a full (I) and a partial (II) agonist in that they produce responses in the same dose range, but the partial agonist produces a smaller maximum response. Or curves I and II could represent the effects of a noncompetitive antagonist in reducing the number of receptors the agonist can react with, thereby reducing the maximal response (Ref. 1, pp. 28−35).

5.28. (C) Sulfamethoxazole and trimethoprim inhibit sequential steps in an obligate enzymatic pathway in bacteria; therefore, their combination is synergistic. Sulfamethoxazole alone is usually bacteriostatic, but the combination with trimethoprim is bactericidal (Refs. 1, pp. 1048−1049, 1108, 1116−1119; 2, pp. 532−533, 570−573; 3, pp. 737, 767−768; 4, pp. 1721−1722, 1733−1742).

5.29. (D) Although the mechanism of action of cardiac glycosides has not been completely elucidated, most evidence suggests that at therapeutic concentrations cardiac glycosides inhibit Na^+-K^+ exchange due to the sodium pump. Increased intracellular Na^+ results in an increase in its exchange for extracellular Ca^{2+} by a Na^+-Ca^{2+} pump mechanism (Ref. 1, pp. 732−734).

5.30. (B) Phenytoin, primidone, and phenobarbital are not effective in the treatment of absence seizures and may increase the frequency of their occurrence. Mephobarbital requires higher doses than phenobarbital and most of its actions can be attributed to its metabolite phenobarbital (Refs. 1, pp. 448−471; 3, pp. 900−908).

5.31. (A) Corticosteroid hormones exhibit a wide range of activities. The glucocorticoids show relatively greater potencies for liver glycogen disposition than potencies of the mineralocorticoids for sodium retention (Refs. 1, pp. 1470−1493; 2, pp. 353−364).

5.32. (C) The patient's symptoms are those of propranolol overdose and represent widespread β-receptor blockade. In addition to β-blocking action propranolol also has quinidinelike actions on the heart. Propranolol is also indicated for migraine. Diazepam is a sedative; amitriptylene, a tricyclic antidepressant; methysergide, an ergot alkaloid used in migraine; and diphenhydramine, an antihistamine (Refs. 1, pp. 188−194, 418−427, 436−442, 622−629, 946−947; 2, pp. 98−102, 183−196, 226−241, 295−307).

5.33. (A) The treatment for propranolol overdose is atropine to improve AV conduction (Refs. 1, p. 193; 3, pp. 254−255, 478−479).

5.34. (E) The child has symptoms of muscarinic-blocker poisoning. The anticholinesterase physostigmine is the drug of choice because it is able to cross the blood-brain barrier and reverse the central effects of the belladonna poisoning. Acetylcholine would be hydrolyzed too rapidly. The other anticholinesterases are either too toxic (isoflurophate) or unable to cross the blood—brain barrier (Refs. 1, pp. 100—128; 2, pp. 61—78).

5.35. **(B)** Urinary and/or plasma catecholamines levels are usually diagnostic, but in some patients urinary catecholamines may be normal; therefore, release of catecholamines may be stimulated by injection of histamine or tyramine. Blood pressure and urinary and blood catecholamines should be monitored. Phentolamine should be available in case of a large rise in blood pressure (Refs. 1, pp. 186—187; 3, pp. 175—179).

5.36. **(B)** To allow improvement of the cardiovascular function of the patient, persistent α-blockade is used. Phenoxybenzamine is the choice for its long duration of action. *After* α-blockade, propranolol may be added to block the β actions of the circulating catecholamines on the heart (Refs. 1, pp. 186—187; 3, pp. 175—179).

References

1. Gilman A.G., Goodman L.S., and Gilman A. (eds.): *Goodman and Gilman's The Pharmacological Basis of Therapeutics*, 6th Ed., Macmillan, New York, 1980.

2. Meyers, F.H., Jawerz, E., and Goldfien, A.: *Review of Medical Pharmacology*, 7th Ed., Lange Medical Publications, Los Altos, CA, 1980.

3. Melmon, K.L. and Morrelli, H.F. (eds.): *Clinical Pharmacology: Basic Principles in Therapeuticals*, 2nd Ed., Macmillan, New York, 1978.

4. *AMA Drug Evaluations*, 5th Ed., American Medical Association, Chicago, 1983.

6

Physiology
James L. Poland, Ph.D.

DIRECTIONS: Each of the questions or incomplete statements below is followed by five suggested answers or completions. Select the **one** that is best in each case.

6.1. Given the following ECG complexes as recorded from the indicated leads (Figure 16), determine whether the major QRS vector is directed anteriorly (toward the sternum) or posteriorly (toward the spine); inferiorly (toward the feet) or superiorly (toward the head); to the right (toward the subject's right arm) or to the left (toward the subject's left arm).
   A. Posteriorly, superiorly, to the left
   B. Posteriorly, superiorly, to the right
   C. Anteriorly, superiorly, to the left
   D. Anteriorly, superiorly, to the right
   E. Posteriorly, inferiorly, to the left

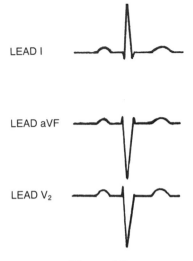

LEAD I

LEAD aVF

LEAD V$_2$

Figure 16

6.2. Figure 17 represents a graduated centrifuge tube containing
10 ml of heparinized blood following centrifugation. Which
of the following is the best combination of hematocrit value
and probable donor?

A. 7 ml, healthy subject living at sea level
B. 70%, healthy subject living at sea level
C. 3 ml, healthy subject living at high altitude
D. 30%, healthy subject living at high altitude
E. 30%, anemic subject living at sea level

Figure 17

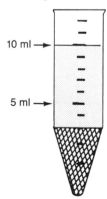

10 ml →

5 ml →

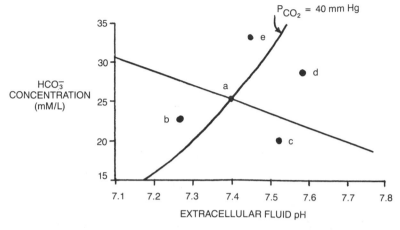

Figure 18

6.3. On the pH-HCO_3^- diagram (Figure 18) which point represents respiratory compensation of metabolic alkaloses?
  A. a
  B. b
  C. c
  D. d
  E. e

6.4. A membrane permeable to water but not to Na^+ or Cl^- separates compartments A and B in Figure 19. With pure water on side B and a NaCl solution on side A initially
  A. the volume of fluid on side B will increase
  B. the concentration of NaCl on side A will increase
  C. a hydrostatic pressure applied to side A could prevent osmosis
  D. the osmolarity of side B is greater than that of the solution on side A
  E. the movement of water molecules is by diffusion as opposed to bulk flow

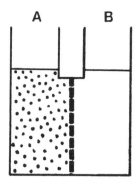

Figure 19

6.5. Surface tension forces within the alveoli of a normal healthy lung:
  A. tend to make the lungs collapse
  B. are increased by the presence of surfactant molecules
  C. are greater at low lung volumes than at high lung volumes in normal lungs
  D. are insignificant compared to the magnitude of the elastic fiber forces within lung tissues
  E. prevent edema

6.6. Absorption readily occurs in all of the following gastrointestinal surfaces EXCEPT
  A. villi
  B. brush border of microvilli
  C. valvulae conniventes
  D. stomach lining
  E. lining of the jejunum

6.7. Severe irritation of the mucosa lining of the small intestine may cause
  A. a stop in the propulsion of chyme
  B. intestinal obstruction
  C. the chyme to move more slowly to reduce the irritation
  D. a "peristaltic rush" to quickly move the chyme into the colon
  E. little or no effect on the movement of chyme

6.8. Carbon dioxide is transported in the blood to the greatest extent as
  A. carbonic anhydrase
  B. carboxyhemoglobin
  C. carbaminohemoglobin
  D. bicarbonate ions
  E. dissolved carbon dioxide

6.9. The rapid repolarization phase of an action potential in a neuron is due to an increase in the permeability of
  A. calcium
  B. sodium
  C. chloride
  D. potassium
  E. magnesium

6.10. Taste buds sensitive to sodium chloride tend to
  A. be concentrated along the lateral margins of the tongue
  B. become increasingly sensitive in old age
  C. be absent on circumvallate papillae
  D. contain taste cells whose life span is about 1 year
  E. persist following their nerve fiber destruction

6.11. Which of the following conditions is NOT associated with diabetes mellitus?
  A. Vascular disease
  B. Acidosis
  C. Dehydration
  D. Ketonuria
  E. Positive nitrogen balance

6.12. While standing the lower portion of the lung, relative to the upper part, has a
  A. smaller blood flow
  B. larger ventilation
  C. higher ventilation−perfusion ratio
  D. higher alveolar PO_2
  E. higher volume for individual alveoli

6.13. In the absence of aldosterone
    A. no sodium is reabsorbed by the proximal tubules
    B. plasma sodium increases
    C. the filtered load of sodium is increased
    D. the distal tubules decrease the reabsorption of sodium
    E. the glomerular filtration rate increases

6.14. A key determinant of the volume of bile generated by the liver is the
    A. number of meals ingested per day
    B. amount of bile salts recycled through the enterohepatic circulation
    C. rate of conjugation of bilirubin
    D. concentration of cholesterol in bile
    E. volume of the gallbladder when fully distended

6.15. A fever is associated with
    A. cold weather activating body heat conservation
    B. inability to regulate body temperature around a set point
    C. elevation of the hypothalamic temperature set point
    D. inactivation of warm receptors in the hypothalamus
    E. inactivation of cold receptors in the skin

6.16. Hypoglycemia will generate
    A. elevated glucagon levels
    B. elevated insulin levels
    C. osmotic diuresis
    D. glycosuria
    E. increased lipid synthesis

DIRECTIONS: Each group of questions below consists of five lettered headings followed by a list of numbered words or statements. For each numbered word or statement, select the **one** lettered heading that is most closely associated with it. Each lettered heading may be selected once, more than once, or not at all.

When contrasting areas of the cardiovascular system, match the most prominent characteristic with the area.

A. Greatest pulse pressure
B. Fastest velocity of blood flow
C. Largest total cross-sectional area
D. Greatest resistance to blood flow
E. Largest volume of blood flow

6.17. Systemic capillaries

6.18. Arterioles

Match the hormone with its site of release.

A. Growth hormone
B. Prolactin
C. Aldosterone
D. Antidiuretic hormone
E. Adrenocorticotropin

6.19. Posterior pituitary

6.20. Adrenal cortex

Match the appropriate changes in alveolar gas composition with the respiratory condition.

A. $\uparrow PO_2$, $\uparrow PCO_2$
B. $\uparrow PO_2$, $\downarrow PCO_2$
C. $\downarrow PO_2$, $\uparrow PCO_2$
D. $\downarrow PO_2$, $\downarrow PCO_2$
E. $\downarrow PO_2$, no change in PCO_2

6.21. Hyperventilation

DIRECTIONS: Each set of lettered headings below is followed by a list of numbered words or phrases. For each numbered word or phrase select

  (A) if the item is associated with A only
  (B) if the item is associated with B only
  (C) if the item is associated with both A and B
  (D) if the item is associated with neither A nor B

Question 6.22:
  A. Type A blood
  B. Type O blood
  C. Both
  D. Neither

6.22. A complete list of possible donors during a transfusion involving a small amount of donor blood for a recipient of type A blood

Question 6.23:
  A. An increase in muscle tension
  B. A decrease in muscle length
  C. Both
  D. Neither

6.23. Isometric contraction of skeletal muscle

Question 6.24:
  A. Cellular immunity will be present
  B. Humoral immunity will be present
  C. Both
  D. Neither

6.24. Removal of the thymus a few years after birth

Question 6.25:
  A. High sodium concentration
  B. High potassium concentration
  C. Both
  D. Neither

6.25. Extracellular fluid (relative to intracellular fluid)

Question 6.26:
    A. Located presynaptically
    B. Located postsynaptically
    C. Both
    D. Neither.

6.26. Synaptic vesicles

DIRECTIONS: For each of the questions or incomplete statements below, **one or more** of the answers or completions given is correct. Select
    (A) if only 1, 2, and 3 are correct
    (B) if only 1 and 3 are correct
    (C) if only 2 and 4 are correct
    (D) if only 4 is correct
    (E) if all are correct

6.27. Lesions of the dorsal–lemniscal system eliminate the ability to
    1. feel touch
    2. localize touch
    3. detect joint location
    4. detect pain

6.28. In normal eyes, accommodation to see an object placed at a short distance (e.g., 50 cm) from the eyes
    1. is enhanced by a concave lens placed in front of each eye
    2. involves pupillary constriction
    3. involves flattening of the lens
    4. involves convergence of the eyes

6.29. The gastrointestinal system is controlled by
    1. parasympathetic innervation
    2. its own intrinsic nervous system
    3. sympathetic innervation
    4. hormonal action

6.30. The sarcoplasmic reticulum
1. releases calcium to initiate contraction
2. is a storage site for calcium between contractions
3. actively removes calcium from the sarcoplasm to bring about relaxation
4. provides a pathway for the inward spread of electrical activity from the sarcolemma

6.31. Potentially detrimental effects of hypertension include
1. coronary arteriosclerosis
2. vascular hemorrhages
3. damage to the retina
4. cardiac atrophy

DIRECTIONS: This section of the test consists of situations, each followed by a series of questions. Study each situation and select the **one** best answer to each question following it.

Questions 6.32−6.33: Given the following data for inulin and substances "X" and "Y" (all the same size):

Inulin concentration in urine	200 mg/100 ml
Inulin concentation in plasma	2.0 mg/100 ml
Concentration in urine for substance "X"	15 mg/100 ml
Concentration in plasma for substance "X"	1.5 mg/100 ml
Concentration in urine for substance "Y"	200 mg/100 ml
Concentration in plasma for substance "Y"	1.0 mg/100 ml

6.32. Which of the following would explain the renal handling of substance "X"?
A. "X" is freely filtered but neither secreted nor reabsorbed
B. "X" is not freely filtered but is reabsorbed
C. "X" is not freely filtered but is secreted
D. "X" is freely filtered and partially reabsorbed
E. "X" is freely filtered and additionally secreted

6.33. Which of the following would explain the renal handling of substance "Y"?
   A. "Y" is freely filtered but neither secreted nor reabsorbed
   B. "Y" is not freely filtered but is reabsorbed
   C. "Y" is not freely filtered but is secreted
   D. "Y" is freely filtered and partially reabsorbed
   E. "Y" is freely filtered and additionally secreted

Question 6.34: The following data were reported for a man of large size (2 m^2 = body surface area) during exercise:
   Oxygen consumption = 1200 ml O$_2$/min
   Arterial oxygen concentration = 20 ml%
   Mixed venous oxygen concentration = 10 ml%
   Heart rate = 120 beats/min

6.34. From this information, which of the following statements is true?
   A. 0.1 ml of oxygen is removed from each 100 ml of circulating blood
   B. Cardiac output = 6 L/min
   C. Cardiac index = 12 L/min
   D. Stroke volume = 100 ml/beat
   E. None of the above

Question 6.35: By mistake a 1-L bottle containing hypertonic saline (1500) mOsm NaCl/L) was administered intravenously to a patient rapidly, instead of using isotonic saline. The patient's body had before infusion:
   12 L = extracellular fluid
   23 L = intracellular fluid
   300 mOsm/L = plasma osmolarity

6.35. Because intracellular water diffuses out osmotically, the new plasma osmolarity, after osmotic equilibrium has been reached, will be
   A. 320 mOsm/L
   B. 333 mOsm/L
   C. 343 mOsm/L
   D. 348 mOsm/L
   E. 352 mOsm/L

Question 6.36: Examination of a patient with a bullet wound that damaged the spinal cord showed suppression of motor function and touch sensation on the right lower extremity, plus the loss of pain and temperature on the left side.

6.36. The diagnosis is likely to be
  A. total transection of the spinal cord at lumbar segment I
  B. compression by a clot over the anterior roots of lumbar segment I
  C. hemorrhage of the anterior horns of the gray matter
  D. traumatic polyneuritis
  E. Brown-Sequard syndrome

Answers and Comments

6.1. (A) The positive (upward) deflection of the QRS wave in lead I indicates that the major QRS vector is directed toward the left arm (upward deflection occurs when the left arm electrode is positive). The negative (downward) deflection of the aVF lead indicates the QRS vector is oriented superiorly rather than inferiorly. The negative (downward) deflection in lead V_2 indicates a posteriorly directed QRS vector (Ref. 1, pp. 180–185).

6.2. (E) Of the total blood sample (10 ml), 3 ml of the volume is red blood cells. Thus the hematocrit (% of whole blood made up of red blood cells) is 30%. This low hematocrit value (normal ~45%) suggests the source could have been an anemic individual. A subject at a high altitude tends to have an elevated hematocrit because the hypoxia stimulates red blood cell production (Ref. 1, pp. 206–207).

6.3. (E) Metabolic alkalosis increases pH, moving the body's equilibrium point from its normal position (point a) up and to the right along the normal CO_2 concentration line. Ventilation is depressed by the low $[H^+]$. Retaining CO_2 partially restores the pH by moving from the normal CO_2 concentration line along an imaginary buffer line (with the same slope as that buffer line through point a) to point e. Compensation is incomplete because some error must remain to depress the ventilation. Renal compensation more slowly restores the body's pH to normal (Ref. 1, pp. 460–461).

6.4. (C) The higher osmolarity of side A drawing water from side B (osmosis via bulk flow) can be offset by a hydrostatic pressure applied to side A (Ref. 1, pp. 47−49).

6.5. (A) Surface tension forces account for about two-thirds of the recoil force of the lungs. The presence of surfactant molecules lowers surface tension force and makes it volume dependent with surface tension forces being greater at higher lung volumes when surfactant is less concentrated. Surface tension forces tend to generate edema, but the presence of surfactant minimizes this action (Ref. 1, 477−478).

6.6. (D) The intestinal mucosa has many folds called valvulae conniventes. This folded surface is covered with millions of small villi. The epithelial cells lining each villus have a brush border of microvilli. These folds, villi and microvilli, increase the absorptive power of the intestine about 600-fold. The stomach, however, is not so designed and thus is a poor absorptive area (Ref. 1, p. 820).

6.7. (D) Some infections can cause a very intense irritation of the intestine which elicits a powerful peristaltic wave that travels long distances. Such a phenomenon is called a "peristaltic rush" (Ref. 1, p. 795).

6.8. (D) The greatest amount of carbon dioxide is transported in the blood as bicarbonate ions. The generation of these ions is facilitated by the enzyme carbonic anhydrase. Smaller quantities of carbon dioxide are transported as dissolved carbon dioxide or carbaminohemoglobin. Carboxyhemoglobin is the name given to hemoglobin with carbon monoxide attached (Ref. 1, pp. 512−513).

6.9. (D) Repolarization occurs when sodium, calcium, and chloride conductance are low but potassium permeability is increased (Ref. 1, p. 109).

6.10. (A) Many taste buds rapidly degenerate after age 45, causing the taste sensation to become less sensitive with age. Taste buds also degenerate when their taste nerve fibers are destroyed. A large number of taste buds, including those sensing salt, are associated with the circumvallate papillae. Taste buds for salt are highly concentrated along the lateral margins of the tongue. Taste cells have a life span of about 10 days (Ref. 1, pp. 776–777).

6.11. **(E)** Diabetes mellitus causes an increase in protein catabolism (*negative* nitrogen balance) in addition to dehydration generated by the high blood glucose and associated polyuria. The shift from carbohydrate to fat metabolism in diabetes causes ketonuria, acidosis, and atherosclerosis (Ref. 1, p. 969).

6.12. **(B)** When standing, the effects of gravity are such that both ventilation and perfusion are greater in the lower part of the lung than in the apex. However, since perfusion is affected more than ventilation the ventilation–perfusion ratio is lower at the base of the lung than at the apex. Since the ventilation–perfusion ratio is lower at the base (relatively hypoventilated area) the PO_2 will also be lower. Individual alveoli are compressed to a smaller volume at the lung's base (Ref. 1, p. 502).

6.13. **(D)** The action of aldosterone is to increase the reabsorption of sodium in the distal tubules. Thus its absence decreases this reabsorption generating decreased plasma sodium levels. Other renal processes are unaltered (Ref. 1, p. 426).

6.14. **(B)** Over 90% of the bile salts secreted in bile are reabsorbed and are used again in the formation of bile. The normal volume of bile produced by the liver is highly dependent on the recycling of bile salts (Ref. 1, p. 872).

6.15. **(C)** A fever is produced by the elevation of the hypothalamic temperature set point. The activity of warm and cold receptors as well as the ability of the body to regulate body temperature around a set point are maintained (Ref. 1, pp. 895–896).

6.16. **(A)** Low blood glucose levels (hypoglycemia) will cause insulin to decrease and glucagon to increase. Since blood glucose levels are low, none would be expected to escape reabsorption by the kidney. Thus glucosuria is unlikely and since the number of glucose particles in the urine does not increase there is no tendency for an osmotic diuresis to occur (Ref. 1, p. 968).

6.17. (C) The systemic capillaries are small in size but so numerous that their collective cross-sectional area is larger than that of any other area of the cardiovascular system. Since velocity of flow is related to cross-sectional area, velocity is slowest in the capillaries. Additionally, there is very little pulse in the capillaries and their resistance to flow is much less than that of arterioles. The venous side of the systemic circulation contains the largest volume of blood of any area in the cardiovascular system (Ref. 1, pp. 219–221).

6.18. (D) The greatest resistance to blood flow, as indicated by a drop in pressure, occurs in the arterioles. The pulse pressure is dampened considerably in the arterioles and virtually disappears in the capillaries (Ref. 1, pp. 219–221).

6.19. (D) The anterior pituitary releases growth hormone, prolactin, and adrenocorticotropin, while ADH comes from the posterior pituitary (Ref. 1, pp. 919–920).

6.20. (C) Of the hormones listed only aldosterone comes from the adrenal cortex (Ref. 1, p. 944)

6.21. (B) Hyperventilation supplies oxygen to the alveoli at an enhanced rate (PO_2) and blows off carbon dioxide at an increased rate (PCO_2) (Ref. 1, p. 495).

6.22. (C) The danger during a transfusion involving a relatively small amount of donor blood is that the recipient's antibodies will cause agglutination of the donor's red blood cells. Thus the recipient must contain no antibodies against the donor's cells. Therefore, a type A recipient (having anti-B) could receive A or O type blood, but not B or AB type (Ref. 1, pp. 85–88).

6.23. (A) An isometric contraction involves an increase in developed tension but no change in muscle length (Ref. 1, p. 132).

6.24. (C) Since the T lymphocytes for cellular immunity are pre-processed by the thymus before birth, removal of the thymus gland after birth does not impair the T-lymphocytic immune system. B lymphocytes, which account for humoral immunity, are also pre-processed before birth but the thymus gland is not likely to be involved. Thus removal of the thymus would not affect humoral immunity (Ref. 1, p. 76).

6.25. **(A)** Relatively high extracellular sodium and low extracellular potassium concentrations are established by the cell membrane's active sodium—potassium pump extruding sodium and pumping potassium into the cell (Ref. 1, p. 3).

6.26. **(A)** Synaptic vesicles, containing a transmitter substance, are found in presynaptic "knobs." Transmission of a signal across a synaptic cleft is in one direction, with the postsynaptic neuron containing no vesicles (Ref. 1, p. 565).

6.27. **(A)** The dorsal—lemniscal system transmits sensations of touch and helps localize touch as well as indicate joint position. Sensations of pain and temperature are transmitted via the antero-lateral spinothalamic system (Ref. 1, p. 600).

6.28. **(C)** Accommodation to see an object placed at a short distance from the eye involves convergence of the eyes, pupillary constriction to minimize spherical aberrations, and bulging of the lens to increase its refractive power. A convex lens placed in front of the eye will supplement the refractive power of the lens to assist accommodation (Ref. 1, pp. 728—729).

6.29. **(E)** The gastrointestinal tract has an intrinsic nervous system but is additionally innervated by both parasympathetic (stimulatory) and sympathetic (inhibitory) nerves. Several hormones also influence gastrointestinal performance (Ref. 1, pp. 786—787).

6.30. **(A)** The sarcoplasmic reticulum releases calcium in response to electrical activity propagated inward from the sarcolemma via the T tubules. This release of calcium initiates contraction which is then terminated by the active uptake of calcium by the sarcoplasmic reticulum, in which it is stored until the next stimulus (Ref. 1, pp. 129—131).

6.31. **(A)** Hypertension increases the workload of the left ventricle causing hypertrophy, causes hemorrhage of vessels including those of the retina, and generates coronary arteriosclerosis (Ref. 1, p. 272).

6.32. **(D)** Inulin is freely filtered but neither secreted nor reabsorbed, resulting in inulin becoming 100 times more concentrated in the urine (200 mg/100 ml) than in the plasma (2.0 mg/100 ml). For substance "X" to be concentrated by the kidney to a lesser extent (1.5–15 mg/100 ml), "X" must be freely filtered and then partially reabsorbed (Ref. 1, p. 418).

6.33. **(E)** Inulin is freely filtered but neither secreted nor reabsorbed by the kidney tubules, resulting in inulin becoming 100 times more concentrated in the urine than in the plasma. For substance "Y" to become 200 times more concentrated (1.0–200 mg/100 ml), "Y" must be freely filtered (since it is the same size as inulin) and then additional "Y" secreted by the tubules (Ref. 1, p. 418).

6.34. **(D)** Cardiac output $=$ $\dfrac{O_2 \text{ uptake by the lungs (ml/min)}}{\text{Arteriovenous } O_2 \text{ difference}}$
(L/ml) $\quad\quad\quad\quad\quad\quad$ (ml/L of blood)

$$= \frac{1200 \text{ ml/min}}{200 \text{ ml/L} - 100 \text{ ml/L}}$$

$$= \frac{1200 \text{ ml/min}}{100 \text{ ml/L}^*}$$

$(^*100 \text{ ml/L} = 10 \text{ ml } O_2 \text{ removed/}$
$100 \text{ ml blood})$

Cardiac output $= 12$ L/min

Cardiac index $=$ Cardiac output/body surface area

$$= \frac{12 \text{ L/min}}{2 \text{ m}^2}$$

$$= \frac{6 \text{ L/min}}{\text{m}^2}$$

Stroke volume $= \dfrac{\text{Cardiac output}}{\text{Heart rate}} = \dfrac{12 \text{ L/min}}{120 \text{ beats/min}}$

$= 0.1$ L/beat or 100 ml/beat

(Ref. 1, pp. 274, 286–287).

6.35. **(B)** See Table 1 for explanation (Ref. 1, p. 401).

TABLE 1

	Extracellular Fluid			Intracellular Fluid			Total Body Water		
	Vol. (L)	Concentration (mOsm/L)	Total (mOsm)	Vol. (L)	Concentration (mOsm/L)	Total (mOsm)	Vol. (L)	Concentration (mOsm/L)	Total (mOsm)
Initial	12.0	300.00	3600	23.0	300.0	6900	35	300.0	10,500
Solution added	1.0	1500.0	1500	—	—	—	1	1500.0	1,500
Instantaneous effect	13.0	392.3	5100	23.0	300.0	6900	36	No equilibrium	12,000
After osmotic equilibrium	15.3	333.3	5100	20.7	333.3	6900	36	333.3	12,000

6.36. (E) The Brown-Sequard syndrome occurs when only one side of the spinal cord is transected. In this situation motor functions are blocked on the side of the transection below the level of the transection. Many sensations, including touch, are lost on the same side as the transection and the sensations of pain, heat, and cold are lost on the opposite side (Ref. 1, p. 621).

Reference

1. Guyton, A.C.: *Textbook of Medical Physiology*, 6th Ed., W.B. Saunders, Philadelphia, 1981.

CLINICAL
MEDICINE

Cardiology

Louis E. Grenzer, M.D., P.A.

DIRECTIONS: Each of the questions or incomplete statements below is followed by five suggested answers or completions. Select the **one** that is best in each case.

7.1. Which of the following is true of Prinzmetal's variant angina?
  A. Good medical prognosis
  B. ST depression is the characteristic ECG finding
  C. Propranolol is contraindicated
  D. Ventricular arrhythmias are common
  E. Most patients have spasm but otherwise normal coronary arteries

7.2. Which of the following is NOT characteristic of hyperkalemia on the ECG?
  A. Tall peaked T waves
  B. Widening of the QRS complex
  C. Reduction in P wave amplitude
  D. Prominent U waves
  E. Ventricular fibrillation

. Which of the following is NOT seen in over 50% of patients with pulmonary embolism?
   A. Hemoptysis
   B. Tachypnea
   C. Dyspnea
   D. Pleuritic chest pain
   E. Cough

7.4. All of the following apply to IHHS EXCEPT
   A. rapid carotid upstroke
   B. Valsalva maneuver increases murmur
   C. propranolol is contraindicated
   D. syncope is common
   E. left ventricular hypertrophy

7.5. The major element of the American diet that contributes to excessive cholesterol and saturated fat is
   A. red meat
   B. eggs
   C. milk
   D. butter
   E. cheese

7.6. All of the following are seen as a normal response to exercise EXCEPT
   A. vasodilation in the exercising muscles
   B. marked increase in stroke volume with light to moderate exercise
   C. increase in systolic blood pressure
   D. increased venous return
   E. sinus tachycardia

7.7. All of the following are true of scleroderma EXCEPT
   A. endocardial involvement common
   B. cardiac involvement is a frequent cause of death
   C. pericarditis is common in the absence of uremia
   D. cardiac tamponade may occur
   E. hypertension is common

7.8. Which of the following drugs acts by inhibiting converting enzyme?
   A. Aldomet
   B. Propranolol
   C. Guanethidine
   D. Apresoline
   E. Captopril

7.9. All of the following are characteristic cardiac findings in hyperthyroidism EXCEPT
   A. Means-Lerman murmur
   B. decreased coronary blood flow
   C. atrial fibrillation
   D. mitral valve prolapse
   E. loud first heart sound

7.10. A holosystolic murmur which gets louder with inspiration is characteristic of
   A. mitral insufficiency
   B. tricuspid insufficiency
   C. aortic stenosis
   D. pulmonic stenosis
   E. none of the above

7.11. Which of the following characteristically produces a loud first heart sound?
   A. First degree AV block
   B. Mitral insufficiency
   C. Aortic stenosis
   D. Left bundle branch block
   E. Mitral stenosis

7.12. Which of the following is associated with an Austin-Flint murmur?
   A. Mitral insufficiency
   B. Aortic stenosis
   C. Aortic insufficiency
   D. Pulmonary stenosis
   E. None of the above

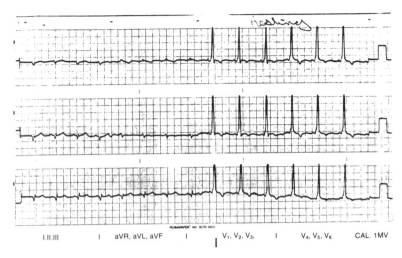

I,II,III   I   aVR, aVL, aVF   I   V₁, V₂, V₃,   I   V₄, V₅, V₆   CAL. 1MV

Figure 20

7.13. Figure 20 shows
   A. left bundle branch block
   B. Wolff-Parkinson-White syndrome
   C. right bundle branch block
   D. acute myocardial infarction
   E. normal ECG

7.14. A short PR interval with a normal QRS complex in association with paroxysmal tachycardias is known as
   A. Lown-Ganong-Levine syndrome
   B. Barlow's syndrome
   C. Wolff-Parkinson-White syndrome
   D. Bartter's syndrome
   E. none of the above

7.15. Which of the following is characteristic of Barlow's syndrome?
   A. Ejection click
   B. Early systolic murmur
   C. Mid-systolic click
   D. Normal echocardiogram
   E. Mitral stenosis

7.16. Which of the following is NOT a cause of paradoxical splitting of the second heart sound?
- **A.** Left bundle branch block
- **B.** Large patent ductus arteriosus
- **C.** Aortic stenosis
- **D.** Severe aortic regurgitation
- **E.** Right bundle branch block

7.17. Which of the following is NOT true of sarcoid heart disease?
- **A.** Corticosteroids are contraindicated
- **B.** Premature ventricular beats are common
- **C.** Heart block occurs characteristically
- **D.** Perfusion defects occur in the resting thallium-201 cardiac scan
- **E.** Sudden death is common

7.18. Which of the following is NOT characteristic of severe aortic stenosis?
- **A.** Angina pectoris
- **B.** Syncope
- **C.** Heart failure
- **D.** Sudden death
- **E.** Hypertension

7.19. A patient with a systolic ejection murmur in the pulmonic area and fixed splitting of the second heart sound most likely has
- **A.** pulmonic stenosis
- **B.** atrial septal defect
- **C.** an innocent murmur
- **D.** aortic stenosis
- **E.** patent ductus arteriosus

7.20. Bronchial breath sounds and egophony in a patient with pericardial effusion is called
- **A.** Levine's sign
- **B.** Kussmaul's sign
- **C.** Treppe phenomenon
- **D.** Ewart's sign
- **E.** Hill's sign

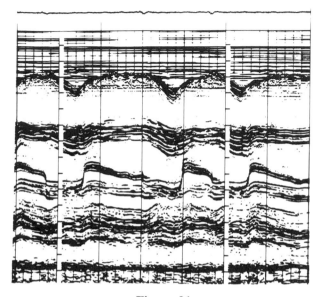

Figure 21

7.21. Figure 21 shows
   A. IHHS
   B. mitral stenosis
   C. Barlow's syndrome
   D. no abnormality
   E. no evidence of pericardial effusion

7.22. Which of the following is LEAST likely to occur in ankylosing spondylitis?
   A. Presence of HLA-B27 antigen
   B. Aortic insufficiency
   C. Mitral regurgitation
   D. Atrioventricular block
   E. Loud aortic second sound when aortic insufficiency first develops

7.23. Which of the following is NOT characteristic of a right ventricular infarction?
  A. Hypotension
  B. Pulmonary edema
  C. Kussmaul's sign
  D. Elevated jugular venous pressure
  E. Pulsus paradoxicus

7.24. Which of the following is NOT a cause of an elevated resting cardiac output?
  A. Hyperkinetic heart syndrome
  B. Arteriovenous fistula
  C. Mitral stenosis
  D. Anemia
  E. Thyrotoxicosis

7.25. The most common cause of new heart failure in the elderly (over 75 years) is
  A. coronary artery disease
  B. amyloidosis
  C. calcific aortic stenosis
  D. hypertension
  E. calcification of the mitral annulus

7.26. Which of the following is NOT a branch of the right coronary artery?
  A. Conus branch
  B. Right ventricular branch
  C. Acute marginal
  D. Sinus node branch
  E. Obtuse marginal

7.27. Which of the following is a loop diuretic?
  A. Furosemide
  B. Hydrochlorothiazide
  C. Spironolactone
  D. Triamterene
  E. None of the above

7.28. Which of the following is LEAST helpful in the treatment of adult respiratory distress syndrome (shock lung)?
  A. Tracheal intubation
  B. Oxygen at concentrations of less than 60%
  C. Large amounts of intravenous albumin
  D. PEEP
  E. Furosemide intravenously

7.29. What causes the Y descent in the jugular venous pulse?
  A. Atrial relaxation
  B. Atrial contraction
  C. Rapid flow into the right ventricle when the tricuspid valve opens
  D. Right ventricular contraction
  E. None of the above

DIRECTIONS: Each group of questions below consists of five lettered headings followed by a list of numbered words or statements. For each numbered word or statement, select the **one** lettered heading that is most closely associated with it. Each lettered heading may be selected once, more than once, or not at all.

Questions 7.30–7.34:
  A. Group I antiarrhythmic drugs
  B. Group II antiarrhythmic drugs
  C. Group III antiarrhythmic drugs
  D. Group IV antiarrhythmic drugs
  E. Group V antiarrhythmic drugs

7.30. Propranolol

7.31. Quinidine

7.32. Verapamil

7.33. Lidocaine

7.34. Bretylium tosylate

Questions 7.35–7.39:
- **A.** Paradoxically split second sound
- **B.** Widely split second heart sound
- **C.** Loud first heart sound
- **D.** Fixedly split second heart sound
- **E.** First heart sound varies in intensity

7.35. Right bundle branch block

7.36. Mitral stenosis

7.37. Mobitz I block

7.38. Atrial septal defect

7.39. Left bundle branch block

DIRECTIONS: Each set of lettered headings below is followed by a list of numbered words or phrases. For each numbered word or phrase select
- **(A)** if the item is associated with (A) only
- **(B)** if the item is associated with (B) only
- **(C)** if the item is associated with both (A) and (B)
- **(D)** if the item is associated with neither (A) nor (B)

Questions 7.40–7.42:
- **A.** Low renin hypertension
- **B.** High renin hypertension
- **C.** Both
- **D.** Neither

7.40. 60% of patients with uncomplicated essential hypertension

7.41. Percentage increases as the age of the population increases

7.42. Relatively low incidence of myocardial infarction and stroke

118 / Clinical Medicine

Questions 7.43–7.45:
  A. Straight back syndrome
  B. Athletic heart syndrome
  C. Both
  D. Neither

7.43. Systolic murmur

7.44. Cardiac enlargement by chest x-ray

7.45. Cardiac arrhythmias including second-degree heart block

---

DIRECTIONS: For each of the questions or incomplete statements below, **one or more** of the answers or completions given is correct. Select
  (A) if only 1, 2, and 3 are correct
  (B) if only 1 and 3 are correct
  (C) if only 2 and 4 are correct
  (D) if only 4 is correct
  (E) if all are correct

7.46. Abnormal Q waves on the ECG can occur in
  1. left anterior hemiblock
  2. left bundle branch block
  3. Wolff-Parkinson-White syndrome
  4. emphysema

7.47. Regarding aortic stenosis
  1. atrial fibrillation usually occurs early
  2. the proximal aorta is usually small on the chest x-ray
  3. the murmur is usually loudest in advanced disease
  4. fourth heart sounds are common

7.48. Regarding calcification of the mitral annulus
  1. antibiotic prophylaxis for dental procedures is not necessary
  2. heart block may occur
  3. it is more common in men
  4. systolic murmurs are common

7.49. Left atrial myxoma may present which of these findings?
1. Fever
2. Arthralgias
3. Peripheral emboli
4. Elevated sedimentation rate

7.50. Regarding central alveolar hypoventilation
1. there is daytime hypersomnolence
2. many patients are not obese
3. most patients are males between the ages of 40 and 60
4. there is tachycardia during sleep

7.51. Regarding dissecting aneurysm of the aorta
1. in women, pregnancy increases the incidence
2. aortic insufficiency is common in type III
3. the angiogram may be misleading
4. heart failure is most common in type III

7.52. Regarding ruptured chordae tendineae
1. most cases occur with previously abnormal valves
2. fourth heart sound is frequent
3. marked left atrial enlargement is usual
4. there is sudden onset of exertional dyspnea

7.53. Primary aldosteronism may present which of these findings?
1. Hypokalemia
2. Twenty-four-hour urinary potassium excretion of less than 30 milliequivalents
3. Low stimulated plasma renin
4. In Conn's syndrome there is bilateral adrenal hyperplasia

7.54. Regarding verapamil
1. it acts by β blockade
2. it is a useful drug in sick sinus syndrome
3. tachycardia is a common side effect
4. it is very useful in paroxysmal supraventricular tachycardia

7.55. Regarding clonidine
1. it acts on the central nervous system to decrease sympathetic output
2. rebound hypertension may occur when the drug is stopped
3. it may cause severe sedation
4. bradycardia may occur

DIRECTIONS: This section of the test consists of a situation followed by a series of questions. Study the situation, and select the **one** best answer to each question following it.

Question 7.56: A 52-year-old white man is admitted to the hospital with an acute anterior myocardial infarction. Three days later, a grade IV out of VI holosystolic murmur develops at the left lower sternal border. There is a palpable thrill in that area.

7.56. Cardiac catheterization is most likely to show
  A. giant V waves in the left atrium
  B. a normal pulmonary capillary wedge pressure
  C. marked elevation of the pulmonary capillary wedge pressure
  D. a higher oxygen content in pulmonary artery blood than in right atrial blood
  E. no abnormality

Questions 7.57–7.58: A 60-year-old white man is admitted to the hospital because of the sudden onset of chest pain radiating through to the back. The blood pressure is low in the left arm and the left femoral pulse is not palpable. A left pleural effusion is noted on chest x-ray. The ECG shows left ventricular hypertrophy.

7.57. Which of the following is most likely to confirm the diagnosis?
  A. Cardiac isoenzymes done serially
  B. Aortic angiography
  C. Echocardiography
  D. Serum amylase
  E. A thallium scan

7.58. If the patient dies, which is most likely to be found at autopsy?

    A. Cystic medial necrosis of the aorta

    B. A recent myocardial infarction

    C. An aneurysm of the left ventricle

    D. A perforated peptic ulcer

    E. Acute bacterial endocarditis

Question 7.59: A 25-year-old black woman has a history of previous acute rheumatic fever. She has been followed for many years because of heart murmurs and now complains of increasing dyspnea. Her chest x-ray is shown in Figure 22.

Figure 22

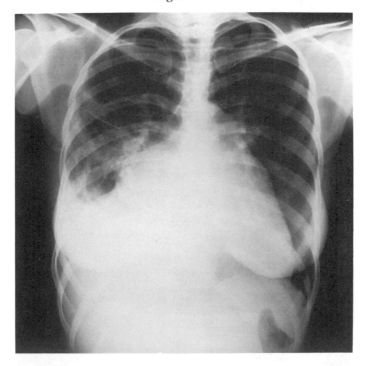

7.59. Which of the following is likely to be her predominant valvular lesion?
  A. Mitral stenosis
  B. Aortic stenosis
  C. Aortic insufficiency
  D. Mitral insufficiency
  E. Pulmonic insufficiency

Question 7.60: A 54-year-old black woman is admitted to the hospital because of dyspnea. A loud decrescendo diastolic murmur is noted. Her chest x-ray is shown in Figure 23.

7.60. Which of the following tests is most likely to be abnormal?
  A. Antinuclear antibody
  B. ASO titer
  C. STS
  D. Urinary VMA
  E. Blood culture

Figure 23A

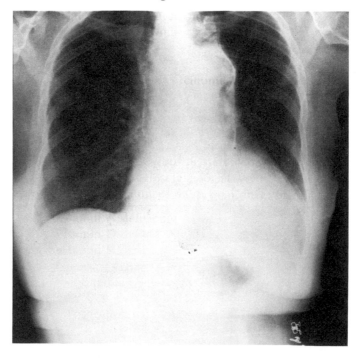

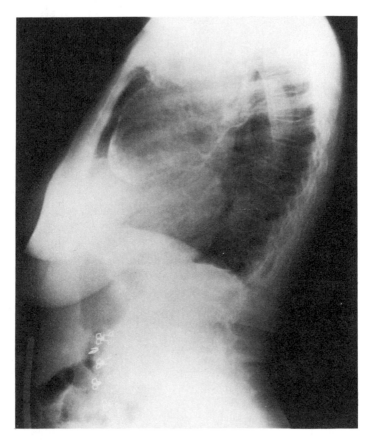

Figure 23B

Questions 7.61–7.63: A 52-year-old white man gives a history of vomiting after a heavy meal. He presents to the emergency room with dyspnea and epigastric pain. Physical exam shows him to be diaphoretic and cyanotic. The temperature is 102° F. Auscultation over the heart reveals a crunching sound in systole. There is dullness and absent breath sounds at the left base.

7.61. Which of the following treatments is most likely to be successful?
  A. Surgery
  B. Digitalis and oxygen
  C. Ligation of the inferior vena cava
  D. Pericardiocentesis
  E. Thoracentesis

7.62. Which of the following tests is LEAST likely to be helpful?
  A. Measurement of the pH of the pleural fluid
  B. Chest x-ray
  C. Pulmonary angiogram
  D. Upper gastrointestinal series
  E. X-ray of the soft tissues of the neck

7.63. The name for the crunching sound on cardiac auscultation is
  A. Hamman's sign
  B. Ewart's sign
  C. Ashman's phenomenon
  D. Hill's sign
  E. Branham's sign

Question 7.64: A 25-year-old black woman is noted to have a loud holosystolic murmur at the apex. The electrocardiogram shown in Figure 24 is obtained.

7.64. Which of the following is NOT true regarding her ECG?
  A. There is right axis deviation
  B. There is left atrial abnormality
  C. The tracing suggests right ventricular hypertrophy
  D. The arm electrodes have been transposed
  E. There is normal sinus rhythm

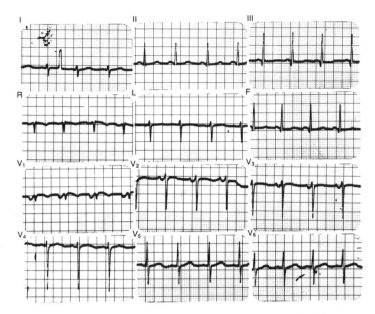

Figure 24

Question 7.65: A 29-year-old white woman has a mitral valve Bjork-Shiley prosthesis.

7.65. Which of the following would NOT be correct if the patient becomes pregnant?

A. Oral anticoagulation can be begun immediately after delivery but breast feeding is then contraindicated

B. Subcutaneous heparin is preferred especially in the first trimester and the last three weeks of pregnancy

C. The female sex steroids do not affect the anticoagulant dose

D. The fetal mortality rate is high (over 10%)

E. Heparin does not cross the placenta

Answers and Comments

7.1. (D) Prinzmetal's angina is characterized by a poor medical prognosis, ST elevation, and ventricular arrhythmias. Propranolol could theoretically make the condition worse but in practice is either helpful or has no effect. Only 15% of patients have normal coronary arteries (Ref. 1, pp. 304–305, 373).

7.2. (B) Prominent U waves are characteristic of hypokalemia (Ref. 4, p. 236).

7.3. (A) Hemoptysis is seen in only 34% of patients. Pulmonary embolism remains a frequently missed diagnosis (Ref. 4, p. 390).

7.4. (C) Propranolol is the drug of choice. Verapamil may be of benefit also (Ref. 1, pp. 648–661).

7.5. (A) Undue emphasis has been placed on eggs and dairy products (Ref. 1, p. 408).

7.6. (B) However, during MAXIMAL treadmill exercise, stroke volume may double (Ref. 4, pp. 440–442).

7.7. (A) Endocardial involvement is rare. The primary clinical manifestations are those of pericarditis and congestive heart failure (Ref. 4, pp. 1663–1664).

7.8. (E) Blocks conversion of angiotensin I to angiotensin II (Ref. 1, p. 945).

7.9. (B) Coronary blood flow, cardiac and stroke volume index, and mean systolic ejection rate are all increased (Ref. 4, p. 1728).

7.10. (B) This is called Carvallo's sign (Ref. 1, p. 446).

7.11. (E) All of the others produce a soft first heart sound (Ref. 2, pp. 181–186).

7.12. (C) The Austin-Flint murmur is an apical diastolic rumble imitating the murmur of mitral stenosis but caused by the regurgitant stream from aortic insufficiency striking the mitral valve (Ref. 2, p. 375).

7.13. (B) The features are: short PR interval, prolonged QRS, and a delta wave (Ref. 1, pp. 134–135).

7.14. (A) This is a form of preexcitation (Ref. 1, p. 148).

7.15. (C) Also called the mitral valve prolapse syndrome (MVPS). There is frequently an associated late systolic murmur (Ref. 1, pp. 505–506).

7.16. (E) Right bundle branch block, of course, causes wide splitting of the second heart sound (Ref. 2, pp. 220–221).

7.17. (A) Corticosteroids may be helpful although their use is controversial (Ref. 1, pp. 634–635).

7.18. (E) Hypertension is unusual but by no means excludes the diagnosis, especially in the elderly (Ref. 1, pp. 471–472).

7.19. (B) The second heart sound should be carefully evaluated in patients with a pulmonic systolic murmur (Ref. 1, pp. 787–788).

7.20. (D) See the index of reference 1 for the other four if you do not recognize them (Ref. 1, p. 667).

7.21. (B) Note the diminished E–F slope and anterior movement of the posterior leaflet as well as the thickening of the mitral valve. There is a large anterior and posterior pericardial effusion as well (Ref. 1, p. 1008).

7.22. (C) Mitral regurgitation is infrequent and usually insignificant. As the aortic insufficiency progresses, the second sound may disappear as the valve cusps become sclerosed (Ref. 4, pp. 1656–1658).

7.23. (B) The wedge pressure is normal or only mildly elevated. Intravascular volume expansion is indicated (Ref. 1, p. 327).

7.24. (C) Patients with the hyperkinetic heart syndrome most commonly present for evaluation of a heart murmur (Ref. 1, p. 14).

7.25. (A) This accounts for one to two-thirds of the cases (Ref. 1, pp. 82–83).

7.26. (E) This is a branch of the circumflex (Ref. 1, p. 1077).

7.27. (A) Ethacrynic acid is also a loop diuretic (Ref. 1, p. 78).

7.28. (C) The use of albumin is fraught with difficulty because of the rapidity with which it leaves the circulation and enters the pulmonary interstitium and alveoli (Ref. 4, pp. 584–585).

7.29. (C) This is the descending limb of the V wave (Ref. 2, p. 95).

7.30. (C) The β-adrenergic blockers are group III drugs (Ref. 1, p. 180).

7.31. (A) Also included in group I are procainamide and disopyramide (Ref. 1, p. 178).

7.32. (E) The calcium antagonists also include nifedipine (Ref. 1, p. 180).

7.33. (B) Also included in group II is phenytoin (Ref. 1, p. 178).

7.34. (D) This drug has an antiadrenergic effect (Ref. 1, p. 180).

7.35. (B) P2 is delayed because of the electrical delay of activation of the right ventricle (Ref. 2, p. 206).

7.36. (C) The valve is closing from a wide open position because of the delayed emptying of the left atrium. Also, the first sound is delayed and since the ventricle "accelerates as it contracts," the ventricle is contracting more forcefully (increased dp/dt). There is a gradient at the end of diastole that requires the ventricle to reach a higher pressure before it closes the valve (Ref. 2, pp. 185–186).

7.37. (E) As the PR interval increases, the first sound gets softer (the valve is closing from a less wide open position). This is not a constant finding as discussed in the reference (Ref. 2, p. 184).

7.38. (D) Because of the communication between the atria, the increase in flow on the right is compensated for by a decrease in the left to right shunt during inspiration. Therefore flow is increased through both the mitral and the tricuspid valves during inspiration (both components of the second sound are thus delayed to an approximately equal degree) (Ref. 2, p. 211).

7.39. (A) There is a prolongation of isovolumic contraction time (Ref. 2, p. 221).

7.40. (D) Thirty percent low, 60% normal, 10% high (Ref. 4, p. 869).

7.41. (A) This probably just represents a progressive decline in functioning juxtaglomerular cells or in their responsiveness, a process that occurs in normal subjects as well but is accentuated in hypertensive individuals, in whom nephrosclerosis is usually more advanced (Ref. 4, p. 869).

7.42. (D) Although one study seemed to show a low incidence of these complications in low renin hypertension, more recent studies have failed to document a good prognosis in low renin hypertension. There may be an increase in renin levels after a vascular complication (Ref. 4, p. 871).

7.43. (C) Those with the straight back syndrome also occasionally have early diastolic murmurs (Ref. 1, pp. 11–14).

7.44. (C) Note the globular "pancake" appearance of the cardiac silhouette in the straight back syndrome (Ref. 1, pp. 11–14).

7.45. (B) Sinus bradycardia also occurs probably related to vagotonia (Ref. 1, pp. 11–14).

7.46. (E) See the chart in the reference for other causes of "coronary mimicry" (Ref. 1, p. 15).

7.47. (D) Atrial fibrillation should prompt a search for associated mitral valve disease or coronary artery disease. Poststenotic dilation of the proximal aorta usually occurs. The murmur may be soft as the disease worsens and flow decreases (Ref. 1, pp. 473–475).

7.48. (C) Endocarditis is very difficult to eradicate in these patients. The incidence in women is twice that in men. Fifty-five percent had systolic murmurs in one series (Ref. 1, pp. 512–513).

7.49. (E) These findings may suggest acute rheumatic fever or bacterial endocarditis (Ref. 1, pp. 442−443).

7.50. (A) Bradycardia occurs during sleep (Ref. 1, pp. 926−927).

7.51. (B) Heart failure usually results from aortic insufficiency which is not a feature of type III (Ref. 1, pp. 961−966).

7.52. (C) Over half involve previously normal valves. Because the mitral regurgitation is acute, the left atrium is not massively enlarged and a fourth sound is common (Ref. 1, pp. 502−503).

7.53. (B) The urinary potassium is greater than 30 in spite of the hypokalemia. There is a benign adrenal adenoma in Conn's syndrome (Ref. 1, pp. 947−948).

7.54. (D) Verapamil acts by blocking the slow inward current carried primarily by calcium. It is contraindicated in sick sinus syndrome and bradycardia is a common side effect (Ref. 1, p. 188).

7.55. (E) Clonidine is rapidly replacing guanethidine as the drug of choice in severe hypertension (Ref. 1, p. 952).

7.56. (D) This is a typical history for rupture of the interventricular septum. A left to right shunt develops. The pulmonary capillary wedge pressure usually is only moderately elevated (Ref. 1, pp. 355−356).

7.57. (B) This is a typical history for a dissecting aneurysm of the aorta. Angiography confirms the diagnosis but as noted in the text, is not foolproof (Ref. 1, pp. 966−968).

7.58. (A) Note the relation of hypertension, Marfan's syndrome, and the Ehlers-Danlos syndrome (Ref. 1, p. 961).

7.59. (D) The x-ray shows a giant left atrium. Note the extreme enlargement to the right, the convexity just below the main pulmonary artery on the left which represents the left atrial appendage, and perhaps hard to see on the photograph, the elevation of the left main stem bronchus. Marked enlargement of the left atrium is more compatible with mitral insufficiency than with stenosis, and is not characteristic of the other three mentioned lesions (Ref. 1, p. 444).

7.60. **(C)** There is a large aortic aneurysm. The linear calcification in the wall of the ascending aorta is characteristic of luetic etiology (Ref. 3, pp. 1665–1666).

7.61. **(A)** This is a classic case of spontaneous rupture of the esophagus (Boerhaave's syndrome) (Ref. 3, pp. 1184–1185).

7.62. **(C)** The pH of the pleural fluid would be acid. Air can be seen in the soft tissues of the neck, often on the chest x-ray and crepitus can be noted on palpation of the neck (Ref. 3, pp. 1184–1185).

7.63. **(A)** Consult the index of the reference if you do not know the other four signs (Ref. 3, p. 1185).

7.64. **(D)** This ECG is from the patient whose chest x-ray is shown in Figure 22 and whose ECG is shown in Figure 24. The large negative component of the P wave in lead V1 is characteristic of left atrial hypertrophy. The large S wave in lead 1 is because of the right axis deviation. If the arm electrodes were transposed, the P wave would be inverted in lead 1. The right axis and deep S waves in the left precordial leads suggests right ventricular hypertrophy (Ref. 3, p. 1008).

7.65. **(C)** The fetal mortality was 28% in one series of 50 pregnancies. Oral anticoagulants are excreted in the milk and do cross the placenta. The patient whose x-ray is shown in figure 24 and whose ECG is shown in Figure 24 later did have a Bjork-Shiley valve inserted. She did not reliably take her anticoagulants and developed a clot on the valve necessitating surgery during a pregnancy. The valve was replaced with a pig valve. The infant was delivered successfully but developed hydrocephalus (Ref. 3, pp. 1729–1730).

References

1. Johnson, R.A., Haber, E., and Austen, W.G.: *The Practice of Cardiology*, Little, Brown, Boston, 1980.
2. Constant, J.: *Bedside Cardiology*, 3rd Ed., Little, Brown, Boston, 1985.
3. Hurst, J.W.: *The Heart*, 4th Ed., McGraw-Hill, New York, 1978.
4. Braunwald, E.: *Heart Disease: A Textbook of Cardiovascular Medicine*, W.B. Saunders, Philadelphia, 1984.

8

Endocrinology

Leonard J. Kryston, M.D.

DIRECTIONS: Each of the questions or incomplete statements below is followed by five suggested answers or completions. Select the **one** that is best in each case.

8.1. Which of the following laboratory tests is the most sensitive indicator of primary hypothyroidism?
  A. T_4 (thyroxine)
  B. T_3 resin uptake (T_3RU)
  C. T_3 by RIA (radioimmunoassay)
  D. TSH (thyroid-stimulating hormone)
  E. Radioiodine uptake

8.2. Which of the following studies is most helpful in evaluating a pregnant patient for thyrotoxicosis?
  A. T_4
  B. TSH
  C. Free thyroxine index calculated from T_4 and T_3RU
  D. T_3 by RIA
  E. Radioiodine uptake

8.3. All of the following are present in a seriously ill patient with the euthyroid sick syndrome EXCEPT
  A. low serum T_4
  B. low T_3RU
  C. low T_3 by RIA
  D. elevated reverse T_3 (rT_3)
  E. normal free thyroxine (FT_4)

132

8.4. Which of the following is the most useful screening test for occult medullary carcinoma of the thyroid in family members of a patient with this disease?
- **A.** Soft tissue x-ray of the neck
- **B.** Calcitonin level following pentagastrin
- **C.** Antimicrosomal antithyroid antibody titer
- **D.** Thyroglobulin level
- **E.** Radioiodine uptake and thyroid scan

8.5. Which of the following has the greatest effect on enhancing calcium absorption from the gastrointestinal tract?
- **A.** 1,25-Dihydroxycholecalciferol
- **B.** 24,25-Dihydroxycholecalciferol
- **C.** 25-Hydroxycholecalciferol
- **D.** Parathyroid hormone
- **E.** Calcitonin

8.6. Which of the following is characteristic in a patient with Klinefelter's syndrome?
- **A.** XY karyotype
- **B.** Hypospadias
- **C.** Webbed neck and short stature
- **D.** Low serum testosterone and elevated luteinizing hormone (LH)
- **E.** Small, soft, immature testes on biopsy

8.7. Growth hormone secretion from the anterior pituitary is inhibited by
- **A.** a rise in blood glucose (hyperglycemia)
- **B.** arginine infusion
- **C.** insulin-induced hypoglycemia
- **D.** L-dopa administration
- **E.** none of the above

8.8. The best screening test for Cushing's syndrome is
- **A.** 8 AM and 4 PM plasma cortisol levels
- **B.** 24-hour urinary 17-hydroxycorticosteroid excretion
- **C.** 24-hour urinary 17-ketosteroid excretion
- **D.** overnight dexamethasone (1 mg) suppression test
- **E.** plasma ACTH level

8.9. The most specific diagnostic test for Addison's disease is the
  A. 8 AM plasma cortisol level
  B. 24-hour urinary 17-hydroxycorticosteroid excretion
  C. cosyntropin (synthetic ACTH) stimulation test
  D. metyrapone test
  E. insulin tolerance test

8.10. All of the following are useful in the acute treatment of hypercalcemia EXCEPT
  A. hydration using intravenous saline solution
  B. furosemide
  C. hydrochlorothiazide
  D. mithramycin
  E. calcitonin

8.11. All of the following factors would make one suspect thyroid carcinoma in a patient with a thyroid nodule EXCEPT
  A. history of irradiation to the head, neck, or chest
  B. solitary nodule in a 30-year-old man
  C. cold nodule on radioiodine scanning
  D. hoarseness
  E. thyrotoxicosis

8.12. All of the following are present in patients with Kallman's syndrome EXCEPT
  A. XXY sex chromosome pattern
  B. anosmia
  C. delayed onset of puberty in a 19-year-old man
  D. low luteinizing hormone (LH) level
  E. low serum testosterone level

8.13. Which of the following buccal smears and sex chromosome patterns would you expect to find in a patient with Turner's syndrome?
  A. Chromatin-positive smear; XXY sex chromosomes
  B. Chromatin-negative smear; XO sex chromosomes
  C. Chromatin-negative smear; XYY sex chromosomes
  D. Chromatin-negative smear; XXY sex chromosomes
  E. Chromatin-positive smear; XO sex chromosomes

8.14. All of the following clinical and laboratory findings are characteristic of the glucogonoma syndrome EXCEPT
   A. increased fasting serum alanine
   B. elevated fasting plasma glucagon level
   C. weight loss
   D. necrolytic migratory erythema
   E. hyperglycemia

8.15. All of the following are favorable prognostic indicators of a probable long-term remission of thyrotoxic Graves' disease following treatment by antithyroid drugs EXCEPT
   A. small initial size of goiter
   B. decreased size of goiter during treatment
   C. normalization of T_4 during treatment
   D. normalization of TRH stimulation
   E. positive tests for thyroid stimulating immunoglobulin (TSI) and thyrotropin binding stimulating immunoglobulin (TBII)

8.16. All syndromes listed below result from target tissue insensitivity to hormone action EXCEPT
   A. Reifenstein's syndrome
   B. pseudohypoparathyroidism
   C. testicular feminization syndrome
   D. Refetoff's syndrome
   E. Turner's syndrome

8.17. The low-dose (10 U infusion/hr) insulin treatment of diabetic ketoacidosis offers an advantage over the classical high-dose (50–100 U IV/2hr) method. Which of the following is the most significant advantage?
   A. Decreased mortality
   B. Shortened period of ketoacidosis
   C. Less chance of hypoglycemia
   D. Total mean insulin dose is lower
   E. Less hypokalemia

8.18. All of the following are characteristic of the inappropriate antidiuretic-hormone secretion (SIADH) EXCEPT
  A. low plasma osmolality (275 mOsm/kg)
  B. low serum sodium (130 mEq/L)
  C. increased urine osmolality (500 mOsm/kg)
  D. low plasma cortisol level (5 μg/dl)
  E. mental confusion

8.19. All of the following are potential causes of the syndrome of inappropriate antidiuretic-hormone (SIADH) secretion EXCEPT
  A. bronchogenic carcinoma of the oat-cell type
  B. chlorpropramide
  C. clofibrate
  D. pulmonary tuberculosis
  E. craniopharyngioma

8.20. All of the following are characteristic findings in Nelson's syndrome EXCEPT
  A. bitemporal hemianopsia
  B. increased skin pigmentation
  C. enlargement of sella on skull x-ray
  D. galactorrhea
  E. markedly elevated plasma ACTH level

8.21. The following drugs are useful in the management of Cushing's syndrome due to recurrence of adrenal carcinoma EXCEPT
  A. aminoglutethamide
  B. mitotane (o, p' - DDD)
  C. cyproheptadine
  D. metyrapone
  E. none of the above

8.22. Which of the following normally results from metyrapone administration?
  A. Decreased plasma 11-deoxycortisol level
  B. Increased plasma cortisol level
  C. Increased urinary cortisol excretion
  D. Increased urinary 17-hydroxycorticosteroid excretion
  E. Decreased ACTH secretion

8.23. Which of the following is characteristic of a woman with an andrenogenital syndrome due to a 21-hydroxylase deficiency?
  A. Hypertension
  B. Elevated urinary 17-hydroxycorticosteroids
  C. Elevated urinary pregnanetriol level
  D. Low urinary 17-ketosteroids
  E. Elevated urinary tetrahydro-compound-S excretion

8.24. All of the following disorders may be found in a patient with the multiple endocrine adenomatosis syndrome type II EXCEPT
  A. medullary carcinoma of the thyroid
  B. parathyroid hyperplasia
  C. pheochromocytoma
  D. Cushing's syndrome with bilateral adrenal hyperplasia
  E. insulinoma

8.25. Which of the following agents is used as a provocative test for pheochromocytoma?
  A. Phentolamine (Regitive)
  B. Phenoxybenzamine (Dibenzyline)
  C. Propranolol (Inderal)
  D. Tyramine
  E. α-methyltyrosine (Metyrosine)

8.26. Which of the following tests best evaluates the overall long-term control of diabetes in a patient with type I (insulin-dependent) diabetes mellitus?
  A. A fasting glucose determination
  B. A 2-hour postprandial blood glucose level
  C. A determination of the hemoglobin AIC concentration (glycosylated hemoglobin)
  D. A record of the fractional urine glucose levels
  E. None of the above

8.27. All of the following abnormalities occur in newborn infants of a diabetic mother EXCEPT
  A. macrosomia
  B. respiratory distress syndrome
  C. congenital heart disease
  D. hyperglycemia
  E. hypoglycemia

8.28. All of the following characterize the state of insulin resistance EXCEPT

   A. nonobese patient requiring more than 200 U insulin daily
   B. develops in patients who use insulin intermittently
   C. antibodies are IgG type
   D. switching to monocomponent highly purified pork insulin is often helpful
   E. antibodies are IgE type

8.29. All of the following drugs are useful in the treatment of a 28-year-old woman with known thyrotoxicosis admitted to the emergency room with high fever, marked tachycardia, restlessness, and delirium EXCEPT
   A. propranolol
   B. hydrocortisone
   C. potassium iodide
   D. propylthiouracil
   E. chlorpromazine

DIRECTIONS: Each group of questions below consists of five lettered headings or a diagram with lettered components, followed by a list of numbered words or statements. For each numbered word or statement, select the **one** lettered heading that is most closely associated with it. Each lettered heading may be selected once, more than once, or not at all.

For each set of laboratory findings, indicate the disorder most likely to be found.
   A. Bilateral adrenal hyperplasia due to Cushing's disease
   B. Adrenal adenoma causing Cushing's syndrome
   C. Adrenal carcinoma causing Cushing's syndrome
   D. Adrenal hyperplasia due to ectopic ACTH production from an oat-cell carcinoma of the bronchus
   E. None of the above

8.30. Markedly elevated plasma ACTH level

8.31. High-normal level of plasma ACTH

8.32. Greater than 50% decrease in 17-hydroxycorticosteroid excretion during high-dose dexamethasone administration

8.33. Responsive to exogenous ACTH administration in only 50% of cases

For each disorder, indicate the most likely pathogenic mechanism.

A. Type I, insulin-dependent diabetes mellitus
B. Type II, noninsulin-dependent diabetes mellitus
C. Diabetes mellitus associated with chronic pancreatitis
D. Diabetes mellitus associated with acanthosis
E. Diabetes mellitus associated with obesity

8.34. Significantly increased frequency of certain HLA antigens (DR3 and DR4) is identified in patients with this type of diabetes mellitus

8.35. Antireceptor antibodies to insulin may be present in such patients

8.36. Inherited susceptibility to environmental factors such as viruses (coxsackie B4) has been identified in some patients with this type of diabetes mellitus

For questions 8.37–8.39, refer to Figure 25.

For each disorder, indicate the most appropriate TSH response to the intravenous infusion of thyrotropin-releasing hormone (TRH).

8.37. Thyrotoxicosis due to Graves' disease

8.38. Hashimoto's thyroiditis and primary hypothyroidism

8.39. Hypopituitarism due to a pituitary adenoma

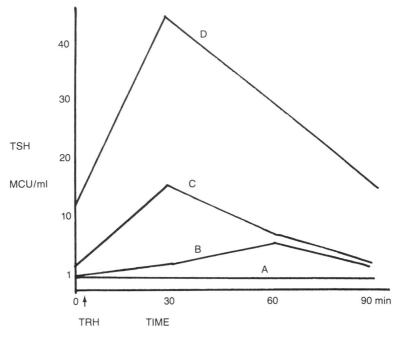

Figure 25

DIRECTIONS: Each set of lettered headings below is followed by a list of numbered words or phrases. For each numbered word or phrase select

   (A) if the item is associated with A only
   (B) if the item is associated with B only
   (C) if the item is associated with both A and B
   (D) if the item is associated with neither A nor B

   A. Advanced bone age
   B. Small testes
   C. Both
   D. Neither

8.40. Pseudoprecocious puberty in a male patient

8.41. True precocious puberty in a male patient

A. Hypertension
B. Low urinary 17-hydroxycorticosteroid excretion
C. Both
D. Neither

8.42. Pseudohermaphroditism due to 21-hydroxylase deficiency

8.43. Pseudohermaphroditism due to 11B-hydroxylase deficiency

    A. Synthetic ACTH (cosyntropin) fails to elicit a rise in cortisol excretion even after repeated administration
    B. Plasma ACTH levels are low
    C. Both
    D. Neither

8.44. Sheehan's syndrome

8.45. Addison's disease

8.46. Conn's syndrome

    A. Low serum calcium
    B. Low serum phosphorus
    C. Both
    D. Neither

8.47. Osteomalacia

8.48. Osteoporosis

8.49. Primary idiopathic hypoparathyroidism

DIRECTIONS: For each of the questions or incomplete statements below, **one or more** of the answers or completions given is correct. Select
(A) if only 1, 2, and 3 are correct
(B) if only 1 and 3 are correct
(C) if only 2 and 4 are correct
(D) if only 4 is correct
(E) if all are correct

8.50. Which of the following are characteristic features of idiopathic hypoparathyroidism?
1. Hypocalcemia
2. Hyperphosphatemia
3. Convulsions
4. Vitamin D deficiency

8.51. Which of the following are characteristic of pseudohypoparathyroidism?
1. Hypocalcemia
2. Elevated serum parathormone
3. Hyperphosphatemia
4. Shortened metacarpal bones on x-ray of the hands

8.52. Which of the following characterize osteomalacia due to poor intake of vitamin D?
1. Hypocalcemia
2. Hypophosphatemia
3. Elevated serum alkaline phosphatase
4. Low parathyroid horome levels

8.53. Which of the following laboratory tests would be consistent with the diagnosis of primary hyperparathyroidism due to a parathyroid adenoma?
1. Hypercalcemia
2. Hypophosphaturia
3. Elevated serum alkaline phosphatase
4. Elevated serum parathormone

8.54. The multiple endocrine adenomatosis syndrome (MEA) type I results in tumors of which of the glands listed below?
1. Pituitary
2. Adrenal medulla
3. Pancreas
4. Gonads

8.55. Which of the following features characterize the MEA type II syndrome?
1. Pheochromocytoma
2. Medullary carcinoma of the thyroid
3. Hyperparathyroidism
4. Multiple neuromas of the lips

8.56. A 24-year-old woman is being evaluated for postpill amenorrhea after having taken oral contraceptives for 6 years. Galactorrhea is noted on physical examination. Which of the following would be helpful in the workup of this problem?
1. Serum prolactin level
2. Tomograms of the sella
3. CT scan with coronal views
4. B-hCG titer

8.57. Which of the following endocrine abnormalities causes osteoporosis?
1. Cushing's disease
2. Thyrotoxicosis
3. Hypogonadism
4. Hyperparathyroidism

8.58. Which of the following laboratory findings are present in a patient with T_3 thyrotoxicosis?
1. Normal T_4
2. Elevated T_3RIA
3. Absent TSH response to TRH
4. Elevated T_3RU

8.59. Which of the following may be used to treat Paget's disease?
1. Calcitonin
2. Calcium carbonate
3. Etidronate
4. Bedrest

8.60. Primary amenorrhea may be seen in which of the following conditions?
1. Imperforated hymen
2. Turner's syndrome
3. Anorexia nervosa
4. Craniopharyngioma

DIRECTIONS: This section of the test consists of situations, each followed by a series of questions. Study each situation and select the **one** best answer to each question following it.

Question 8.61: A 40-year-old woman is found to have a sudden appearance of a nodular enlargement over the right lobe of the thyroid. She has no history of prior irradiation to the area of the head or neck. There is no lymphadenopathy, no hoarseness or dysphagia. T_4 and T_3RU are normal. Ultrasound is demonstrated in Figure 26.

Figure 26

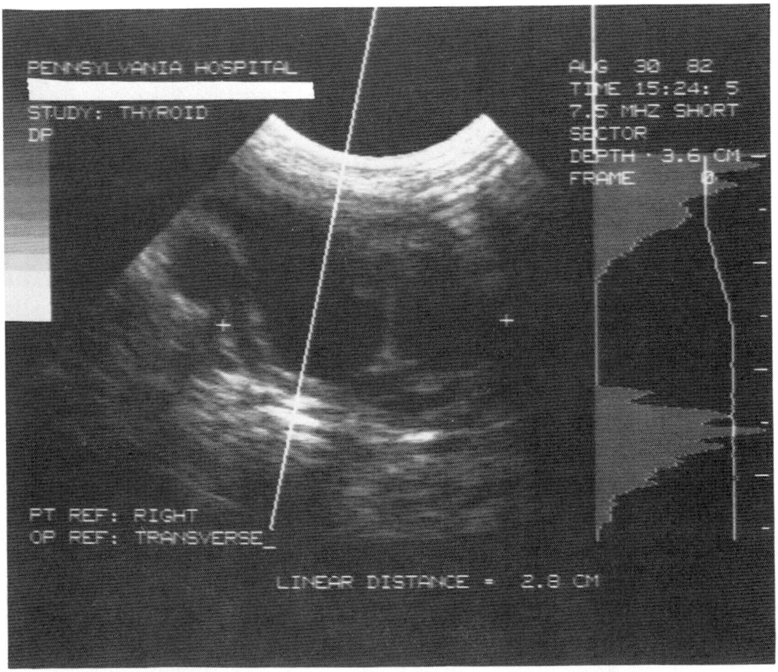

8.61. What would your recommendation be based on the findings?
  A. Observation of the nodule at yearly intervals
  B. Place the patient on L-thyroxine (0.15 mg daily) for suppression of the nodule
  C. Aspirate the nodule and do a cytologic examination of the aspirate
  D. Recommend an excisional biopsy of the nodule by right lobectomy and removal of the isthmus
  E. Recommend a radioiodine scan of the thyroid

Question 8.62: A 30-year-old man is found to have a 2.5-cm thyroid nodule over the right lobe of thyroid during a routine physical examination. There is no history of prior irradiation to the area of the head or neck. T_4 and T_3RU are normal. Thyroid scan is shown in Figure 27. Ultrasound reveals a solid nodule.

Figure 27

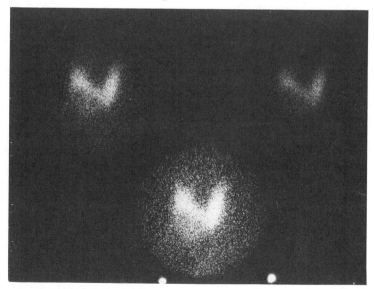

8.62. What would your next recommendation be based on these findings?
  A. Observation of the nodule at yearly intervals
  B. Place the patient on L-thyroxine (0.15 mg daily) for suppression of the nodule
  C. Aspirate the nodule and do a cytologic examination of the aspirate
  D. Recommend an excisional biopsy of the nodule with a right lobectomy and isthmusectomy
  E. Recommend a total thyroidectomy

Question 8.63: A 28-year-old woman has a history of irradiation to the area of the neck for swollen glands at age 8. The thyroid gland is not palpable. There is no lymphadenopathy, no hoarseness or dysphagia. T_4 and T_3RU are normal. Thyroid scan is normal.

8.63. What recommendation would you give the patient based on the information above?
  A. Observation of the gland at yearly intervals
  B. Place the patient on L-thyroxine (0.15 mg daily) to suppress the thyroid
  C. Aspirate the gland and do a cytologic examination of the aspirate
  D. Recommend a subtotal thyroidectomy
  E. Recommend a total thyroidectomy

Questions 8.64–8.65: A 40-year-old man is found to have a palpable nodule in the lateral portion of each thyroid lobe. Lymph nodes are not palpable. Chest x-ray is normal. T_4 and T_3RU are normal. Thyroid scan shows cold nodules over the lateral portion of each lobe. Fine needle aspiration of the nodules reveals possible malignancy and shows a positive stain for amyloid. SMA 12 and plasma catecholamines are normal.

8.64. What recommendation would you give the patient based on this information?
  A. Place the patient on thyroid suppression using L-thyroxine (0.15 mg daily)
  B. Ablate the thyroid using radioiodine
  C. Ablate the thyroid by external radiation
  D. Recommend a subtotal thyroidectomy
  E. Recommend a total thyroidectomy and removal of all palpable nodes

8.65. Close relatives of the previous patient should be examined for thyroid nodules and undergo screening tests. Which of the following tests should be done on these relatives?
  A. Thyroid scan
  B. Thyroid autoantibodies
  C. Thyrocalcitonin levels stimulated by pentagastrin or calcium infusion
  D. Gastrin levels
  E. T_4 and T_3RU

Answers and Comments

8.1. (D) The serum TSH is the most sensitive indicator of primary hypothyroidism. It is elevated in the mildest case of hypothyroidism even before the serum T_3 and T_4 falls to a subnormal range. The radioiodine uptake may vary markedly in hypothyroidism. While it is usually subnormal, the 24-hr uptake may occasionally be normal or even elevated in the early phase of Hashimoto's thyroiditis and hypothyroidism (Ref. 1, pp. 131, 138).

8.2. (C) Both the T_4 and T_3RIA levels are elevated during pregnancy due to the estrogen-induced increase in thyroxine-binding globulin (TBG) production. T_3RU is normally low during pregnancy as a result of the increased TBG. Both T_4 and T_3RU are elevated if thyrotoxicosis is present, resulting in an elevated free thyroxine index calculated from the T_4 and T_3RU values. TSH measurement is of little value in the diagnosis of thyrotoxicosis except when measured in response to thyrotropin-releasing hormone (TRH). Radioiodine uptake is contraindicated during pregnancy (Ref. 1, pp. 120–121).

8.3. **(B)** Seriously ill patients often have markedly low serum T_4 concentrations due to abnormalities in T_4 binding and increased metabolic clearance. Inhibition of T_4 binding results in an elevated T_3RU. Free T_4 levels are normal as thyroid function is maintained. There is decreased conversion of T_4 to T_3 in peripheral tissues resulting in low T_3 by RIA. This is accompanied by increased reverse T_3 (rT_3) due to decreased metabolic clearance of rT_3 (Ref. 2, pp. 726−727).

8.4. **(B)** Medullary carcinoma of the thyroid develops from the parafollicular cells or calcitonin-producing cells of thyroid. Since the potential for developing such a tumor is inherited as an autosomal dominant trait, family members are screened by measuring calcitonin levels after calcium or pentagastrin infusion. If basal levels of calcitonin are elevated or the calcitonin level rises significantly, occult medullary carcinoma must be suspected. Thyroid scan and soft tissue x-rays of the neck are only useful in patients with *clinically palpable* thyroid nodules revealing cold areas over the nodules and dense homogeneous calcifications. Thyroglobulin levels are useful only in following the course of thyroid carcinomas other than medullary carcinoma (Ref. 1, pp. 166−167).

8.5. **(A)** 1,25-Dihydroxycholecalciferol is produced in the kidney and is the active form of vitamin D. The principal action of this hormone is to increase calcium absorption from the gut. Parathyroid hormone affects calcium absorption only indirectly by increasing conversion of 25-hydroxycholecalciferol to the more active 1,25-dihydroxycholecalciferol. There is no indication that calcitonin affects calcium absorption from the gut (Ref. 1, pp. 171−173).

8.6. **(D)** Low serum testosterone and elevated LH levels indicate primary testicular failure due to hypergonadotropic hypogonadism such as seen in Klinefelter's syndrome. This syndrome results from nondisjunction of the sex chromosomes leading to an XXY pattern. Testes are small and firm, and biopsy reveals Leydig cell hyperplasia and sclerosis of the seminiferous tubules. Skeletal anomalies, such as radioulnar synostosis and craniofacial defects, may be present and the patient is usually tall in stature (Ref. 1, p. 214).

8.7. **(A)** Hyperglycemia will normally suppress growth hormone secretion and has become an important diagnostic test for acromegaly. On the other hand, hypoglycemia stimulates growth hormone secretion and is a useful diagnostic test for hypopituitarism. Arginine fusion and L-dopa administration have also been used to evaluate pituitary reserve and growth hormone secretion by normally stimulating their release (Ref. 1, pp. 8, 13, 21).

8.8. (D) The overnight dexamethasone suppression test utilizing 1 mg at bedtime is the best screening test for Cushing's syndrome. Only rarely do false-positive results occur requiring further clarification by the more definitive 2-mg dexamethasone suppression test. Urinary measurements of 17-hydroxycorticosteroids are less reliable being frequently elevated in obesity. There is a loss of the usual diurnal secretion of cortisol in Cushing's syndrome with both the morning and evening levels higher than normal but this is not a reliable indicator of Cushing's syndrome. Urinary 17-ketosteroid excretion is not a diagnostic test of Cushing's syndrome and is useful only when considering the causes of this disorder. The plasma ACTH measurement is in the same category being useful only for diagnosis of the cause of Cushing's syndrome. The highest levels are found in patients with the ectopic ACTH syndrome while the lowest levels are seen in patients with adrenal tumors (Ref. 1, pp. 56−57).

8.9. (C) Addison's disease results from primary adrenocortisol insufficiency. The measurement of plasma cortisol and the 24-hr urinary excretion of 17-hydroxycorticosteroid are below normal in patients with Addison's disease as well as in patients with pituitary insufficiency. While useful in evaluating adrenal function, a low level is not diagnostic of Addison's disease. The cosyntropin stimulation test evaluates the adrenocortical response to ACTH. Failure to increase cortisol levels on repeated stimultion by ACTH is diagnostic of Addison's disease. The metyrapone stimulation test and the insulin tolerance test are tests of endogenous ACTH production and more useful in the diagnosis of pituitary insufficiency (Ref. 1, pp. 63−71).

8.10. (C) Rehydration with intravenous saline can rapidly lower serum calcium levels in patients with hypercalcemic crisis. Sodium diuresis enhances calcium excretion and the combination of saline infusion and furosamide 100 mg/2 hr is effective in the acute treatment of this problem. Hydrochlorothiazide is contraindicated. Thiazides increase renal calcium reabsorption and may aggravate hypercalcemia. Mithromycin inhibits osteoclast activity and bone resorption and a dose of 25 μg/kg may correct hypercalcemia within 24—48 hr. Repeated doses may be used provided there is no significant bone marrow suppression, liver or kidney failure. Calcitonin also inhibits bone resorption and is most effective in hypercalcemia caused by hyperparathyroidism, malignancy, and vitamin D intoxication (Ref. 2, pp. 982—983, 989).

8.11. **(E)** There is a markedly increased incidence of thyroid carcinoma in those patients having a previous history of irradiation to the head, neck, or chest during childhood or adolescence. Palpable abnormalities develop in 27% of these patients whereas carcinoma occurs in approximately 7% of those irradiated. Solitary cold nodules must be suspected of harboring malignancy in a young adult patient. Local metastasis must be considered if there are palpable nodes or if hoarseness is present, suggesting involvement of the recurrent laryngeal nerve. Carcinoma rarely occurs in a hot nodule causing thyrotoxicosis (Ref. 1, pp. 161—162).

8.12. **(A)** Patients with Kallman's syndrome have a normal XY sex chromosome pattern. This syndrome presents as delayed onset of puberty. It is associated with various congenital anomalies,, deafness, harelip, cleft palate, certain skeletal defects causing craniofacial asymmetry, and anosmia or hyposmia. Testes are immature. Serum LH, FSH, and testosterone are low due to an absence of hypothalamic secretion of gonadotropin-releasing hormone (GN-RH) causing hypogonadotropic hypogonadism (Ref. 2, pp. 328—329).

8.13. **(B)** Cytologic examination of the epithelial cells of the buccal mucosa for chromatin (Barr bodies) provides the physician with a practical method of determining the number of X chromosomes present. Chromatin-positive cells indicate that there are more than one X chromosome. The sex chromosome pattern in Turner's syndrome is XO and the X chromatin pattern is negative (Ref. 2, pp. 316, 455—459).

8.14. **(A)** Glucogonomas arise from the α cells of the pancreatic islets. The tumors are often malignant and secret morbidly increased amounts of glucagon causing protein wasting, malnutrition, weight loss, and dermatitis characterized by necrolytic migratory erythema. Glucose intolerance is present and hypoaminoacidemia results from the markedly high glucagon levels (Ref. 1, pp. 208–209; 2, pp. 837).

8.15. **(E)** The likelihood of long-term remission therapy following a course of antithyroid drug therapy of thyrotoxic Graves' disease increased when the goiter is initially small and reduces in size during treatment. Remissions are also more likely when T_3-toxicosis is noted on initial presentation or when other thyroid function tests return to normal on decreasing doses of antithyroid drug. The TSH response to TRH normalizes in such patients. The thyroid stimulating immunoglobulin (TSI) and the thyrotropin binding inhibiting immunoglobulin (TBII) disappear from the serum when patients go into remission and is a favorable prognostic sign (Ref. 2, p.760).

8.16. **(E)** Reifenstein's syndrome results from a reduction in androgen cytosol receptors. This leads to incomplete virilization producing varying degrees of hypospadias. Chromosomes are normally XY. Testosterone is normal or high and LH is elevated. Refetoff's syndrome results from apparent resistance of the peripheral tissue to the action of thyroid hormone. T_4 and T_3 levels are increased in the presence of a normally detectable TSH concentration. Exogenous T_4 and T_3 administration does not completely suppress thyroid function. Deaf-mutism, skeletal anomalies, goiter, and a clinically euthyroid state have been found in such patients. Pseudohypoparathyroidism results from an inherited disorder leading to hypocalcemia and certain other phenotypic anomalies, particularly shortened metacarpal bones. Hypocalcemia results from a lack of end-organ responsiveness to the effects of parathormone (PTH). PTH concentration is elevated and urinary cAMP and phosphate fail to rise upon stimulation by exogenous PTH. Testicular feminization syndrome results from complete androgen insensitivity. These are genetic males who develop as females phenotypically and show typical female gender identity (Refs. 1, pp. 189, 215; 2, pp. 160, 222, 648).

8.17. **(C)** Significant hypoglycemia occurs in 25% of the patients treated by the high-dose method, but this is not a problem using the low-dose regimen. The period of ketoacidosis may actually be prolonged during low-dose treatment and overall mortality remains the same using either method of treatment. While the total mean insulin dose is significantly lower (46 U compared to 263 U) with the low-dose method, this is only an advantage with respect to preventing hypoglycemia (Ref. 1, pp. 278–279).

8.18. **(D)** SIADH results from the continued secretion of vasopressin (antidiuretic hormone) without regard to the plasma osmolality. Patients are unable to excrete a dilute urine so that the extracellular fluid volume expands and dilutional hyponatremia develops. Patients develop symptoms of water intoxication, namely weakness, confusion, and convulsions, and may even slip into coma resulting from cerebal edema. Renal function and adrenal function are normal (Ref. 1, pp. 51–51).

8.19. **(E)** Craniopharyngiomas are tumors that arise from remnants of Rathke's pouch. They occur in the suprasellar area often causing hypopituitarism and diabetes insipidus. SIADH occurs in 50% of patients with oat-cell carcinoma of the bronchus by producing ectopic antidiuretic hormone (ADH). Other carcinomas are also capable of secreting ADH, namely duodenal and pancreatic carcinoma, lymphoma, and ureteral carcinoma. Medications such as chlorpropamide and clofibrate also cause SIADH. These do so by enhancing the renal tubular effect of ADH as well as increasing ADH release from the posterior pituitary. Injury to the central nervous system from skull fracture, subdural hematoma, subarachnoid hemorrhage, cerebral vascular thrombosis or hemorrhage often results in SIADH. Encephalitis, tuberculosis, meningitis, pulmonary tuberculosis, and lung abscess can also produce SIADH (Ref. 1, pp. 45, 49–50).

8.20. **(D)** Nelson's syndrome occurs in 10–38% of patients who have bilateral adrenalectomy for treatment of Cushing's's disease. It results from rapid enlargement of a previously existing basophilic microadenoma of the pituitary. Sella is enlarged and the tumor is often invasive causing headache, chiasmal compression, and visual-field defects. ACTH secretion increases markedly and patients become hyperpigmented. Galactorrhea is not commonly present in patients with basophil adenomas. Hyperprolactinemia and galactorrhea more commonly occur in the galactorrhea-amenorrhea syndrome due to prolactinomas or in acromegaly due to acidophil adenomas of the pituitary (Refs. 1, pp. 23, 27, 31, 61; 2, p. 101).

8.21. (C) Mitotane (o, p' - DDD) is an adrenolytic agent used to treat nonresectable adrenal carcinoma selectively destroying adrenal tissue. It causes regression in tumor size in one-third of patients and a reduction in cortisol production in another third. Metyrapone and aminoglutethamide block cortisol production and are useful when the patients are debilitated by their hypercortisolism. Cyroheptadine is an antiserotonin agent and decreases the output of pituitary ACTH in some patients with Cushing's disease due to pituitary microadenoma (Refs. 1, pp. 61−62; 2, p. 271).

8.22. (D) Metyrapone blocks 11-hydroxylation of 11-deoxycortisol, lowering plasma cortisol and increasing endogenous ACTH secretion. Plasma 11-deoxycortisol levels are elevated and cortisol levels fall. Urinary excretion of 17-hydroxycorticosteroids rises as a result of the increased urinary excretion of tetrahydro-11-deoxycortisol (compound-S) which is measured as a 17-hydroxycorticosteroid (Ref. 1, p. 15).

8.23. (C) The 21-hydroxylase deficiency is the most commonly found form of the adrenogenital syndrome. It affects both cortisol and mineralocorticoid production and, if severe, leads to hyponatremia, dehydration, hypotension, and shock. Both urinary and 17-hydroxycorticosteroids are decreased and ACTH secretion is increased. Increased adrenal production of androgens leads to virilization and in the female to pseudohermaphroditism. Urinary excretion of 17-ketosteroids is increased. There is excess secretion of 17-α progesterone above the enzymatic block and increased excretion of pregnanetriol (Ref. 2, p. 287).

8.24. (E) The potential for developing medullary carcinoma of the thyroid may be inherited as an autosomal dominant trait as part of the syndrome of multiple endocrine adenomatosis type II. Pheochromocytoma may also be present in the same patient or sometimes precede the development of the medullary carcinoma. Hypercalcemia due to parathyroid hyperplasia is often present. The medullary carcinoma also has the potential to secrete ectopic ACTH causing Cushing's syndrome. Other clinical features of the MEA-II syndrome may include mucosal neuromas, marphanoid habitus, pes cavus, poor enamel, absent facial and axillary hair, visible corneal nerves, and thickened eyelids (Ref. 1, p. 167).

8.25. (D) Phentolamine is a short-acting, α-adrenergic blocking agent. It is used to lower the blood pressure in life-threatening hypertensive crisis or as a pharmacologic test for pheochromocytoma lowering the blood pressure promptly by at least 35/25 mm. It may be used in the preparation of patients for surgery or for the treatment of hypercrisis during surgery or the induction of anesthesia. Phenoxybenzamine is a longer acting α-adrenergic blocking agent useful in the preparation of the patient for surgery producing smooth control of blood pressure. It is also useful in the long-term control of blood pressure in patients with malignant pheochromocytoma. Propranolol is a β-adrenergic blocking agent useful in controlling tachycardia and arrhythmia. It should not be used alone in the preparation of patients for surgery but rather in combination with an α-blocking agent to prevent onset of a hypertensive crisis due to α-receptor stimulation. α-Methyltyrosine (Metyrosine) is a tyrosine hydroxylase inhibitor blocking catecholamine synthesis. It is useful in the preparation of patients for surgery and in the management of patients with inoperable or recurrent malignant pheochromocytoma. Tyramine (0.1 mg IV) is a provocative test for pheochromocytoma and raises the blood pressure within 1−2 min in patients with pheochromocytoma. Phentolamine must be available to treat excessive or prolonged hypertension resulting from tyramine injection. Propranolol should be available to treat arrhythmias. Other provocative tests are glucagon (1 mg IV) and histamine (10−25 μg IV). Since the provocative tests can precipitate a hypertensive crisis or arrhythmia, they should be used only in patients with strong clinical evidence of pheochromocytoma and normal catecholamine determinations (Ref. 1, pp. 91−97).

8.26. (C) Approximately 5−7% of hemoglobin is normally glycosylated forming an irreversible bond with glucose. In the poorly controlled patient the blood glucose levels are elevated allowing glycosylation of a greater percentage of hemoglobin. Since the normal life span of the red blood cell is approximately 120 days, the percentage of glycosylated hemoglobin gives a quantitative index of the level of blood glucose control. Glucose levels vary from day to day according to insulin dosage, physical activity, and dietary intake. These are very useful, however, if measured under a system of glucose self-monitoring of capillary blood samples by chemstrip BG or Dextrostix. The monitoring of fractional urine for glucose is less useful since the renal threshold for glucose reabsorption varies widely and often does not give an accurate estimate of blood glucose levels (Ref. 1, pp. 275).

8.27. **(D)** Macrosomia is the most common abnormality in the newborn infant of a diabetic mother. When the mother's diabetes is poorly controlled, the resultant hyperglycemia and elevated amino acid concentrations stimulate excessive insulin secretion and secretion of other growth factors. This stimulates fetal growth resulting in large birth weight, increased body fat, hypertrophy of most organs, islet cell hyperplasia, and hyperinsulinism. The hyperinsulinism places the newborn at risk for developing hypoglycemia during the first hours and days of life. Respiratory distress syndrome is increased in offspring of diabetic mothers until the 38th week of gestation. Congenital heart disease with atrial and septal defects, coarctations of the aorta and transposition of the great vessels occur more commonly in these infants (Ref. 2, pp. 1055–1056).

8.28. **(E)** Insulin resistance is present in patients requiring over 200 U insulin daily provided there is no infection, obesity, or other medical or endocrine disorder causing the increased insulin need. Antibodies of the IgG type are produced and bind the insulin. Resistance often occurs when insulin is reinstituted after a period of nonuse. Both beef and pork insulin are capable of stimulating antibody formation but beef insulin is more antigenic. Switching to purified pork or human insulin is often helpful in alleviating the insulin resistance. If this fails, high-dose prednisone may be used (Ref. 1, pp. 278–279; 2, p. 1061).

8.29. **(E)** The high fever, restlessness, and delirium in a patient with thyrotoxicosis suggest that the patient is in thyrotoxic crisis or storm. This requires immediate treatment since the mortality can be quite high. Hydration and temperature control are essential. Precipitating factors are identified and treated, particularly infections. Hydrocortisone is started immediately since the patients are in a state of relative adrenal insufficiency. Tachycardia is controlled by propranolol. Potassium iodide blocks release of thyroid hormones from the gland while propylthiouracil blocks further hormone synthesis and the conversion of thyroxine to triiodothyronine (Ref. 1, p. 122).

8.30. **(D)** The oat-cell carcinoma of the bronchus is the most common nonendocrine tumor secreting ACTH. The highest levels of plasma ACTH are found in patients with nonendocrine neoplasms secreting ectopic ACTH while ACTH production in Cushing's disease is either normal or only slightly elevated. ACTH secretion is suppressed in patients with adrenal tumors (Ref. 1, pp. 56−58).

8.31. **(A)** Cushing's disease results from secretion of inappropriately excessive amounts of ACTH from a basophilic pituitary adenoma. Plasma ACTH levels are either normal or only slightly elevated in Cushing's disease and are suppressed or low in patients whose Cushing's syndrome is due to an adrenal tumor (Ref. 1, pp. 26−28).

8.32. **(A)** The dexamethasone suppression test is an important diagnostic test useful in separating normal patients from those with Cushing's syndrome and can be very helpful in the differential diagnosis of this disorder. Low-dose dexamethasone (2 mg/day) fails to cause adequate suppression of 17-hydroxycorticosteroid excretion in patients with Cushing's disease due to pituitary ACTH production, while high-dose dexamethasone (8 mg/day) produces definite suppression of 17-hydroxycorticosteroid excretion. Patients with adrenal tumors or those with nonendocrine tumors secreting ACTH fail to suppress on either low-dose or high-dose dexamethasone (Ref. 1, pp. 56−57).

8.33. **(B)** The ACTH stimulation test is also helpful in the differential diagnosis of Cushing's syndrome. Patients with Cushing's disease due to pituitary adenomas have an excessive response. Adrenal carcinomas are totally autonomous and unresponsive. Patients with the ectopic ACTH syndrome also fail to respond since their adrenal glands are already being maximally stimulated by the excessive ACTH from their nonendocrine tumors. Adrenal adenomas respond to ACTH stimulation in approximately 50% of cases (Ref. 1, p. 58).

8.34. **(A)** Type I diabetes mellitus develops mainly in children and young adults resulting in a state of insulin deficiency due to destruction of the pancreatic islets. Studies have suggested that the initial damage to the β cells is by a virus mediated immune mechanism leading to ileitis. Certain HLA antigens, namely DR3 and DR4, are significantly increased in frequency in patients with type I diabetes mellitus. Over 90% of white type I diabetic patients have either D3-DR3 or D4-DR4 antigens. Fifty-five to 60% have both DR3 and DR4 antigens. This suggests that these individuals are susceptible to environmental factors such as viruses which induce an autoimmune reaction in the islets (Ref. 1, pp. 258–260; 2, p. 1022).

8.35. (D) Defective receptor binding of insulin occurs in patients with acanthosis. Two types of patients have been identified. One group of patients has a decreased number of insulin receptors. These patients are young and have features of excess androgen-hormone production leading to hirsutism, polycystic ovaries, and accelerated growth. The other group of patients are older and have features of an autoimmune disease. Antireceptor antibodies are present which displace the insulin from its receptor leading to a state of marked hyperglycemia and insulin resistance. Patients will often have a positive ANA, increased sedimentation rate, increased gamma globulin, neutropenia, proteinuria, and alopecia (Ref. 1, p. 262).

8.36. (A) The coxsackie-B4 virus has been isolated from the pancreas of a newly diagnosed diabetic child and this virus was found to have caused ilitis and insulin-dependent diabetes mellitus in the experimental animal (Ref. 1, p. 258).

8.37. (A) The TSH response to TRH is blunted in thyrotoxicosis due to negative feedback inhibition of TSH secretion by the normal pituitary (Ref. 1, p. 103).

8.38. (D) In primary hypothyroidism TSH secretion is increased and there is TSH hyperresponsiveness to TRH administration (Ref. 1, p. 134).

8.39. (A) There is an absent TSH response to TRH infusion in patients with hypopituitarism due to an expanding pituitary adenoma. There is destruction of the normal pituitary gland by the adenoma through local pressure and loss of pituitary function (Ref. 1, p. 14).

8.40. (C) Both advanced bone age and small testes are found in a male with pseudoprecocious puberty due to the adrenogenital syndrome. Pseudoprecocious puberty results from hormonal secretions from either gonadal or adrenal sources. The patient is taller than his peers because of increased linear growth stimulated by the increased androgen secretion. Bone age is advanced but the accelerated linear growth terminates earlier due to premature closure of the epiphyses. Secondary sex characteristics develop. The penis enlarges but the testes remain small (Ref. 1, pp. 245, 250).

8.41. (A) True precocious puberty in a man causes increased linear growth, advanced bone age, growth of axillary and pubic hair, beard, and body hair. Increased penile size and maturation of the testes occur as a result of stimulation of the testes by LH and FSH (Ref. 1, p. 246).

8.42. (B) A 21-hydroxylase deficiency leads to virilization and pseudohermaphroditism in women. It is the most common enzymatic defect in cortisol synthesis leading to congenital adrenal hyperplasia. Both partial and complete forms of the enzymatic deficiency occur. The more complete forms lead to both deficient cortisol and mineralocorticoid secretion causing hypotension, hyponatremia, and adrenocortical insufficiency (Ref. 1, pp. 82—83).

8.43. (C) A deficiency of 11B-hydroxylase leads to adrenocortical insufficiency, virilization, and hypertension. Virilization results from excessive adrenal androgen production leading to pseudohermaphroditism in women. Plasma cortisol secretion is diminished since this enzyme controls the final step in cortisol synthesis. 11-Deoxycortisol secretion is increased as a result of this blockade resulting in the increased excretion of its metabolite tetrahydro-11-deoxycortisol which may be measured as a 17-hydroxycorticosteroid. Hypertension results from the excessive secretion of desoxycorticosterone (DOC), a potent mineralocorticoid (Ref. 1, p. 84).

8.44. (B) Sheehan's syndrome is usually caused by infarction of the anterior pituitary at the time of delivery as a result of obstetrical complications such as hemorrhage or hypotension. Hypopituitarism develops leading to amenorrhea, failure to lactate, and features of panhypopituitarism, including hypothroidism. Plasma ACTH secretion is low and cortisol production falls. Repeated infusion of synthetic ACTH given over 3—5 days will stimulate the adrenal secretion of cortisol since the adrenal glands are still intact (Ref. 1, pp. 64—69).

Endocrinology / 159

8.45. (A) Addison's disease results from primary adrenal insufficiency. Basal cortisol secretion is diminished and the adrenal reserve is low. Adrenal reserve is best tested by the ACTH stimulation test. Patients with Addison's disease fail to respond even after repeated administration of ACTH. Plasma ACTH levels are elevated in Addison's disease (Ref. 1, p. 69).

8.46. (D) Conn's syndrome is due to an adrenal adenoma causing primary hyperaldosteronism and resulting in hypertension, hypokalemia, increased aldosterone secretion, and suppressed renin activity. Cortisol production is not affected. ACTH secretion is normal as is the cortisol response to exogenous ACTH administration (Ref. 1, pp. 72, 75).

8.47. (C) Osteomalacia in the elderly may be caused by poor dietary intake of vitamin D. The vitamin D deficiency leads to poor absorption of calcium and phosphorus from the gastrointestinal tract. Secondary hyperparathyroidism develops as a result of the hypocalcemia. The increased parathyroid hormone secretion causes phosphaturia and further lowers serum phosphorus (Ref. 2, p. 1236).

8.48. (D) Idiopathic osteoporosis in women is defined as a state of reduced bone mass and occurs in approximately 25% of white women over the age of 60. Wedge fractures of the thoracic vertebrae may be observed. The cause for the condition has not been clearly determined. Serum calcium, phosphorus, and alkaline phosphatase levels are normal, the alkaline phosphatase rising only transiently after a recent fracture (Ref. 2, pp. 1006–1010).

8.49. (A) Idiopathic hypoparathyroidism is a rare clinical condition usually beginning during childhood and often associated with diseases of autoimmune cause. Serum calcium is low and phosphate elevated. Serum alkaline phosphatase is usually normal or slightly low (Ref. 1, pp. 187, 188).

8.50. (A) Idiopathic hypoparathyroidism probably results from autoimmune hypoparathyroidism often associated with other autoimmune disorders (Addison's disease, Hashimoto's thyroiditis, pernicious anemia). The decreased secretion of parathyroid hormone leads to hypocalcemia and hyperphosphatemia. The hypocalcemia is often severe leading to muscle cramps, tetany, mental retardation, and convulsions in children with this disorder. While these patients are not vitamin D-deficient, high doses of cholecalciferol (25,000−100,000 U daily) are required to raise their serum calcium to normal (Ref. 1, pp. 184−188).

8.51. (E) Pseudohypoparathyroidism is a rare genetic disorder inherited as an X-linked dominant trait. There is end-organ unresponsiveness to parathyroid hormone leading to hypocalcemia and hyperphosphatemia. Parathormone levels are elevated. Patients with this disorder have certain phenotypic abnormalities. The most characteristics are short stature and shortening of the metacarpal bones (Ref. 1, p. 189).

8.52. (A) Vitamin D deficiency may be caused by lack of exposure to sunlight, poor dietary intake, or altered metabolism of vitamin D from the intestine. Rickets occurs in children. Osteomalacia is present in the adult. Hypocalcemia and hypophosphatemia result from poor absorption of these elements from the intestine. The hypophosphatemia is aggravated by the increased secretion of parathyroid hormone leading to phosphaturia. Alkaline phosphatase is elevated (Ref. 1, p. 194).

8.53. (E) Primary hyperparathyroidism results either from parathyroid adenoma, carcinoma, or from hyperplasia of all parathyroid glands. Parathyroid secretion is elevated leading to hypercalcemia. Hypophosphatemia results from increased renal losses of phosphorus. Alkaline phosphatase becomes elevated if significant bone loss is present (Ref. 1, pp. 176−177).

8.54. (B) The MEA-I syndrome (Wermer's syndrome) is inherited as an autosomal dominant, causing tumors, usually benign, of multiple tissues often with associated hypersecretion of their hormones. Primary hyperparathyroidism is a common feature and adenomas of other endocrine glands occur less often. Pancreatic islet tumors secreting gastrin, insulin, glucagon, and vasoactive polypeptides may occur. Pituitary adenomas, lipomas, adrenocortical tumors, carcinoid tumors, and even thyroid adenomas may also occur (Refs. 1, p. 89; 2, p. 1275).

8.55. (E) The MEA-II syndrome (Sipple's syndrome) is inherited as an autosomal dominant, causing tumors of the adrenal medulla and the c cells of the thyroid. Pheochromocytoma and medullary carcinoma of the thyroid may be present in the same patient. Some kindred exhibit a characteristic propensity for developing mucosal neuromas and ganglioneuromas. Such patients have a marphanoid habitus and represent what has been termed MEA-IIb syndrome. While hyperparathyroidism commonly occurs in patients with the MEA-II syndrome, it is rarely present in patients with the MEA-IIb syndrome (Refs. 1, p. 89; 2, p. 1279).

8.56. (E) One must first be sure that the patient is not pregnant before embarking on a full workup of postpill amenorrhea. This is best accomplished by the B-hCG determination. If the patient is not pregnant, she may have the galactorrhea-amenorrhea syndrome and may even have a pituitary microadenoma. Prolactin levels would be elevated in such patients and you may be able to visualize a focal area of erosion on tomograms of the sella. Coronal sections of the sella by CT scanning are also useful in visualizing such tumors (Ref. 1, pp. 31, 35, 230, 239).

8.57. (B) Osteoporosis is state of reduced bone mass with a normal mineral to matrix ratio. The most common form is that of senile or postmenopausal osteoporosis seen in 25% of white females over 60 years of age. Estrogen is an important factor leading to osteoporosis in these women. Bone loss declines rapidly after menopause whether it occurs naturally or is induced surgically. Secondary forms of osteoporosis occur from cortisol excess as in Cushing's disease, thyrotoxicosis, hypogonadism, hyperprolactinemia, hyperparathyroidism, and diabetes mellitus (Ref. 2, pp. 1241, 1247−1248.)

8.58. (A) T_3 thyrotoxicosis results from disproportionately increased production of T_3 in preference to thyroxine. Serum T_4 and T_3RU are normal. T_3RIA is elevated. Radioiodine uptake may be normal or only slightly elevated and fails to suppress with T_3 (Cytomel) administration. TSH is suppressed and fails to rise following TRH administration (Ref. 1, p. 118).

8.59. **(B)** Paget's disease results in disordered bone remodeling. Indications for treatment include pain, neurological complications, fractures, hypercalcemia due to immobilization, and high output cardiac failure. Treatment with calcitonin results in inhibition of bone resorption often producing rapid relief of pain and reversal of neurological complications. Etidronate also may induce a remission in Paget's disease which may persist for long periods after discontinuation of the drug (Ref. 2, 1240–1241).

8.60. **(E)** The imperforate hymen obstructs the patency of the vaginal tract leading to cryptomenorrhea. Turner's syndrome results in ovarian dysgenesis. There is primary amenorrhea and poorly developed secondary sex characteristics as well as characteristic phenotypic features such as webbed neck, short stature, and other congenital anomalies. Anorexia nervosa often begins during adolescence. The marked weight loss and emaciation interferes with onset of menarche. The critical body weight initiating puberty is never attained. Craniopharyngioma occurs in the area of the pituitary stalk leading to hypopituitarism. Onset is often in childhood. Skull x-ray and CT scan will show suprasellar calcification and cyst formation (Ref. 1, pp. 234, 239).

8.61. **(C)** Ultrasound shows that there are large cystic areas with septae. The sudden enlargement of such a nodule results from hemorrhage into a degenerating adenoma. Aspiration of the cystic nodule will produce immediate collapse. Fluid removed should be examined by cytology for malignant change. Fluid may reaccumulate and may be removed by repeated aspiration. Excision is only recommended if the cytology suggests malignant changes or if the cyst reaccumulates after repeated aspiration (Ref. 1, p. 161).

8.62. **(C)** The nodule is a solitary nodule which is cold on thyroid scan and solid on ultrasound. Such a nodule in a young man carries a significant risk for thyroid carcinoma. A biopsy should be performed. Aspiration biopsy of such a nodule offers a simple means of obtaining a sample of tissue for cytologic examination with relatively little risk to the patient. An experienced pathologist can identify those patients with possible or probable malignant cells so that excisional biopsy can be performed on these selected patients (Ref. 1, pp. 161, 163).

8.63. (A) Thyroid nodules develop in about 27% of those patients exposed to irradiation to the area of the head or neck. Thyroid carcinoma develops in about 7% of such patients. There is a long lag period (average 28 years) between exposure to irradiation and development of the thyroid nodule. Every patient with a history of irradiation should be examined for thyroid nodules and have a thyroid scan. If no abnormalities are detected, they should be reexamined for nodules on a yearly basis. Thyroid suppression is indicated for those patients with diffusely enlarged glands or for those patients with abnormal scans and no palpable nodules. Biopsy is recommended for patients with palpable nodules (Ref. 1, pp. 161–162, 165).

8.64. (E) The patient has medullary carcinoma of the thyroid. This occurs in the parafollicular cells of the thyroid located in the middle third of each thyroid lobe. Tumors are multifocal and often bilateral so that total thyroidectomy is recommended. Tumors are easily recognized by their amyloid deposits (Ref. 1, pp. 166–167).

8.65. (C) The parafollicular cells of the thyroid secrete calcitonin and the calcitonin levels in patients with medullary carcinoma are markedly elevated. The disease is a genetic disorder inherited as an autosomal dominant trait so that all family members must be examined. Calcitonin levels are an early marker for this disorder rising markedly upon stimulation by either pentagastrin or calcium infusion (Ref. 1, pp. 166–167).

References

1. Kryston, L.J.: *Endocrine Disorders: Focus on Clinical Diagnosis*, Medical Examination Publishing, New York, 1981.

2. Williams, R.H.: *Textbook of Endocrinology*, 6th Ed., W.B. Saunders, Philadelphia, 1981.

3. Wilson, J.D., and Foster, D.W.: *Williams Textbook of Endocrinology*, 7th Ed., W.B. Saunders, Philadelphia, 1985.

9

Gastroenterology
William A. Sodeman, Jr., M.D.

DIRECTIONS: Each of the questions or incomplete statements below is followed by five suggested answers or completions. Select the **one** that is best in each case.

9.1. The characteristics of the ascitic fluid can be of great help in differential diagnosis of the cause of ascites. A fluid with a specific gravity of 1.010 and a protein of 2.1 g/100 ml, straw-colored and without red or white cells is likely to come from
  A. metastatic carcinoma
  B. pancreatic pseudocyst
  C. tuberculous peritonitis
  D. cirrhosis
  E. none of the above

9.2. All of the following chronic diseases are associated with the development of duodenal ulcers EXCEPT
  A. systemic mastocytosis
  B. chronic pancreatitis
  C. chronic lung disease
  D. chronic renal failure
  E. cirrhosis of the liver

9.3. In a 55-year-old patient with a presentation that includes postprandial cramping pain, weight loss, and loss of appetite, but without a history of prior surgery or medical therapy for gastrointestinal disease, which of the following is the most likely?
A. Gastric ulcer
B. Gastric carcinoma
C. Regional ileitis
D. Intestinal angina
E. Carcinoma of the colon

9.4. In a patient with prolonged diarrhea as a result of lactose malabsorption which of the following is NOT likely to be present?
A. Distension
B. Flatulence
C. Weight loss
D. Cramping discomfort
E. Watery stools

9.5. Which of the following is the most useful screening test for atrophic gastritis?
A. Gastric analysis
B. Upper gastrointestinal exam
C. Endoscopy
D. Shilling test
E. Parietal-cell antibody determinations

9.6. Many laboratory tests are available to help differentiate malabsorption (sprue) from maldigestion (pancreatic disease). All of the following are abnormal in malabsorption EXCEPT
A. duodenal fluid
B. small intestinal x-ray
C. D-xylose absorption
D. urinary indican
E. small bowel biopsy

9.7. All of the following have been associated with chronic duodenal ulcer EXCEPT
   A. burns
   B. hyperparathyroidism
   C. Zollinger-Ellison syndrome
   D. chronic pulmonary insufficiency
   E. APUD cell tumor

9.8. Acute erosive gastritis is best diagnosed by
   A. history
   B. gastric analysis
   C. endoscopy
   D. double-contrast (air-contrast) upper GI
   E. capsule biopsy

9.9. A patient with a past history of acid-peptic disease presents with recent worsening of his symptomatology. He complains of pain on arising in the morning which now is poorly relieved by antacid. There also is bloating and postprandial emesis. The most likely cause is
   A. posterior penetration of a duodenal ulcer
   B. Zollinger-Ellison syndrome
   C. hyperparathyroidism
   D. outlet obstruction
   E. missed carcinoma of the stomach

9.10. Acute elevation of amylase may be found with all of the following EXCEPT
   A. salpingitis
   B. mesenteric infarction
   C. chronic renal insufficiency
   D. diabetic ketoacidosis
   E. Crohn's disease of the stomach

9.11. The use of tests for tissue antibodies (smooth muscle antibodies, mitochondrial antibodies, and nuclear antibodies) may be helpful in differentiation of some varieties of chronic hepatitis. Mitochondrial antibodies are characteristic of
   A. chronic active hepatitis
   B. primary biliary cirrhosis
   C. postnecrotic cirrhosis
   D. acute hepatitis A
   E. acute hepatitis B

9.12. In the evaluation of patients with fulminant hepatic failure, it ·is important in establishing the prognosis to separate acute fulminant hepatitis with liver failure from acute deterioration of chronic liver disease. All of the following suggest acute failure EXCEPT
   A. short history
   B. good nutrition
   C. no palpable liver
   D. no palpable spleen
   E. spiders

9.13. In a patient who presents with acute upper gastrointestinal hemorrhage the initial therapy usually will arrest the hemorrhage. During that nonbleeding interval the first diagnostic maneuver should be
   A. upper gastrointestinal examination
   B. panendoscopy
   C. angiography
   D. surgery
   E. none of the above

9.14. In the United States hepatoma (hepatocellular carcinoma)
   A. is the most common liver tumor
   B. is well visualized on gallium scan
   C. only occasionally produces fetoprotein
   D. is associated with hemachromatosis
   E. is unassociated with hepatitis B infection

9.15. The early (presenting) finding in primary biliary cirrhosis is usually
  A. jaundice
  B. pruritus
  C. esophageal varices
  D. splenomegaly
  E. bleeding

9.16. All of the following drugs are capable of producing a hepatitislike reaction in the liver EXCEPT
  A. halothane
  B. tetracycline
  C. INH
  D. aspirin
  E. oxycicillin

9.17. Long-term therapy with cimetidine for duodenal ulcer may produce all of the following adverse side effects EXCEPT
  A. gynecomastia
  B. SGOT and SGPT elevation
  C. chronic active hepatitis
  D. granulocytopenia
  E. mental confusion

9.18. All of the following are etiologies for conjugated hyperbilirubinemia EXCEPT
  A. Dubin-Johnson syndrome
  B. methyltestosterone ingestion
  C. Rotor's syndrome
  D. Gilbert's syndrome
  E. carcinoma of the ampulla of Vater

9.19. Adult celiac disease (nontropical sprue) is worsened by ingestion of all of the following EXCEPT
  A. wheat
  B. rye
  C. rice
  D. oats
  E. barley

9.20. In the management of acute cholecystitis all of the following are indications for prompt surgical intervention EXCEPT
   A. toxicity, impending gallbladder rupture
   B. nondiagnostic radionucleotide scan
   C. palpable tender gallbladder
   D. empyema of the gallbladder
   E. perforation of the gallbladder

9.21. Which of the following tests could be ordered to diagnose the presence of peptic esophagitis?
   A. Barium swallow
   B. Esophageal manometry
   C. Esophageal pH measurement
   D. Endoscopy
   E. Capsule biopsy

9.22. All of the following are risk factors in the development of carcinoma of the colon EXCEPT
   A. inflammatory bowel disease
   B. carcinoma of the breast
   C. ameba infection
   D. familial polyposis
   E. immunodeficiency disease

9.23. In the diagnosis of malabsorption syndrome a small intestinal biopsy can confirm the diagnosis in all of the following EXCEPT
   A. Whipple's disease
   B. blind-loop syndrome
   C. gluten-sensitive enteropathy (celiac disease)
   D. eosinophilia gastroenteritis
   E. tropical sprue

9.24. Differentiation of delirium tremens from hepatic precoma is essential in the evaluation of the acute alcoholic. All of the following suggest delirium tremens EXCEPT
   A. the patient is alert
   B. the patient has slurring of the speech
   C. the patient is anxious
   D. the patient has tachycardia
   E. the patient has a fine tremor

DIRECTIONS: Each group of questions below consists of several lettered headings followed by a list of numbered words or statements. For each numbered word or statement, select the **one** lettered heading that is most closely associated with it. Each lettered heading may be selected once, more than once, or not at all.

    A. Defective intraluminal digestion
    B. Mucosal defect
    C. Postabsorptive transport (not transit) defects

9.25. Whipple's disease

9.26. Blind-loop syndrome

9.27. Lymphangiectasia

9.28. Cystinuria

Evaluation of the gallbladder and the biliary tree for stone may be done by a variety of invasive and noninvasive tests. Select the test which seems most appropriate in each of the following situations.

    A. Oral cholecystography
    B. Ultrasound
    C. Endoscopic retrograde cholangiography
    D. Intravenous cholangiography
    E. Radionucleotide scan of the biliary tree

9.29. Suspect acute cholecystitis

9.30. Evaluate for asymptomatic gallstones

9.31. Common duct stone

Match the diagnosis with the assorted signs or symptom(s).

    A. Carcinoma of the head of pancreas
    B. Carcinoma of the ampulla of Vater

9.32. Fever and chills

9.33. Occult blood in the stool

9.34. Weight loss before jaundice

Knowledge concerning the response or squeeze of the lower esophageal sphincter is essential to selecting therapy for motor disorders of the esophagus. Each of the following motor problems in the esophagus indicate whether the lower esophageal sphincter (LES) pressure is hyper- or hypotonic.

    A. Hypertonic
    B. Hypotonic

9.35. Diffuse esophageal spasm

9.36. Achalasia

9.37. Scleroderma

DIRECTIONS: Each set of lettered headings below is followed by a list of numbered words or phrases. For each numbered word or phrase select
    (A) if the item is associated with A only
    (B) if the item is associated with B only
    (C) if the item is associated with both A and B
    (D) if the item is associated with neither A nor B

    A. Crohn's disease
    B. Chronic ulcerative colitis
    C. Both
    D. Neither

9.38. Arthritis, both peripheral and spondylitis

9.39. Pyoderma gangrenosum

9.40. Erythema nodosum

    A. Crohn's disease
    B. Chronic ulcerative colitis (CUC)
    C. Both
    D. Neither

9.41. Intestinal obstruction

9.42. Suppression of relapse with sulfasalazine (Azulfidine)

9.43. Iritis and episcleritis

DIRECTIONS: For each of the questions or incomplete statements below, **one or more** of the answers of completions given is correct. Select
    (A) if only 1, 2, and 3 are correct
    (B) if only 1 and 3 are correct
    (C) if only 2 and 4 are correct
    (D) if only 4 is correct
    (E) if all are correct

9.44. A 45-year-old male patient has a single 1 cm polyp visualized at the time of sigmoidoscopy. This is biopsied and reported as an adenomatous polyp. The next step in management should include
    1. air-contrast barium enema
    2. anterior resection of the involved colon
    3. fiberoptic colonoscopic polypectomy
    4. repeat test for occult blood

9.45. The initial treatment of a known cirrhotic who develops ascites should include which of the following?
    1. Salt (Na^+) restriction
    2. Fluid restriction
    3. Aldactone
    4. Thiazide diuretics

9.46. Primary carcinoma of the gallbladder
1. commonly presents with jaundice
2. is generally a disease of older women
3. is well treated surgically
4. seems related to gallbladder presence

9.47. In a patient presenting with frank diarrhea, abdominal cramping pain, and gross blood in the stools, which of the following is the likely diagnosis?
1. Enterotoxigenic *Escherichia coli*
2. *Yersinia* infection
3. *Campylobacter* enteritis
4. *Vibrio parahemolyticus*

9.48. Which of the following will cause presinusoidal portal hypertension?
1. Schistosomiasis
2. Venoocclusive disease
3. AV fistula involving the portal veins
4. Budd-Chiari syndrome

9.49. Hepatic granulomas have been reported in association with many diseases. Which of the following does NOT have this association?
1. Whipple's disease
2. Infectious mononucleosis
3. Brucellosis
4. Hepatitis A virus

9.50. The histologic pattern of chronic active hepatitis (chronic active liver disease) can be produced by
1. hepatitis B virus
2. methyldopa
3. INH
4. Wilson's disease

9.51. Carcinoma of the stomach is
1. decreasing in incidence
2. higher in incidence in the United States for blacks than whites
3. more common in men than women
4. a sequela of benign gastric ulcer

DIRECTIONS SUMMARIZED

A	B	C	D	E
1,2,3	1,3	2,4	4	All are
only	only	only	only	correct

9.52. Which of the following are features of the Zollinger-Ellison syndrome?
   1. Duodenal ulcer
   2. Age 40
   3. Diarrhea
   4. Abdominal pain

DIRECTIONS: This section of the test consists of situations, each followed by a series of questions. Study each situation and select the **one** best answer to each question following it.

Questions 9.53–9.56: A 51-year-old white man presents with a history of recent onset of substernal burning pain with some radiation to the left shoulder and arm. This discomfort is not clearly related by history to exercise or is it particularly characteristic of peptic discomfort in terms of timing and relief. The accompanying x-ray (Figure 28) was obtained as part of an upper gastrointestinal examination. The results of an electrocardiogram were normal. The concern is to differentiate esophageal pain from cardiac pain. Prior to a stress test, the esophagus is to be evaluated. The full range of radiologic as well as gastroenterologic procedures is yours to order. Which test would you select to determine each of the following conditions?

   A. Capsule biopsy of the esophagus
   B. Esophageal manometry
   C. Bernstein test
   D. Intraesophageal pH following an acid load
   E. Barium syphonage by x-ray

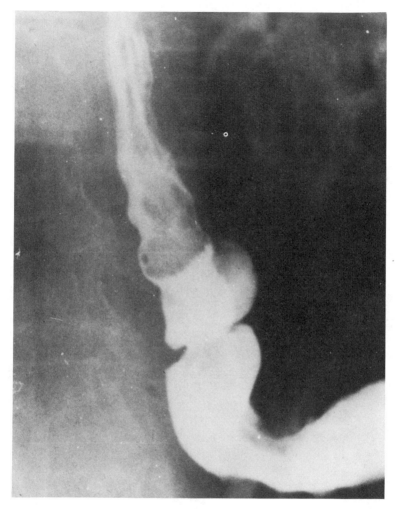

Figure 28

9.53. Acid-sensitive esophagus

9.54. Esophagitis

9.55. Competent lower esophageal sphincter

9.56. Reflux

Questions 9.57–9.58: A 45-year-old man presents with a history of recent onset of upper abdominal discomfort described as indigestion. This is partially relieved by food and somewhat better relieved by antacid. There has been no vomiting or melena. There is no past history of acid-peptic disease. The accompanying film (Figure 29) was obtained as part of an upper gastrointestinal series.

9.57. A pentagastrin-stimulated gastric analysis would show
    A. normal volume, decreased acid concentration
    B. increased volume, increased acid concentration
    C. normal volume, increased acid concentration
    D. decreased volume, normal acid concentration
    E. decreased volume, decreased acid concentration

Figure 29

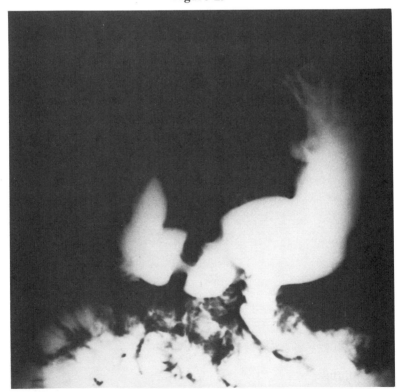

9.58. The next diagnostic maneuver should be
  A. gastric cytology
  B. gastroscopy
  C. therapeutic trial of cimetidine and antacid
  D. surgery
  E. gastric radiation

Questions 9.59 – 9.60: A 52-year-old woman presents with cramping abdominal pain and alternating diarrhea and constipation. She has occasional blood-streaking of her stool and a history of hemorrhoids. On examination she is afebrile and there is a tender left lower quadrant mass. The examination of the stool by guaiac for blood is negative. Sigmoidoscopy shows only internal hemorrhoids. The accompanying film (Figure 30) is taken from barium enema. There is no anemia, leukocytosis, or left shift.

Figure 30

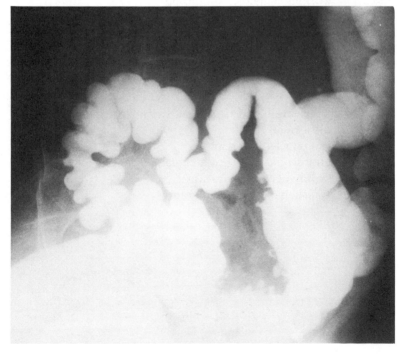

9.59. The most likely diagnosis is
 A. diverticulosis
 B. diverticulitis
 C. paracolic abscess
 D. carcinoma of the colon
 E. adenomatous polyp

9.60. The first therapeutic endeavors should be
 A. high-residue diet
 B. low-residue diet
 C. colomyotomy
 D. segmental resection and colostomy
 E. irradiation

Questions 9.61–9.62: A 50-year-old black man presents with a recent onset of upper midabdominal pain and weight loss. The accompanying x-ray (Figure 31) was taken from his upper gastrointestinal series.

9.61. The working diagnosis should be
 A. gastric ulcer
 B. duodenal ulcer
 C. chronic pancreatitis
 D. carcinoma of the pancreas
 E. gastritis

9.62. To further evaluate this patient the next test should be
 A. ultrasound
 B. radionucleotide scan
 C. endoscopic retrograde cholangiopancreatography
 D. skinny needle aspiration
 E. transhepatic cholangiogram

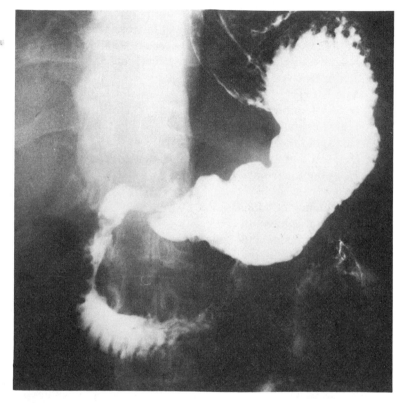

Figure 31

Questions 9.63−9.65: A 22-year-old white woman presents with a history of chronic ulcerative colitis diagnosed at age 10. She has had intermittent exacerbations and was treated with steroids on two occasions in the past. At present, she has noticed some fresh blood in her stool and an occasional cramping pain. She is on no medication at this time.

9.63. Her initial evaluation should include
  A. sigmoidoscopy
  B. barium enema
  C. both
  D. neither

9.64. Evaluation demonstrates that there is total colonic involvement but while there is friability of mucosa there is no ulceration or exudate at the time of endoscopy and little evidence of active disease. This relapse is mild and the appropriate therapy includes
   A. ACTH
   B. systemic steroids in doses equivalent to 40 mg of prednisone daily
   C. sulfasalazine
   D. rest and a low-residue diet
   E. none of the above

9.65. Recommended management is
   A. total colectomy
   B. partial sphincter-sparing colectomy
   C. sulfasalazine maintenance therapy
   D. yearly CEA
   E. none of the above

Answers and Comments

9.1. (D) Tumors and infections increase both the protein and the cell count. Amylase levels are most helpful in separating ascitic fluid secondary to pseudocysts. With pseudocysts most of the values are quite variable (Ref. 2, p. 210).

9.2. (B) Although an association between chronic pancreatitis and duodenal ulcer disease is often alluded to, there is no real evidence for a relationship (Ref. 5, p. 644).

9.3. (D) Ulcer and carcinoma do give rise to peptic pain relieved by food. Ileitis would be the second choice (Ref. 2, p. 1759).

9.4. (C) Malabsorption of single selective nutrients generally does not lead to weight loss (Ref. 2, p. 1734).

9.5. (E) Parietal-cell antibodies are either easiest or least invasive of the list. If present, they indicate atrophic gastritis. It is possible to be antibody-negative and still have atrophic gastritis (Ref. 4, p. 234).

9.6. **(A)** Bile salts are unaffected by either sort of nutritional problem. Indican is elevated in sprue (Ref. 2, p. 1724).

9.7. **(A)** Burns cause acute stress ulcers rather than chronic acid-peptic disease (Ref. 4, p. 423).

9.8. **(C)** These people are usually acute bleeders. Endoscopy remains the best bet for diagnosis (Ref. 4, p. 243).

9.9. **(D)** With outlet obstruction there is a significant shift in the pain pattern. One gets morning pain and the volume of retained secretion is so large that antacids tend to be relatively ineffective (Ref. 4, p. 388).

9.10. **(E)** Elevated amylase occurs readily with many diverse inflammatory and noninflammatory conditions. There is no amylase in the gastric mucosa (Ref. 5, p. 1473).

9.11. **(B)** Ninety percent of patients with primary biliary cirrhosis have mitochondrial antibodies. Otherwise, tissue antibodies do not seem to be of great diagnostic help (Ref. 3, p. 279).

9.12. **(E)** Spiders take time to form and are not a feature of acute fulminant hepatic failure (Ref. 3, p. 108).

9.13. **(B)** Every case must be individualized but endoscopy is probably the most sensitive tool. Angiography is most helpful *during* bleeds (Ref. 1, p. 793).

9.14. **(D)** Hepatoma is rare in the United States. Gallium will not show the tumor but colloid scans will. Usually it does produce fetoprotein and even in the United States hepatitis B is a positive association (Ref. 1, p. 849).

9.15. **(B)** Pruritus usually preceds other overt manifestations of liver disease in primary biliary cirrhosis. Varices, bleeding, and splenomegaly are late features (Ref. 1, p. 838).

9.16. **(B)** Tetracycline generally produces a fatty liver (Ref. 1, p. 821).

9.17. **(C)** While enzymes do go up, hepatitis as such has not been a feature of cimetidine therapy (Ref. 1, p. 688).

9.18. **(D)** Gilbert's syndrome is an unconjugated hyperbilirubinemia due to impaired uptake and/or conjugation (Ref. 2, p. 206).

9.19. **(C)** Gluten of many but not all grains is toxic to sprue patients. Rice gluten is well tolerated (Ref. 1, p. 733).

9.20. **(B)** These scans are sensitive indicators of gallbladder function and disease. A nondiagnostic scan makes the diagnosis of acute cholecystitis suspect (Ref. 1, p. 858).

9.21. **(E)** Only biopsy or a Bernstein test will show an inflamed or acid sensitive esophagus and make the diagnosis (Ref. 5, p. 456).

9.22. **(C)** Ameba infection has not been associated with carcinoma of the colon. In tropical areas where ameba infection is frequent, colon carcinoma is rare (Ref. 1, p. 765).

9.23. **(B)** Small bowel culture rather than biopsy is necessary to confirm the diagnosis of blind-loop syndrome with bacterial overgrowth. Such mucosal changes as do occur in biopsy are nonspecific (Ref. 1, p. 726).

9.24. **(B)** Speech is rapid but not slurred. Tremor is fine but not flapping. Both tachycardia and flushing tend to be present in delirium tremens (Ref. 3, p. 339).

9.25. **(B)**
9.26. **(A)**
9.27. **(C)**
9.28. **(B)** Blind-loop syndrome with deconjugation of bile acids is a digestive problem. The mucosal cell is defective because of infection in Whipple's disease and because of inborn error in cystinuria. Transport of nutrient after absorption is impaired in lymphangiectasia (Ref. 1, p. 722).

9.29. **(E)** While both ultrasound and intravenous cholangiography have proven useful, scans after intravenous injection of radioactive compounds excretable in the biliary tree seem to be the safest and most reliable tool (Ref. 1, p. 854).

9.30. **(A)** If the intestinal absorption is normal and liver function is intact, oral cholecystography is still the most reliable and least invasive approach (Ref. 1, p. 854).

9.31. **(C)** Transhepatic cholangiography can also be used. Both have some hazards and require experience as well as backup (Ref. 1, p. 854).

9.32. **(B)**
9.33. **(B)**
9.34. **(A)** Ductular obstruction and bleeding give rise to fever and occult blood with ampullary tumors even when they are small. More bulky tumors in the head of the pancreas can lead to weight loss, but the tiny ampullary tumors tend not to do this (Ref. 2, p. 1846).

9.35. **(A)**
9.36. **(A)**
9.37. **(B)** Pressure or squeeze by the LES is impaired in scleroderma. Squeeze is normal to high in diffuse esophageal spasm and elevated in untreated achalasia (Ref. 1, p. 673).

9.38. **(C)**
9.39. **(B)**
9.40. **(C)** Many of the complications of inflammatory bowel disease occur in association with both chronic ulcerative colitis and Crohn's disease. Pyoderma gangrenosum seems limited to a relationship with chronic ulcerative colitis (Ref. 1, p. 744).

9.41. **(A)**
9.42. **(B)**
9.43. **(C)** The fibrotic reaction in the wall of the intestine in Crohn's disease may lead to obstruction. The mucosal involvement in CUC does not. Azulfidine does seem to prevent relapse of CUC but not Crohn's. Eye lesions are more common with CUC but also occur with Crohn's (Ref. 5, p. 1000).

9.44. **(B)** Air-contrast barium enema will aid in identifying additional polyps. In most instances an endoscopic polypectomy coupled with complete evaluation of the colon would be the next test in order. Examination for occult blood as a screening test offers little advantage after polyps have been identified. Anterior resection is a last resort (Ref. 2, p. 1761).

184 / Clinical Medicine

9.45. **(A)** It is unwise to use potent oral diuretics like the thiazides as initial therapy in cirrhotic ascites. The risk of precipitating hepatorenal syndromes is high. They may be employed cautiously after observation of response to other measures (Ref. 2, p. 1814).

9.46. **(C)** Jaundice is usually a terminal event. Survivals by any therapy are at the 3% level (Ref. 2, p. 1828).

9.47. **(D)** *V. parahemolyticus* can rarely give bloody stools. Bloody stools are not a regular feature of any of the infections except *Campylobacter* (Ref. 5, p. 944).

9.48. **(B)** AV fistula results in high flow which because of vascular resistance in the liver will give rise to portal hypertension. Schistosome eggs give rise to granulomas which occlude portal venules. They are too large to reach the sinusoides (Ref. 1, p. 842).

9.49. **(D)** Hepatic granulomas are associated with few viral infections. Neither hepatitis A or B have been noted to produce granulomas (Ref. 1, p. 831).

9.50. **(E)** It is only an occasional pattern in Wilson's disease, but it does occur. Reactions of the liver parenchyma are limited in scope (Ref. 1, p. 824).

9.51. **(A)** Benign gastric ulcer is not a precancerous lesion. The problem is the initial differentiation of benign from malignant gastric ulcers (Ref. 1, p. 697).

9.52. **(E)** Abdominal pain is the most common clinical feature. Ulcers are mostly duodenal. All age groups can be involved, but the 30−50 yr group predominates (Ref. 1, p. 696).

9.53. **(C)**
9.54. **(A)**
9.55. **(B)**
9.56. **(D)** The film shows a hiatal hernia with a Schatzki's ring. Hiatus hernia is present in approximately one-half of the population in the United States. To determine if reflux is present, acid loading of the stomach followed by measurement of intraesophageal pH is most sensitive. Manometry is the best direct measure of sphincter

competence. The Bernstein test with intraesophageal infusion of acid will tell if the mucosa is acid-sensitive. Esophagitis is a biopsy diagnosis. Barium syphonage, while easy to perform, is unreliable (Ref. 2, p. 1689).

9.57. **(E)** This appears to be a benign gastric ulcer. These patients do secrete acid but volumes are low as is total acid secreted (Ref. 2, p. 1378).

9.58. **(B)** Gastroscopy and biopsy or brush cytology under direct vision can confirm the benign nature of the lesion. It offers the best balance of yield versus complications and missed diagnosis (Ref. 2, p. 1704).

9.59. **(A)** This is probably just massed diverticulosis. There is no evidence of inflammation (white blood count, shift to the left, or fever). X-ray does not suggest a tumor although after some therapy colonoscopy might be in order (Ref. 2, p. 1755).

9.60. **(A)** Bulk in the form of cellulose is the first maneuver to try. Colonic rest is not necessary in the absence of inflammation (Ref. 2, p. 1756).

9.61. **(D)** The duodenal loop is enlarged. This could be a result of chronic pancreatitis or carcinoma of the pancreas. Operationally, it is the question of carcinoma which needs to be addressed urgently (Ref. 1, p. 779).

9.62. **(A)** There is no calcification in the pancreatic mass. If the bile ducts are dilated, endoscopic retrograde cholangiopancreatography or transhepatic cholangiography is in order. If bile ducts are normal, skinny needle aspiration should be next. Ultrasound or CT scans will not only tell if bile ducts are dilated, but also help define the mass (Ref. 1, p. 779).

9.63. **(C)** Activity is determined by the presence or friability in the mucosa which is an endoscopic finding. The extent is best assessed by barium enema (Ref. 1, p. 740).

9.64. **(C)** Steroids are best reserved for moderate or severe attacks. Some bulk (cellulose) in the diet is likely to be helpful, thus a low-residue diet would not be indicated (Ref. 1, p. 740).

9.65. (B) The risk of cancer development is highest in disease which has its onset in childhood, causes total involvement, and persists for 10 or more years. This patient has a significant risk of carcinoma of the colon. Sphincter-saving operations are effective (Ref. 1, p. 740).

References

1. Wyngaarden, J.B. and Smith, L.H., Jr.: *Cecil Textbook of Medicine*, 17th Ed., W.B. Saunders, Philadelphia, 1985.

2. Petersdorf, R.G., Adams, R.D., Braunwald, E., Isselbacher, K.J., Martin, J.B., and Wilson, J.D.: *Harrison's Principles of Internal Medicine*, 19th Ed., McGraw-Hill, New York, 1983.

3. Sherlock, D.S.: *Diseases of the Liver and Biliary System*, 6th Ed., Blackwell Scientific Publications, London, 1981.

4. Sprio, H.M.: *Clinical Gastroenterology*, 3rd Ed., Macmillan, New York, 1983.

5. Sleisenger, M.H. and Fordtran, J.S.: *Gastrointestinal Disease*, 3rd Ed., W.B. Saunders, Philadelphia, 1983.

10
Hematology
Peter C. Ungaro, M.D.

DIRECTIONS: Each of the questions or incomplete statements below is followed by five suggested answers or completions. Select the **one** that is best in each case.

10.1. Which of the following would be most likely in the patient with sickle-cell trait and no other hematologic disorder?
A. Splenomegaly
B. Hyposthenuria
C. Reticulocytosis
D. Anemia
E. Thrombocytopenia

10.2. Which of the following laboratory tests would be expected to be *abnormal* in a patient with von Willebrand's disease?
A. Factor IX level
B. Platelet aggregation with ADP (adenosine diphosphate)
C. Factor VI level
D. Platelet aggregation with risotocetin
E. Platelet count

10.3. Which of the following would be LEAST likely to result in a prolonged bleeding time?
  A. Thrombocytopenia
  B. von Willebrand's disease
  C. Hemophilia A
  D. Aspirin ingestion
  E. Scurvy

10.4. Which of the following would be LEAST likely to be associated with macrocytosis?
  A. Thalassemia
  B. Phenytoin (Dilantin) therapy
  C. Folic acid deficiency
  D. Reticulocytosis
  E. Liver disease

10.5. Which of the following neurologic abnormalities would be LEAST likely to be found in a patient with vitamin B_{12} deficiency?
  A. Impaired temperature sensation
  B. Positive Romberg sign
  C. Presence of clonus
  D. Decreased vibration sensation
  E. Hypokinesia and muscle stiffness

10.6. Which of the following would be LEAST likely to be a cause of the anemia of chronic disease?
  A. Osteomyelitis
  B. Subacute bacterial endocarditis
  C. Pancreatic cancer without metastasis to bone
  D. Cushing's disease
  E. Rheumatoid arthritis

10.7. Which of the following would be anticipated in a patient with chronic lymphocytic leukemia?
  A. Low LAP (leukocyte alkaline phosphatase) score
  B. Elevated serum vitamin B_{12} level
  C. Presence of Philadelphia chromosome
  D. Lymphadenopathy
  E. Erythrocytosis

10.8. Which of the following would NOT be an appropriate treatment for a patient with aplastic anemia who was to have bone marrow transplantation?
  A. Administration of glucocorticoids
  B. Administration of androgens
  C. Prophylactic platelet transfusions to keep the platelet count at 60,000 or higher
  D. Use of penicillin or penicillin-related antibiotics in treatment of infection
  E. Administration of immunosuppressive drugs prior to transplantation

10.9. Which of the following is LEAST characteristic of Waldenstrom's macroglobulinemia?
  A. Lytic bone lesions
  B. Anemia
  C. Hyperviscosity
  D. Lymphadenopathy
  E. Hepatosplenomegaly

10.10. The patient with the serum protein electrophoresis shown in Figure 32 is found to have 40% plasma cells on bone marrow aspirate and generalized osteoporosis on bone films. Which of the following additional laboratory abnormalities would be LEAST likely?
  A. Azotemia
  B. Hypercalcemia
  C. Hyperuricemia
  D. Hypoglobulinemia
  E. Increased erythrocyte sedimentation rate (ESR)

10.11. Which of the following laboratory abnormalities would be most helpful in establishing the presence of a hemolytic anemia?
  A. Low haptoglobin level
  B. Megathrombocytes on peripheral smear
  C. Low erythropoietin level
  D. Elevated serum-transferrin level
  E. Presence of hyperuricemia

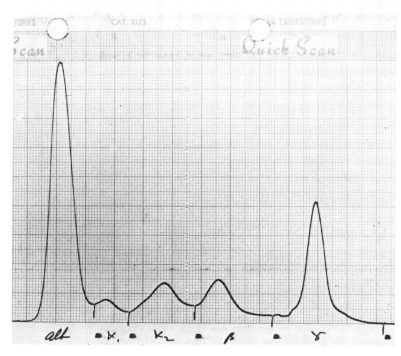

Figure 32

10.12. Which of the following would be LEAST likely to be associated with eosinophilia?
   A. Toxoplasmosis
   B. Hypoadrenocorticism
   C. Loeffler's endocarditis
   D. Allergic vasculitis
   E. Myxedema

10.13. Which of the following would NOT be expected in association with G-6-PD (glucose-6-phosphate dehydrogenase) deficiency?
   A. Increased erythrocyte osmotic fragility
   B. Reticulocytosis with hemolysis
   C. Positive Heinz-body test
   D. Sensitivity to oxidant drugs
   E. Predominance in black males

DIRECTIONS: Each group of questions below consists of five lettered headings followed by a list of numbered words or statements. For each numbered word or statement, select the **one** lettered heading that is most closely associated with it. Each lettered heading may be selected once, more than once, or not at all.

A. Acute myelogenous leukemia (AML)
B. Acute lymphocytic leukemia (ALL)
C. Chronic myelogenous leukemia (CML)
D. Chronic lymphocytic leukemia (CLL)
E. Acute promyelocytic leukemia (APL)

10.14. Occurs predominantly in children with peak incidence at the age of 4

10.15. Busulfan (Myleran) administration is generally considered to be the treatment of choice for patients in the chronic phase

10.16. This leukemia is the most likely to be associated with disseminated intravascular coagulopathy (DIC)

10.17. The malignant cells in thie leukemia are likely to contain cytoplasmic Auer rods

10.18. Autoimmune hemolytic anemia develops in 5–10% of patients with this leukemia

DIRECTIONS: Each set of lettered headings below is followed by a list of numbered words or phrases. For each numbered word or phrase select
(A) if the item is associated with A only
(B) if the item is associated with B only
(C) if the item is associated with both A and B
(D) if the item is associated with neither A nor B

A. Folic acid deficiency
B. Vitamin B_{12} deficiency
C. Both
D. Neither

10.19. Associated with hypersegmented neutrophils on peripheral blood smear

10.20. Serum antibodies to intrinsic factor are found in this condition

10.21. High-dose vitamin C therapy will correct the hematologic abnormalities associated with this disorder, but not the neurologic manifestations

---

DIRECTIONS: For each of the questions or incomplete statements below, **one or more** of the answers or completions given is correct. Select
(A) if only 1, 2, and 3 are correct
(B) if only 1 and 3 are correct
(C) if only 2 and 4 are correct
(D) if only 4 is correct
(E) if all are correct

10.22. Which of the following laboratory determinations would be expected in a patient with iron-deficiency anemia?
  1. Depressed serum-transferrin level
  2. Low serum-ferritin level
  3. Increased corrected reticulocyte count
  4. Elevated free erythrocyte protoporphyrin

10.23. Which of the following would be characteristic of the anemia of chronic disease?
  1. Elevated serum-transferrin level
  2. Hyperchromic macrocytic erythrocyte indices
  3. Elevated serum-iron level
  4. Normal or increased serum-ferritin level

10.24. Which of the following has been associated with erythrocytosis?
  1. Hypernephroma
  2. Uterine fibroids
  3. Hepatoma
  4. Pheochromocytoma

10.25. Which of the following is considered to be a myeloproliferative disorder?
1. Polycythermia rubra vera
2. Agnogenic myeloid metaplasia (myelofibrosis)
3. Chronic myelocytic leukemia
4. Multiple myeloma

10.26. Which of the following coagulation tests would be expected
to be prolonged in association with congenital Factor VII
deficiency?
1. Partial thromboplastin time
2. Euglobulin lysis time
3. Thrombin time
4. Prothrombin time

DIRECTIONS: This section of the test consists of a situation,
followed by a series of questions. Study the situation and select the
one best answer to each question following it.

Questions 10.27–10.30: The chest x-ray shown in Figure 33 is from
a young woman with Hodgkin's disease. Biopsy of a supraclavicular
lymph node established a diagnosis of the nodular sclerosis variant.
The patient's weight has not dropped and she denies night sweats.
There is no evidence of disease below the diaphragm after lymphan-
giogram and laparotomy with liver biopsy, splenectomy, open bone
marrow biopsy, and extensive lymph node sampling. The only palpable lymph nodes are in the right supraclavicular area.

10.27. What is the patient's stage?
A. Stage IB
B. Stage IIA
C. Stage IIIB
D. Stage IVA
E. Stage IVB

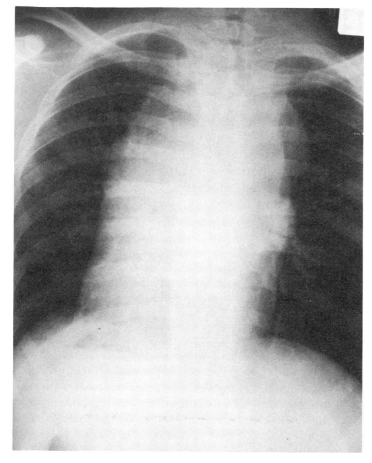

Figure 33

10.28. Which of the following laboratory abnormalities would be LEAST likely in this patient?

A. Elevated sedimentation rate
B. Normochromic normocytic anemia
C. Pancytopenia
D. Eosinophilia
E. Elevated serum copper

10.29. Even if the patient is cured of her Hodgkin's disease, she will be at increased risk for certain infectious complications due to her splenectomy. Which of the following might be a particular problem?
A. *Salmonella* osteomyelitis
B. Rocky mountain spotted fever
C. Pneumococcal septicemia
D. Bacillary dysentery
E. Nocardiosis

10.30. If a patient with this disease is treated with both radiation and combination chemotherapy, which of the following would be LEAST likely to be a consequence?
A. Ovarian dysfunction
B. Acute leukemia
C. Hypothyroidism
D. Impaired spermatogenesis
E. Adrenal insufficiency

Answers and Comments

10.1. (B) Under usual circumstances the individual with sickle-cell trait has normal hematologic studies except for the presence of abnormal hemoglobin. Anemia, reticulocytosis, splenomegaly, and thrombocytopenia are not present. Hyposthenuria, the inability to concentrate urine, is typically encountered in these individuals (Ref. 4, pp. 588–598, 591).

10.2. (D) Patients with this disorder characteristically have a prolonged bleeding time, a low factor VIII level, and defective ristocetin aggregation (Ref. 3, p. 810).

10.3. (C) The bleeding time is prolonged by platelet and vascular abnormalities, and not affected by factor deficiency. Aspirin impairs platelet function and scurvy has an adverse effect on both platelets and vessels (Ref. 3, p. 797).

10.4. (A) In thalassemia the RBCs are hypochromic and microcytic. The other conditions are associated with macrocytosis (Ref. 3, pp. 426, 476).

10.5. **(E)** Hypokinesia and muscle stiffness are characteristic of Parkinson's disease and not vitamin B_{12} deficiency (Ref. 5, p. 571).

10.6. **(D)** Suppression of erythropoiesis occurs with multiple inflammatory disease states and as an indirect effect of neoplasms not involving the bone marrow. Cushing's disease is associated with enhanced erythropoiesis from steroid marrow stimulation (Ref. 5, p. 646).

10.7. **(D)** Low LAP score, elevated vitamin B_{12}, and positive Philadelphia chromosome are all characteristic of chronic myelogenous leukemia but not chronic lymphocytic leukemia. Patients are frequently anemic, and erythrocytosis is not a feature of the disease (Ref. 1, pp. 122–123).

10.8. **(C)** Use of blood products prior to transplantation results in a lower success rate than when they are not used (Ref. 2, p. 537).

10.9. **(A)** Lytic bone lesions are characteristic of multiple myeloma and not macroglobulinemia (Ref. 2, p. 496).

10.10. **(D)** The serum protein electrophoresis shows a monoclonal spike and with the other clinical information establishes a diagnosis of multiple myeloma. The laboratory abnormalities listed would all be expected except hypoglobulinemia (Ref. 5, p. 1747).

10.11. **(A)** The hemoglobin–haptoglobin complex is rapidly removed by the reticuloendothelial system, and a low level suggests hemolysis (Ref. 4, pp. 389–390).

10.12. **(E)** Myxedema would not be expected to be an explanation for eosinophilia. There is an association between myxedema and basophilia (Ref. 4, p. 826).

10.13. **(A)** The osmotic fragility is normal in G-6-PD deficiency. It is primarily abnormal in conditions associated with erythrocyte membrane abnormalities such as hereditary spherocytosis (Ref. 3, pp. 582–586).

10.14. **(B)** ALL is predominantly a childhood malignancy (Ref. 1, p. 147).

10.15. (C) Alkylating agent therapy with busulfan is the treatment most frequently employed with CML (Ref. 5, p. 1577).

10.16. (E) The high incidence of DIC in APL frequency makes it necessary to combine heparin administration with chemotherapy (Ref. 5, p. 1543).

10.17. (A) The presence of Auer rods in blast cells establishes a diagnosis of AML (Ref. 4, p. 723).

10.18. (D) Disordered immunoglobulin synthesis with antibodies to red blood cells develops in many patients with CLL (Ref. 4, pp. 985–987).

10.19. (C) Hypersegmented neutrophils constitute a megaloblastic morphologic abnormality that may be associated with both vitamin B_{12} and folate deficiency (Ref. 1, p. 61).

10.20. (B) Antibodies to intrinsic factor are found in many patients with vitamin B_{12} deficiency due to pernicious anemia (Ref. 1, p. 63).

10.21. (D) Folic acid will mask the hematologic but not the neurologic manifestations of vitamin B_{12} deficiency (Ref. 1, p. 62).

10.22. (C) In iron-deficiency anemia the transferrin or total iron-binding capacity (TIBC) is elevated and there is reticulocytopenia (Ref. 4, pp. 471–472).

10.23. (D) The anemia of chronic disorders is characterized by a normochromic normocytic anemia with low serum-iron and transferrin levels. Sometimes the indices are hypochromic and microcytic (Ref. 5, p. 648).

10.24. (E) All have been associated with inappropriate secondary polycythemia (Ref. 4, pp. 678–681).

10.25. (A) Plasma cell proliferations are not included in the myeloproliferative disorders (Ref. 1, p. 120).

10.26. (D) Only the prothrombin time is prolonged (Ref. 3, pp. 834–835).

10.27. (B) The patient has a disease involving both the supraclavicular area and the mediastinum, the mediastinal involvement being documented on the x-ray. Involvement of two sites above the diaphragm without evidence of disease in parenchymal organs including the liver and bone marrow makes the patient stage II. Absence of 10% weight loss or night sweats makes the patient IIA (Ref. 5, p. 1653).

10.28. (C) Pancytopenia would be expected only in the presence of extensive bone marrow or splenic involvement (Ref. 5, pp. 1657–1658).

10.29. (C) Patients are at increased risk for fatal pneumococcal septicemia following splenectomy (Ref. 2, pp. 436–437).

10.30. (E) Hypothyroidism results from radiotherapy to the gland area. Ovarian dysfunction and impaired spermatogenesis result from chemotherapy with the alkylating agents. Both chemotherapy and radiotherapy have the potential for inducing acute leukemia, a potential that is enhanced by using both together (Ref. 2, pp. 435–436).

References

1. Erslev, A.J. and Gabuzda, T.G.: *Pathophysiology of Blood*, 2nd Ed., W.B. Saunders, Philadelphia, 1979.

2. Fairbanks, V.F. (ed.): *Current Hematology*, Vol. 1, J. Wiley, New York, 1981.

3. Miale, J.B.: *Laboratory Medicine Hematology*, 6th Ed., C.V. Mosby, St. Louis, 1982.

4. Williams, W.J., Beutler, E., Erslev, A.J., and Lichtman, M.A. (eds.): *Hematology*, 3rd Ed., McGraw-Hill, New York, 1983.

5. Wintrobe, M.M., Lee, G.R., Boggs, D.R., Bithell, T.C., Foerster, J., Athens, J.W., and Lukens, J.N.: *Clinical Hematology*, 8th Ed., Lea & Febiger, Philadelphia, 1981.

11

Infectious Diseases
Martin J. Raff, M.D.

DIRECTIONS: Each of the questions or incomplete statements below is followed by five suggested answers or completions. Select the one that is best in each case.

11.1. An 8-year-old child in southern Connecticut is brought by his mother to the physician with a 6-week history of illness beginning as an annular erythematous lesion following a tick bite on the thigh. The lesion had gradually expanded centrifugally with clearing in the center. Following this he had developed a migratory polyarthritis involving his right knee, left ankle, and right elbow. The cutaneous lesions had resolved within 3 to 4 weeks without therapy The arthralgias had been treated with a variety of nonsteroidal antiinflammatory agents and some oral antibiotics of undetermined nature, none of which had been taken for more than 3 to 4 days. He now presents with signs and symptoms suggestive of aseptic meningitis, and choreiform movements. Each of the following statements concerning this illness is correct except

A. this disease is caused by a spirochete.

B. this disease is transmitted by *Ixodes dammini*

C. this disease is treatable with penicillin

D. tests for rheumatoid factor by latex fixation are likely to be strongly positive

E. although there is usually absence of cardiac valvular lesions, significant episodes of arrhythmias and heart block may occur

11.2. Each of the following statements concerning infection with the Epstein-Barr virus are correct EXCEPT

    A. primary infection with the Epstein-Barr virus results in brisk formation of specific antibodies, including IgE and IgM capsular antibodies, transient responses to the early antigen complex, neutralizing antibodies, and antibody to Epstein-Barr nuclear antigen

    B. Epstein-Barr virus is responsible for infectious mononucleosis, a well-recognized disease of adolescent and young adults in populations with advanced sociohygienic standards

    C. reactivation of the chronic carriage state of the Epstein-Barr virus may produce recurrent illnesses characterized by profound fatigue, myalgia, mild pharyngitis, tender adenopathy, and low-grade fever

    D. Epstein-Barr virus may be responsible for nasopharyngeal malignancies and Burkitt's lymphoma

    E. Epstein-Barr virus may be present in the saliva of asymptomatic patients for long periods of time

11.3. A 36-year-old man diagnosed as having leptospirosis was begun on high doses of intravenous ampicillin, following which his temperature rose abruptly from 99° to 103°F and his pulse to 120/min. Following this he remained afebrile. The most probable explanation for this is

    A. drug fever

    B. Jarisch-Herxheimer reaction

    C. incorrect diagnosis

    D. resistant organism

    E. temperature recorded incorrectly

11.4. Granuloma inguinale is characterized by each statement below EXCEPT

    A. it may be transmitted to humans by feline house pets

    B. it is caused by *Calymmatobacterium granulomatis*

    C. the organism multiplies within the cytoplasm of mononuclear cells

    D. the most common extragenital lesions are on lips and oral cavity

    E. the pathognomonic cell is a large mononuclear endothelial cell containing the organisms in intracytoplasmic cystic spaces

11.5. Each of the following manifestations correctly describes tuberculosis EXCEPT
  A. primary tuberculosis is not expressed symptomatically until lesions are quite extensive
  B. late exacerbating tuberculosis is not expressed symptomatically until lesions are quite extensive
  C. symptoms become specific for tuberculosis only late in the course of the disease
  D. most common symptoms are malaise, fatigue, anorexia, weight loss, and fever
  E. temperature is usually maximal in the evening, accompanied by night sweats

11.6. Ludwig's angina was first described in 1836 by von Ludwig and is characterized correctly by each of the following statements EXCEPT
  A. it is invariably caused by a mixed bacterial infection composed of staphylococci and streptococci
  B. it is a rapidly spreading gangrenous cellulitis or phlegma involving both the submaxillary and sublingual spaces
  C. its pathogenesis is usually related to precipitating factors within the oral cavity such as dental infections, foreign bodies, lacerations of the floor of the mouth, and other maxillofacial injuries
  D. an understanding of the potential spaces defined by the deep cervical fascia is essential to the therapeutic approach
  E. therapy must include the provision of an adequate airway, usually in the form of a tracheostomy

11.7. Each statement below is accurately descriptive of nocardial infection EXCEPT
  A. human-to-human and animal-to-human transmission is assuming increasing importance
  B. brain abscesses occur in almost all patients with disseminated disease
  C. acute necrotizing pneumonitis is usually seen in immunosuppressed patients
  D. draining sinuses may result by extension through the pleura from the lungs
  E. most species are acid-fast

11.8. Which of the following statements concerning infection in patients with indwelling uterine devices (IUD) is INCORRECT?

A. The majority of the pelvic infections are due to *Neisseria gonorrheae*

B. Duration of exposure to IUD is an important factor in development of infection

C. There is a high incidence of anaerobic isolates

D. Foul-smelling mucoid discharge on the IUD tail may be the first clue to infection

E. An infection with an IUD requires removal followed by antibacterial therapy

11.9. The following statements concerning guidelines for urinary catheters are correct EXCEPT

A. cleansing of the meatal catheter junction with an antiseptic soap should be done every 72 hours

B. a sterile closed drainage system should always be used

C. normal unobstructed downhill flow must be maintained at all times

D. in patients with urinary catheterization of less than 2 weeks' duration routine catheter changes are not necessary except when obstruction, contamination, or other malfunctions occur

E. catheterized patients should be separated from each other whenever possible, and should not share the same room or adjacent baths

11.10. Each of the following is correct EXCEPT

A. up to 40% of male contacts of women with symptomatic gonorrhea develop asymptomatic urethral infection

B. fluorescent antibody testing is the most sensitive means of detecting asymptomatic male gonococcal urethritis

C. greater than 60% of infected men may be asymptomatic

D. as many as 2% of sexually active men were found to be infected on routine examination

E. asymptomatically infected men constitute a major reservoir for transmission of gonorrhea

11.11. Each of the following statements about serologic tests for syphilis is correct EXCEPT
 A. the VDRL test may be falsely positive
 B. two-thirds of patients with primary and one-third of patients with secondary syphilis have a negative TPI
 C. the TPI is negative in the nonvenereal treponematoses (bejel, pinta, yaws)
 D. the FTA-ABS test is very rarely falsely positive or negative
 E. a reactive FTA-ABS test is a good indication that a patient has had syphilis but does not indicate clinical activity

11.12. Illnesses sometimes mistaken for botulism can be differentiated by each of the statements below EXCEPT
 A. common bacterial food poisoning shows diarrhea in the absence of cranial nerve involvement
 B. mushroom poisoning *(Amanita phalloides)* produces only pyramidal tract signs
 C. atropine poisoning has rapid onset, with facial flushing and bizarre hallucinations
 D. fever usually distinguishes poliomyelitis, meningitis, and encephalitis
 E. Guillain-Barré syndrome has ascending paralysis followed by cranial nerve involvement

11.13. A 23-year-old woman, four days after the onset of menses, presents with low-grade fever, 8 to 10 peripherally distributed skin lesions appearing as small tender papules or petechiae which have quickly evolved into pustules, tenosynovitis of the extensor tendon of the left thumb, and asymmetrical arthralgias. Unroofing and staining of a cutaneous lesion shows intraleukocytic gram-negative diplococci. Each of the following statements about this disease are correct EXCEPT

    A. patients with this disease may lack local symptoms of infection, but will have positive cultures from orogenital, pharyngeal, or rectal sites

    B. the organisms producing disseminated disease are usually very susceptible to penicillin although a few cases due to penicillinase-producing strains have been reported

    C. strains of this organism responsible for disseminated infection are usually resistant to complement-mediated killing by normal human sera

    D. pharyngeal infection is usually acquired by hematogenous extension from disease elsewhere.

    E. rectal involvement usually produces proctitis and there may be rectal discharge and bleeding, anal and rectal pain, tenesmus, and constipation

11.14. Each of the following suggests the presence of a factitious fever EXCEPT

    A. patient usually a woman and in a paramedical profession

    B. pulse–temperature discrepancy

    C. elevation of axillary temperatures

    D. failure of diaphoresis to accompany defervescence

    E. deviation from the usual diurnal temperature variation

11.15. Each of the following is true of thoracic empyema EXCEPT
  A. as many as one-fifth of cases may be due to anaerobes
  B. peptostreptococci and *Bacteroides* are the most common anaerobic organisms isolated
  C. staphylococci, coliforms, streptococci, and pneumococci are the most common aerobes isolated
  D. mortality is exceedingly high in anaerobic empyema drained with thoracocentesis alone
  E. mortality of anaerobic empyema is higher than that of aerobic empyema

11.16. The clinical features of relapsing fever can be correctly described by all of the statements below EXCEPT
  A. conjunctivitis, iritis, and iridocyclitis occur
  B. tongue symptoms including pain, brown staining, atrophy, and ulcerations are frequent
  C. fever terminating by crisis followed by an apyrexial interval and then by relapse is the classic course
  D. rash usually occurs only during the initial pyrexial episode
  E. neurologic complications indicative of CNS involvement occur in about one-third of cases

11.17. A 14-year-old girl presented to her physician with fever, marked weakness, severe sore throat, cervical lymphadenopathy, and respiratory distress. Physical examination revealed a pharyngeal membrane and an impetigenous cutaneous eruption. Each of the following is true EXCEPT
  A. the clinical diagnosis warrants antitoxin therapy
  B. cutaneous lesions are probably due to *Streptococcus pyogenes*, group A
  C. erythromycin is adequate antibacterial therapy
  D. erythromycin is adequate prophylaxis for contacts and carriers
  E. cutaneous lesions may provide a reservoir for the etiologic agent of this disease

11.18. *Yersinia enterocolitica* infections are characterized by each of the following EXCEPT

    A. infections with *Yersinia enterocolitica* and *Yersinia pseudotuberculosis* are similar

    B. fever is one of the most prominent symptoms

    C. diarrhea and nonspecific abdominal pain are common

    D. local tenderness and pain in the right lower quadrant sometimes lead to operation for suspected appendicitis

    E. when the appendix is removed it is usually gangrenous

11.19. Each of the following are factors responsible for culture-negative endocarditis EXCEPT

    A. prior antimicrobial therapy

    B. poor timing in not drawing cultures just prior to a fever spike

    C. nonusage of hypertonic media to detect cell-wall deficient bacteria

    D. nonusage of truly anaerobic growth conditions

    E. less than optimal quantities of blood inoculated into media

11.20. Staphylococci other than *S. aureus* and *S. epidermidis* have been felt to be nonpathogenic. Each of the following statements are, however, true EXCEPT

    A. *S. saprophyticus* is a novobiocin-resistant, coagulase-negative staphylococcus that may be pathogenic for humans

    B. *S. saprophyticus* synthesizes urease, and therefore may be responsible for infection stones in the renal collecting system

    C. *S. saprophyticus* produces urinary tract infection in men but virtually never in women

    D. recurrent infection due to *S. saprophyticus* occurs in approximately 10% of patients after appropriate antimicrobial therapy

    E. infection-induced urinary stones may be a cause of recurrent staphylococcal bacteriuria due to *S. saprophyticus*

11.21. Guidelines for infection control in intravenous therapy include each of the following EXCEPT
  A. indwelling plastic catheters should be used wherever possible
  B. indwelling cannulae should be changed every 48 hours where possible
  C. skin preparation with iodine-containing antiseptics should be used prior to venipuncture
  D. intravenous infusion sites should be inspected daily and dressings changed
  E. antibacterial ointment should be applied to IV puncture sites

11.22. All of the following statements about staphylococcal endocarditis are true EXCEPT
  A. mortality is twice as high in patients over 50 years old than in patients under 50 years old
  B. tricuspid-valve staphylococcal endocarditis is more common in heroin addicts
  C. myocardial abscesses are extremely rare
  D. meningitis and/or brain abscess is a quite frequent complication
  E. Osler nodes, Roth spots, petechiae, and splinter hemorrhages are uncommon in staphylococcal endocarditis

11.23. In meningococcemia all the statements below are correct EXCEPT
  A. consumption coagulation does not occur in the absence of hypotension
  B. heparin therapy appears to reduce mortality in meningococcemic patients with consumption coagulopathy
  C. hypotension and/or shock may follow institution of antibiotic therapy due to sudden release of endotoxin
  D. resolution of pericarditis, arthritis, and hemorrhagic skin lesions is impaired by heparin therapy
  E. early volume expansion may reduce or prevent hypotension and shock in meningococcemia

11.24. Each of the following statements concerning chronic pyelonephritis is true EXCEPT

    A. dilatation of the calyceal region with a chronic inflammatory reaction is a major characteristic feature

    B. most cases are associated with an underlying structural abnormality

    C. urinary tract infection is demonstrable in most cases of end-stage pyelonephritis

    D. renal parenchymal damage may be a result of immunologic reaction to persistent bacterial antigens

    E. the presence of a parenchymal scar over a dilated calyx helps to distinguish chronic pyelonephritis from other causes of end-stage renal disease

11.25. A 49-year-old woman with a history of extensive travel to Africa, India, and South America had spent several weeks in a Central African Republic 9 months prior to the onset of swelling of her left eyelid which lasted 2 days. One month later she had swelling of the other eyelid following which there were episodes of typical urticaria with severe pruritis. On one occasion she noted "strangling" and was told that she had a "swollen throat." Physical examination was unremarkable. There were 11,300 leukocytes/mm^3 with 27.5% eosinophils. Her IgE level was 1660 ng/ml (normal is $\leq$ 780 ng/ml). Stools were negative for ova and parasites and urine negative for schistosomes. Radioallergosorbent tests were negative to 21 antigens including 12 foods; a C1 esterase inhibitor level, and C3, C4, and total complement values were normal. Serologic tests were negative for leishmaniasis, ascariasis, schistosomiasis, and Chagas's disease. Filariasis testing gave a titer of 1:2048 on direct hemagglutination (diagnostic titer is $\geq$ 1:128). Blood specimens were examined for microfilaria by membrane filtration and were negative. Biopsy of a subcutaneous edematous area revealed an adult gravid female *loa loa* worm. Each of the following comments is correct EXCEPT

A. *Loa loa* is a filarial "eye worm"
B. loaisis often presents with "calabar" swellings, thought to be an allergic response to antigens released by the subcutaneous parasite
C. the insect vector of loaisis is the deer fly, *Chrysops*
D. microfilaremia is extremely common, particularly in individuals not native to the endemic region
E. chronic urticaria with eosinophilia and elevated IgE levels could suggest the possibility of parasitic helminthic diseases, such as loaisis, particularly when there has been travel to an endemic area

11.26. Each of the statements below correctly describes the shock associated with bacteremia EXCEPT
  - **A.** gram-negative bacillus bacteremia rarely produces shock in patients under 35 years of age
  - **B.** the pathophysiology is probably the same in shock states induced by gram-negative and gram-positive bacteremias
  - **C.** intraarterial pressure is an unreliable indicator of the severity of the bacterial shock state
  - **D.** early stages of bacteremic shock evidence hyperventilation, respiratory alkalosis, and an increase in cardiac output
  - **E.** late stages of bacteremic shock evidence perfusion failure, metabolic acidosis, and a decrease in cardiac output

11.27. Each of the following statements is true of whooping cough EXCEPT
  - **A.** antispasmodic drugs are effective in abating the cough
  - **B.** antibiotics are unlikely to be effective unless given during the catarrhal stage of illness
  - **C.** seizures may result from anoxia secondary to coughing spasms
  - **D.** spasmodic stages of disease may last as long as 4 weeks
  - **E.** white blood cell counts of 20,000−60,000 cells/mm^3 are not uncommon

11.28. Each of the following is correct concerning Q fever EXCEPT
  - **A.** there are significant numbers of individuals with antibody titers to *Coxiella burnetii* who have never been clinically symptomatic
  - **B.** incubation period is 9−20 days
  - **C.** living within a mile of infected dairy cattle greatly increases individual risk of infection
  - **D.** disease is limited to restricted geographic areas
  - **E.** *Coxiella burnetii* may remain viable outside a host body for months at room temperature

11.29. All of the statements about shigellosis are correct EXCEPT

    A. shigellae are nonlactose-fermenting organisms with four subgroups, each producing a different type of exotoxin

    B. inflammation is usually limited to colon and rectum but may extend to the terminal ileum

    C. ulceration with bleeding usually does not go deeper than the submucosa

    D. blood cultures are almost invariably negative in patients with shigellosis

    E. severe disease with gangrenous colitis is usually due to infection with *Shigellae shigae*, a subtype of the *Shigella dysenteriae* group

11.30. The effectiveness of prophylactic antibiotics in patients undergoing initial induction chemotherapy for acute leukemia in a protected environment unit has significantly reduced the risk of infection in leukemic patients. A recent study showed that each of the following statements were correct EXCEPT

    A. antibiotic prophylaxis decreased the number of patients achieving complete leukemic remission on initial induction chemotherapy

    B. episodes of fever of unknown origin and major infection were significantly more common in patients receiving only parenteral antibiotic prophylaxis

    C. patients receiving oral combined with parenteral antibiotic prophylaxis had a lower incidence of systemic infection than those receiving parenteral prophylaxis alone

    D. frequency of local infection was similar in both groups of patients

    E. oral antibiotics were not well tolerated by some patients, causing nausea, vomiting, and abdominal discomfort

11.31. Current patterns of subphrenic abscess include each statement below EXCEPT
- **A.** primary subphrenic abscesses (occurring via hematogenous dissemination) now account for over 50% of subphrenic abscesses
- **B.** the most common cause of subphrenic abscess in the preantibiotic era was acute appendicitis or perforated ulcer
- **C.** secondary subphrenic abscesses now most commonly occur after surgery
- **D.** the right side is more commonly involved than the left
- **E.** mortality without surgical intervention approaches 100% despite antibiotic therapy

11.32. Each of the following statements concerning *Bacteroides* bacteremia is correct EXCEPT
- **A.** the isolation of *Bacteroides* from blood culture is extremely rare
- **B.** the overall mortality rate associated with *Bacteroides* bacteremia is quite high
- **C.** patients with *Bacteroides* bacteremia without clinical evidence of infection should be suspected of having an intraabdominal source of infection
- **D.** antibiotic theapy alone is inadequate to treat *Bacteroides* bacteremia when a surgically drainable infection with this organism exists
- **E.** most tetracycline derivatives are inappropriate for use in the treatement of severe *Bacteroides* infections

11.33. The following statements concerning brain abscesses are true EXCEPT
- **A.** brain abscesses frequently present as an expanding intracranial lesion with headache and focal neurologic signs rather than as infectious processes
- **B.** fever is frequently absent
- **C.** lumbar puncture usually provides useful information
- **D.** streptococci are the most frequently isolated organisms
- **E.** brain abscesses show a peak incidence in the first two decades of life and in the two decades between 50 and 70 years of age

11.34. Whipple's disease is an infrequently occurring condition characterized by weight loss, diarrhea, arthralgia, and abdominal pain. Each of the following statements concerning Whipple's disease is correct EXCEPT

   A. biopsies of small intestinal mucosa and/or lymph nodes have become practical and reliable procedures for establishing the diagnosis of Whipple's disease

   B. tissues involved in Whipple's disease show large numbers of foamy macrophages with abundant cytoplasm containing clumped periodic acid-Schiff (PAS)-positive, diastase-resistant material

   C. electron microscopic studies show bacilliform structures within macrophages in tissues of patients with Whipple's disease

   D. bacilliform structures in PAS-positive macrophages have not been found in patients with Whipple's disease outside the GI tract and lymph nodes

   E. Whipple's disease is amenable to curative therapy with antibiotics

11.35. Each of the following statements concerning *Pneumocystis carinii* pneumonia is correct EXCEPT

   A. *P. carinii* is probably acquired by the respiratory route

   B. specific serologic tests of high sensitivity for antipneumocystis antibodies make it possible to diagnose infection and to identify potential carriers

   C. pneumocystis attack rates are higher in patients who receive more intensive antileukemic therapy

   D. acquisition and spread of pneumocystis may be related to contact of immunosuppressed patients with factors in the hospital environment

   E. *P. carinii* is a well-known cause of epidemic interstitial pneumonia in premature and debilitated infants

11.36. Each of the following statements concerning septic pulmonary embolization is correct EXCEPT

A. the incidence is high following suppurative pelvic thrombophlebitis

B. the most common site is from primary right-sided endocarditis

C. signs and symptoms may include dyspnea, tachypnea, chest pain, tachycardia, cough, hemoptysis, restlessness, anxiety, and syncope along with shaking chills and high fever

D. roentgenographic findings are helpful but often subtle and may be characterized by small parenchymal densities as the only suggestion of this diagnosis

E. *Staphylococcus aureus* is the most common offending organism in all patient populations except for the patient with thermal injury in which gram-negative organisms predominate

11.37. *Capnocytophaga* is a recently described genus of gram-negative bacilli formerly identified as *Bacteroides ocharaceus* or CDC biogroup DF-1. Each of the following statements about this organism are correct EXCEPT

A. *Capnocytophaga* produces infectious disease only in immunocompromised, predominantly neutropenic hosts

B. *Capnocytophaga* is a capnophilic microaerophilic gram-negative bacillus

C. *Capnocytophaga* is a frequent inhabitant of the oral cavity, and an etiologic agent of juvenile periodontosis

D. *Capnocytophaga* elaborates a toxin that inhibits neutrophil chemotaxis

E. systemic infections, usually in neutropenic hosts, have included bacteremia, pneumonia, meningitis, septic arthritis, and osteomyelitis

11.38. Each of the following statements concerning the pathogenesis of fever in humans is correct EXCEPT

    A. endogenous pyrogen is produced in phagocytic leukocytes in response to exogenous pyrogens

    B. endogenous pyrogen is a protein released from a variety of phagocytic leukocytes and enters the circulation after new messenger RNA and protein are synthesized

    C. fever is caused by an interaction of endogenous pyrogen with specialized receptors on or near thermosensitive neurons in the thermoregulatory center of the anterior hypothalamus

    D. following activation of the anterior hypothalamus information is transmitted through the posterior hypothalamus to the vasomotor center which directs sympathetic nerve fibers to constrict peripheral vessels and decrease heat dissipation

    E. antipyretics such as aspirin decrease the production of endogenous pyrogen from leukocytes, thereby abating fever

11.39. Clinical features of rubella include each of the following EXCEPT

    A. adults may have 2-day mild prodrome with some conjunctivitis

    B. minute palatal red spots (Forchheimer sign) appear

    C. eruption always begins on the cheeks, spreading to the rest of the body within 24 hours

    D. eruption is intensely pruritic and accompanied by a sensation of warmth

    E. adenopathies are almost a constant finding

11.40. The group G streptococcus is an important opportunistic and nosocomial pathogen. Infection with these organisms can be characterized by each of the following statements EXCEPT

A. malignancy, alcoholism, and diabetes are often important host determinants of susceptibility to infection with this organism

B. polymicrobial infection including polymicrobial bacteremia is an important feature of group G streptococcal infection

C. bacteremic patients almost invariably have a clinically apparent primary source of infection from which hematogenous extension occurred

D. therapy is usually most effective with cell wall active antibiotic/aminoglycoside combinations in patients with serious infections such as septic arthritis and acute endocarditis

E. underlying disease processes or the presence of indwelling foreign bodies often predicate the therapeutic outcome of infections with group G streptococci, with resistance to antibiotics being a lesser factor

11.41. Cases of cytomegalovirus mononucleosis in previously normal individuals are characterized by each statement below EXCEPT

A. sore throat is a frequent complaint

B. illness with fever, malaise, myalgia, atypical lymphocytosis

C. negative heterophile agglutination

D. persistent viruria is common

E. exudative pharyngitis is similar to EBV mononucleosis

11.42. Which of the following statements about rhinovirus infections is INCORRECT
- **A.** Rhinovirus infections cause one-third or more of common colds in adults
- **B.** Rhinovirus is shed in exudative material which is coughed or sneezed out from most infected persons
- **C.** Rhinovirus is not commonly transmitted by aerosolization of the virus
- **D.** Rhinovirus is not commonly transmitted by kissing
- **E.** Rhinovirus is transmitted from dried virus transported on fingers to nasal and conjunctival mucosa

11.43. Each of the following statements concerning infectious mononucleosis in the older patient is correct EXCEPT
- **A.** infectious mononucleosis should be considered in older patients who have febrile illnesses accompanied by abnormal liver function tests and lymphocytosis
- **B.** parenteral transmission of Epstein-Barr virus by extracorporeal circulation may produce infectious mononucleosis in the elderly
- **C.** elderly patients with infectious mononucleosis have no clinical differences from younger patients with the same disease, although jaundice and hepatomegaly may occur with increased frequency in the older group
- **D.** heterophil antibody titer is elevated in older patients with infectious mononucleosis
- **E.** laboratory features of infectious mononucleosis are similar in elderly and young patients although not all patients in the former group have lymphocytosis

11.44. Each of the following is true of blastomycosis EXCEPT
- **A.** acute self-limited pulmonary infection may occur
- **B.** it may present with an influenza-like illness with fever, cough, arthralgia, and myalgia
- **C.** it may present as severe pleuritic chest pain with radiographic evidence of pleural involvement
- **D.** sputum smears may show the characteristic budding yeast
- **E.** the blastomycin complement fixation is a reliable means of establishing a diagnosis serologically

11.45. A 30-year-old man developed fevers to 104°F and night sweats. On tetracycline he developed a maculopapular eruption, sparing only the palm and soles. He had a nonproductive cough, abdominal pain, persistent fever, splenomegaly, and the rash. Multiple tests including antinuclear antibody, cold agglutinins, Coombs' tests, Brucella agglutinins, monospot test, and toxoplasmosis titers were negative. Each of the following statements is correct EXCEPT

   A. this clinical picture is compatible with cytomegalovirus (CMV) mononucleosis
   B. cytomegalovirus mononucleosis often resembles EB virus infectious mononucleosis
   C. patients with CMV mononucleosis often have high prolonged fevers (> 3 weeks) and the diagnosis is often unsuspected
   D. many patients with CMV mononucleosis develop extremely severe morbidity and there is a high mortality rate
   E. since cytomegalovirus titers and cultures of this organism from urine, buffy coat, throat washings, or biopsy specimens are easily obtained, this disease should be diagnosed early when suspected

11.46. Pulmonary cryptococcosis can be correctly described by each statement below EXCEPT

   A. most patients will recover without treatment
   B. most patients with proven pulmonary parenchymal disease have other underlying pulmonary diseases
   C. concomitant extrapulmonary disease should be searched for
   D. it may present as a solitary nodule
   E. there is no predominance of involvement of any single pulmonary lobe

11.47. Phycomycosis can be described by each statement below EXCEPT

    A. it frequently occurs in acidotic uncontrolled diabetes

    B. phycomycetes are normally saprophytic and are ubiquitous fungi

    C. it is invariably resistant to amphotericin B therapy, requiring surgery

    D. the rhinocerebral form may present with black necrotic nasal mucosa

    E. the organism has an affinity for blood vessels and grows along the internal elastic lamina of large arteries

11.48. Sporotrichosis is a fungal infection which may become a serious chronic illness. Each of the following is correct EXCEPT

    A. it is acquired by inhalation of dried spores frequently found in the excreta of perched starlings

    B. dissemination may occur via lymphatics and bloodstream

    C. potassium iodide is a successful form of therapy

    D. amphotericin B is the most effective agent in treating systemic sporotrichosis

    E. local heat therapy may be effective in treatment of lymphocutaneous sporotrichosis

11.49. Each of the following statements concerning systemic *Aspergillus* infections occurring in the hospitalized patient is correct EXCEPT

    A. systemic *Aspergillus* infection frequently involves the pulmonary parenchyma

    B. *Aspergillus* mycetomas are extremely unusual in the hospitalized patient

    C. *Aspergillus* pneumonia is almost invariably fatal

    D. almost all patients with *Aspergillus* pneumonia have severe underlying disease predisposing to this complication

    E. the most frequent finding in patients with *Aspergillus* pneumonia is the appearance of a new infiltrate on x-ray that is progressive and often cavitary

11.50. Each of the following correctly describes chronic pulmonary histoplasmosis EXCEPT

A. an acute or subacute illness is often manifested by large segmental chronic lesions which tend to heal and are designated as early lesions

B. there is a chronic disease marked by persistent cavitation, low-grade chronic illness, and a tendency to promote pulmonary fibrosis and progressive pulmonary insufficiency

C. 80% of early lesions heal completely and most would heal spontaneously

D. persistent thick-walled cavities containing the organism produce progressive pulmonary fibrosis particularly in the lung bases, apparently from aspiration of antigenic material

E. amphotericin B is unnecessary in the treatment of the late lesions of chronic pulmonary histoplasmosis

11.51. Which statement about ascariasis is INCORRECT

A. Adults reside in lumen of small bowel

B. Infection results from ingestion of eggs which migrate through lungs as vermicules and mature in small bowel after being swallowed

C. Heavy infestation may result in bowel obstruction

D. Eosinophilia is invariably absent

E. Therapy is with pyrantel pamoate, mebendazole, or piperazine

11.52. Each of the following correctly describes babesiosis EXCEPT

A. *Babesia* are intracellular red cell parasites

B. it is transmitted by ticks

C. it occurs only in splenectomized humans

D. it is difficult to distinguish from acute falciparum malaria

E. it is found in horses, dogs, cats, raccoons, and rodents in the United States

11.53. Each of the following statements concerning thiabendazole treatment of severe *Strongyloides* in a hemodialyzed patient is correct EXCEPT
  A. hyperinfection with *Strongyloides stercoralis* is a well-documented complication of immunosuppression
  B. thiabendazole is the preferred treatment for strongyloidiasis
  C. failures of therapy with thiabendazole have been reported in the hyperinfected patient
  D. since thiabendazole is excreted via the liver it can be given safely to anephric patients
  E. metabolites of thiabendazole have little or no antihelminthic activity

11.54. Toxoplasmosis in humans has each of the following important facts known to be true EXCEPT
  A. neonatal infection produces CNS and eye disorders
  B. cats are the only animals known to shed oocysts
  C. transmission of toxoplasma to humans occurs through raw meat
  D. transplacental infection is known to occur
  E. oocysts are shed continuously from infected cats and are infectious immediately

11.55. Fish tapeworm infection (diphyllobothriasis) can be characterized by each of the following EXCEPT
  A. pernicious anemia results from inhibition of intrinsic factor by the adult worm
  B. humans are infected by eating raw freshwater fish containing spargana
  C. anemia primarily occurs in infection acquired in Finland
  D. adult worms may be 30 feet long and live 30 years
  E. treatment with extracts from the worm will correct the anemia without eradicating the worms

11.56. Indications for surgical management of hepatic amebic abscesses include each of the following EXCEPT
   A. aspiration of greater than 30 cc of purulent material
   B. clinical evidence of persistent abscess with failure of response to drug therapy
   C. failure to obtain clinical response following repeated aspirations
   D. rupture into the peritoneal cavity
   E. large abscess in the left lobe of the liver to prevent rupture into the pericardium

11.57. A 55-year-old white man returns from a fishing trip in Colombia. Two weeks after arriving home he sustains the sudden onset of shaking chills and fever to 105°F. Blood smears stained with Giemsa stain reveal erythrocytes which contain ring forms with a single chromatid dot. Older trophozoites are highly pigmented and ameboid. Mature schizonts fill the RBC, and an average of 16 merozoites is seen. This is most likely due to
   A. *Plasmodium vivax*
   B. *Plasmodium ovale*
   C. *Plasmodium falciparum*
   D. *Plasmodium malariae*
   E. none of the above

11.58. Respiratory abnormalities, usually in association with pulmonary infiltrates, occur in about one-half of patients with acquired immune deficiency syndrome (AIDS). Each of the following statements is correct EXCEPT
   A. most pulmonary parenchymal disease in AIDS patients is due to *Pneumocystis carinii*
   B. cytomegalovirus is a major cause of pneumonitis in AIDS patients
   C. *Mycobacterium avium-intracellulare*, although frequently producing systemic infection with bacteremia in AIDS patients, rarely if ever produces pulmonary infiltrative disease and respiratory insufficiency
   D. Kaposi's sarcoma can produce pneumonitis in AIDS patients
   E. nonspecific pneumonitis and adult respiratory distress syndrome may be seen as causes of pulmonary disease in AIDS patients

11.59. Anaerobic bacteremia is extremely common and has a propensity to cause infection in areas of low oxygen tension that are far removed from the original portal of entry. Each of the following statements is correct EXCEPT

    A. anaerobic bacteremia in patients without a primary focus of infection invariably emanates from the lower gastrointestinal tract

    B. anaerobic bacteremia may occur in patients with pre-existing infections

    C. anaerobic bacteremia is commonly seen from decubitus ulcers

    D. *Bacteroides fragilis* has been reported to cause anaerobic myocardial abscess following myocardial infarction

    E. the risk of superinfection with anaerobic bacteria is enhanced in sites that are anaerobic, in necrotic tissue from tumors, in sites of chronic infection, in areas of vascular insufficiency, or in the presence of foreign bodies

11.60. Each of the following statements concerning measles encephalomyelitis is correct EXCEPT

    A. measles encephalomyelitis is rare under age 2 but complicates about 1 in 1000 measles-virus infections in older children

    B. the mortality rate in measles encephalomyelitis is 10 to 20% and the majority of survivors have neurologic sequelae

    C. measles encephalomyelitis is extremely rare and constitutes only a fraction of demyelinating diseases in humans

    D. patients with postinfectious encephalomyelitis complicating natural measles virus infection seem to exhibit a pathogenesis similar to that of experimental allergic encephalomyelitis

    E. a lack of intrathecal synthesis of antibody against measles virus suggest that measles encephalomyelitis may not be dependent on virus replication within the central nervous system

Answers and Comments

11.1. (D) Although the arthropathy of Lyme disease may resemble that of juvenile rheumatoid arthritis of the monoarticular or pauciarticular type, the rheumatoid factor will not be present (Refs. 5; 50; 65; 66).

11.2. (A) The formation of antibodies to Epstein-Barr virus nuclear antigen is usually, although not always, delayed until later in the course of the disease (Refs. 32; 39; 51; 68).

11.3. (B) The Jarish-Herxheimer reaction occurs most commonly following the onset of therapy for syphilis but may occur with any of the disease processes caused by spirochaetal organisms, including leptospirosis. The patient may experience transient fever and symptoms of malaise, chills, headaches, and myalgia. A transient neutrophilicocytosis occurs at the height of the reaction which subsides within 24 hours and its occurrence is not an indication for discontinuance of treatment (Refs. 10; 71).

11.4. (A) This is a venereal disease of humans which is rare in temperate climates and has a low degree of contagiousness. It is not known to be transmitted from animals to humans (Ref. 33, pp. 512-515).

11.5. (C) Few if any symptoms of tuberculosis are specific for that disease and, in fact, this is one of the great mimickers of medicine (Ref. 33, pp. 318-342).

11.6. (A) The bacteriology in cases of Ludwig's angina usually involves multiple organisms and frequently staphylococci and streptococci are involved. However, gram-negative organisms may be seen including *E. coli* and *Pseudomonas aeruginosa* and anaerobic organisms including *Bacteroides* have also been implicated. Antimicrobial therapy directed at a mixed population is often necessary to cure this illness (Refs. 26; 41).

11.7. (A) Overall, nocardial infections do not appear to be common in humans, and although they have been isolated from infections in a variety of animals, there are no known cases acquired from either human-to-human or animal-to-human transmission (Ref. 33, pp. 356-364).

11.8. **(A)** The majority of pelvic infections occurring in the presence of indwelling uterine devices may be due to mixed flora including a high percentage of anaerobes (Ref. 22).

11.9. **(A)** This article by the Centers for Disease Control establishes general guidelines for the prevention of catheter-associated urinary tract infections. It is recommended that once or twice daily perineal care for catheterized patients should include cleansing of meatal catheter junction with an antiseptic soap and subsequently antimicrobial ointment might be applied (Ref. 64).

11.10. **(B)** The most sensitive means of detecting asymptomatic male gonococcal urethritis is by culture of urethral swabs (Ref. 28).

11.11. **(C)** The TPI is positive in the nonvenereal treponematoses (Ref. 63).

11.12. **(B)** Poisoning with *Amanita phalloides* is predominantly due to the parasympathomimetic alkaloid muscarine, resulting in symptoms related to parasympathetic simulation. Muscular tremors, confusion, excitement, and delirium are common in severe poisoning (Ref. 15).

11.13. **(D)** Pharyngeal gonococcal infection is almost invariably acquired by orogenital contact; specifically usually by fellatio (Ref. 34).

11.14. **(C)** Elevation of axillary temperatures suggests that the fever is not factitious and is probably real (Ref. 54).

11.15. **(E)** Anaerobic thoracic empyema has an extremely low mortality rate (Ref. 69).

11.16. **(D)** The cutaneous macular eruption over the torso occurring during episodes of relapsing fever is not restricted to the initial pyrexial episode (Refs. 33, pp. 1067–1071; 62).

11.17. **(B)** The cutaneous lesions of diphtheria may be confused with those due to *Streptococcus pyogenes*. It is occasionally possible that complicating streptococcal infections may occur but this is less usual. Although cutaneous infections with *C. diphtheria* persist longer than respiratory infections, they usually do not cause systemic toxicity (Ref. 4; 11).

11.18. (E) Many patients with *Y. enterocolitica* infection may present with abdominal symptoms suggestive of appendicitis but when the appendix is removed, it is usually normal. Some patients have mesenteric lymphomatosis or acute ileitis but not appendicitis (Ref. 46).

11.19. (B) Since the bacteremia of endocarditis is a continuous one, the times at which blood culture are drawn should be of little or no importance (Refs. 42; 43; 55; 75).

11.20. (C) Approximately 10% of symptomatic urinary tract infections in young adult women are caused by *Staphylococcus saprophyticus* (Refs. 20; 35; 44).

11.21. (A) Indwelling plastic catheters should be avoided wherever possible. There is a much higher incidence of infection associated with these than with metal needles (Ref. 23).

11.22. (C) Myocardial abscesses occur with some frequency in patients with staphylococcal endocarditis (Ref. 74).

11.23. (D) Therapy with heparin is directed against disseminated intravascular coagulation and will have little or no effect in helping to resolve already existing pathologic changes (Ref. 77).

11.24. (C) Positive urinary cultures very rarely occur in end-stage pyelonephritis (Ref. 7).

11.25. (D) Microfilaremia occurs usually in natives of an endemic area. It occurs during the day, making the detection of microfilaria easy. However, marked allergic symptoms without microfilaremia may be the most common presentation of loaisis in individuals who are not native to the endemic regions (Ref. 72).

11.26. (B) The pathophysiology differs a great deal between gram-negative and gram-positive bacteremia, the features of each being too extensive to discuss here (Ref. 52).

11.27. **(A)** Antispasmodic drugs are ineffective in abating whooping cough (Ref. 37).

11.28. **(D)** Q fever is found all over the world and is not limited to restricted geographic areas (Ref. 1).

11.29. **(A)** Shigellae do not produce an exotoxin (Ref. 31).

11.30. **(A)** There is no influence of the type of antimicrobial prophylaxis utilized on the incidence of patients undergoing initial remission or who sustained complete remission of leukemia following induction chemotherapy (Ref. 6).

11.31. **(A)** Secondary subphrenic abscesses, that is, those occurring as a result of extension from infections elsewhere, account for the great majority of subphrenic abscesses (Ref. 70).

11.32. **(A)** In this series on a surgical service over 5% of all positive blood cultures were due to *Bacteroides*. In other series this has been as high as 15% (Ref. 45).

11.33. **(C)** Of 60 patients with brain abscesses, most presented with signs of an expanding intracranial lesion, and fever was frequently absent. Most brain abscesses originated from otic or paranasal sinus infection, although the majority were of unknown source. In patients with possible brain abscesses, lumbar puncture should be discouraged. Frequently, only minimal information is obtained and the lethal complication of brain herniation has been repeatedly emphasized (Ref. 8).

11.34. **(D)** There has been a unique case of Whipple's disease in a 54-year-old man with chronic cough and gastrointestinal symptoms in whom the initial diagnosis of Whipple's disease was made by lung biopsy. The bacilliform structures of Whipple's disease were demonstrated in the pulmonary parenchyma of this patient (Ref. 78).

11.35. **(B)** There is a low sensitivity and specificity of serologic tests for antipneumocystis antibody, making it difficult to identify potential carriers or individuals with mild-to-subclinical infections. In a recent outbreak there was epidemiologic and serologic evidence to suggest that acquisition and spread of *Pneumocystis carinii* may have been related to contact with the hospital environment but was insufficient to determine whether spread occurred from patient to staff or staff to patient (Ref. 59).

11.36. **(B)** Primary endocarditis of the right side of the heart is uncommon, usually requiring valvular damage, congenital defects, or a left-to-right shunt to nurture a septic process. Secondary right-sided endocarditis is more common and may become the major and persistent focus of pyemia after the inciting cause has been corrected (Ref. 25).

11.37. **(A)** *Capnocytophaga* has now been described as producing 16 infections in nonimmunocompromised hosts. These have included empyema, lung abscess, sinusitis, conjunctivitis, subphrenic abscess, wound infection, osteomyelitis, and bacteremia (Ref. 53; 79).

11.38. **(E)** Antipyretics such as aspirin do not affect production of endogenous pyrogen from leukocytes but rather interfere with prostaglandin synthesis in the hypothalamus. Prostaglandin release is probably an early step in initiation of fever, mediating AMP stimulation of the hypothalamus (Ref. 14).

11.39. **(D)** The cutaneous eruption accompanying rubella infection is seldom pruritic. It usually begins on the face, spreading to the chest and abdomen, and is pink, maculopapular, and not distinctive in appearance (Refs. 13, p. 356; 17).

11.40. **(C)** Many patients with bacteremia due to group G streptococci have no apparent primary source of infection (Ref. 73).

11.41. **(E)** Exudative pharyngitis is not a common feature of cytomegalovirus mononucleosis (Ref. 40).

11.42. **(B)** Rhinovirus concentrations in respiratory secretions from individuals with natural colds are extremely low and there is a relatively poor yield of the virus in saliva or in the aerosols produced by coughing and sneezing as these secretions come primarily from the pool of saliva in the anterior part of the mouth (Refs. 17; 30).

11.43. **(C)** Although malaise, fever, and fatigue are seen in both younger and older patients, there is a striking infrequency of pharyngitis, lymphadenopathy, and splenomegaly in older patients with infectious mononucleosis (Ref. 9).

11.44. **(E)** The blastomycin complement-fixation test is highly unreliable, with false-positive and false-negative tests being the rule rather than the exception (Ref. 60).

11.45. **(D)** Although most patients with cytomegalovirus mononucleosis may have severe systemic manifestations with multiple organs involved, the disease is most often self-limited and there is little mortality (Ref. 12).

11.46. **(B)** There is no necessity for underlying pulmonary disease to have primary pulmonary parenchymal involvement with cryptococci. The disease may be accompanied by cough, scanty mucoid or blood-tinged sputum, low-grade fever, malaise, and weight loss. However, more often the disease is virtually asymptomatic and is manifested only by the accidental finding at autopsy of an encapusulated healed subpleural granuloma (Ref. 27).

11.47. **(C)** Phycomycetes are almost invariably sensitive to amphotericin B (Ref. 41).

11.48. **(A)** The disease acquired by inhalation of dried spores in excreta of perched starlings is usually histoplasmosis. Sporotrichosis is acquired from plants or inanimate objects that penetrate the skin and implant spores subcutaneously (Refs. 56; 57).

11.49. **(B)** *Aspergillus* mycetomas were evident in 16 of 28 patients with systemic *Aspergillus* infection. Of these patients 13 had preexisting pulmonary cavities and 2 had a residual postoperative pleural air space (Refs. 36; 58).

11.50. **(E)** The use of amphotericin B is recommended for all persistent thick-walled cavities and in some circumstances surgical resection may also be indicated. The reason for this is that once established an infected cavity tends to persist, and the organism within then produces antigen which induces a low-grade chronic allergic response resulting in the pathologic changes of this disease (Refs. 24; 36).

11.51. **(D)** Although a moderate eosinophilia is often noted in individuals infected by this worm, the eosinophilia is not constant and may in fact be absent (Refs. 36, pp. 465−471; 47, pp. 547−549).

11.52. **(C)** Babesiosis occurs in nonsplenectomized humans. Splenectomized individuals, however, have a poorer prognosis and the major mortality in this disease occurs in those patients (Ref. 76).

11.53. **(D)** Thiabendazole is rapidly metabolized to 5-hydroxy metabolites which are eliminated predominantly by the kidney. Patients with marked renal impairment can be cautiously treated with thiabendazole at doses of 25 mg/kg of body weight twice daily. However, if extended therapy is needed as for strongyloidiasis hyperinfection, close monitoring of the patient for serum metabolite levels is recommended (Ref. 61).

11.54. **(E)** *Toxoplasma gondii* cysts infect cats who then shed immature oocysts in their feces. The oocysts then sporulate and become infective 1−5 or more days after shedding. Individuals handling kitty litter are particularly susceptible (Refs. 21; 36, pp. 397−403).

11.55. **(A)** The pernicious anemia of diphyllobothriasis is due to competition for vitamin B_{12} by the parasite with the host. The fish tapeworm has been found to contain considerable amounts of vitamin B_{12} (Refs. 3; 36, pp. 597−600).

11.56. **(A)** It will usually be unnecessary to aspirate all but massive lesions due to amebiasis in the liver. The indications for aspiration are listed as the other choices of answers to this question (Refs. 36; 49).

11.57. **(A)** This description is diagnostic of *Plasmodium vivax* infection (Refs. 2; 29; 36; 47, pp. 240−291).

11.58. **(C)** *Mycobacterium avium-intracellulare* is responsible for approximately 10% of the total etiologic causes of pulmonary disease in patients with acquired immune deficiency syndrome and is the third most common cause of infectious pulmonary parenchymal disease in these patients (Ref. 67).

11.59. (A) When anaerobic bacteremia occurs in the absence of a primary focus of infection, the actual source of the organisms is seldom clearly discernible, but may be from any mucous membrane including the oral cavity (Refs. 18; 19).

11.60. (C) Worldwide measles remains a major cause of death and disability, and measles encephalomyelitis remains the most common demyelinating disease in humans (Ref. 38).

References

1. Alkan, W.J., Alkalay, L., Klingberg, W., et al.: A study of Q fever in central Israel. Scand. J. Infect. Dis. 5:17−21, 1973.

2. Barrett-Connor, E.: Malaria. An "imported" disease to be reckoned with in the U.S. Calif. Med. 19−23, 1971.

3. Barrett-Connor, E.: Anemia and infection. Am. J. Med. 52: 242−253, 1972.

4. Belsey, M.A., Sinclair, M., Roder, M.R., et al.: *Corynebacterium diphtheriae* skin infections in Alabama and Louisiana: A factor in the epidemiology of diphtheria. N. Engl. J. Med. 280:135−141, 1969.

5. Berger, B.W., Clemmensen, O.J., and Ackerman, A.B.: Lyme disease is a spirochetosis. Am. J. Dermatopathol. 5:111−124, 1983.

6. Bodey, G.P., Keating, M.J., McCredie, K.B., et al.: Prospective randomized trial of antibiotic prophylaxis in acute leukemia. Am. J. Med. 78:404−416, 1985.

7. Braude, A.: Current concepts of pyelonephritis. Medicine 52: 257−264, 1973.

232 / Clinical Medicine

8. Brewer, N.S., MacCarty, C.S., and Wellman, W.E.: Brain abscess. A review of recent experience. Ann. Intern. Med. 82: 571–576, 1975.

9. Carter, J.W., Edson, R.S., and Kennedy, C.C.: Infectious mononucleosis in the older patients. Mayo Clin. Proc. 53: 146–150, 1978.

10. Centers for Disease Control: Leptospirosis Annual Summary, 1972, issued February, 1974.

11. Centers for Disease Control: Morbidity and Mortality Wkly. Rpt. 22:250–255, 1973.

12. Cohen, J.I. and Corey, G.R.: Cytomegalovirus infection in the normal host. Medicine 64:100–114, 1985.

13. Debre, R. and Celers, J. (eds.): Clinical Virology. The Evaluation and Management of Human Viral Infections, W.B. Saunders, Philadelphia, 1970.

14. Dinarello, C.A. and Wolff, S.M.: Pathogenesis of fever in man. N. Engl. J. Med. 298:607–612, 1977.

15. Donadio, J.A., Gangarosa, E.J., and Faich, G.A.: Diagnosis and treatment of botulism. J. Infect. Dis. 124:108–112, 1971.

16. Emmons, C.W., Binford, C.H., Utz, J.P., and Kwon-Chung, K.J.: Medical Mycology, 3rd Ed., Lea & Febiger, Philadelphia, 1977.

17. Evans, A.S. (ed.): Viral Infections of Humans, Plenum, New York, 1977.

18. Finegold, S.M.: Anaerobic Bacteria in Human Disease. Academic Press, New York, 1977.

19. Finley, R.W. and Marr, J.J.: Anaerobic myocardial abscess following myocardial infarction. Am. J. Med. 78:513–514, 1985.

20. Fowler, J.E., Jr.: *Staphylococcus saprophyticus* as the cause of infected urinary calculus. Ann. Intern. Med. 120:342−343, 1985.

21. Frederick, J. and Braude, A.I.: Anaerobic infection of the paranasal sinuses. N. Engl. J. Med. 290:135−137, 1974.

22. Golditch, I.M. and Huston, J.E.: Serious pelvic infection associated with intrauterine contraceptive device. Int. J. Fertil. 18:156−160, 1973.

23. Goldman, D.A., Maki, D.G., Rhame, F.S., et al.: Guidelines for infection control in intravenous therapy. Ann. Intern. Med. 79:848−850, 1973.

24. Goodwin, R.A., Jr., Owens, F.T., Snell, J.D., et al.: Chronic pulmonary histoplasmosis. Medicine 55:413−452, 1976.

25. Griffith, G.L., Maull, K.I, and Sachatello, C.R.: Septic pulmonary embolization. Surg. Gynecol. Obstet. 144:105−108, 1977.

26. Gross, B.D., Roark, D.T., and Meador, R.C.: Ludwig's angina due to bacteroides. J. Oral Surg. 34:456−460, 1976.

27. Hammerman, K.J., Powell, K.E., Christianson, C.S., et al.: Pulmonary cryptococcosis: Clinical forms and treatment. Am. Rev. Respir. Dis. 108:1116−1123, 1973.

28. Handsfield, H.H., Lipman, T.O., Harnisch, J.P., et al.: A symptomatic gonorrhea in men. Diagnosis, natural course, prevalence and significance. N. Engl. J. Med. 290:117−123, 1974.

29. Heineman, H.S.: The clinical syndrome of malaria in the United States. A current review of diagnosis and treatment for American physicians. Arch. Intern. Med. 129:607−616, 1972.

30. Hendley, J.O., Wenzel, R.P., and Gwaltney, J.M.: Transmission of rhinovirus colds by self-inoculation. N. Engl. J. Med. 288:1361−1364, 1973.

31. Hendrickse, R.G.: Dysentery including amoebiasis. Br. Med. J. 1:669–672, 1973.

32. Henle, G., Henle, W., and Horowitz, C.A.: Antibodies to Epstein-Barr virus associated nuclear antigen in infectious mononucleosis. J. Infect. Dis. 130:123–239, 1974.

33. Hoeprich, P.D. (ed.): Infectious Diseases, 2nd Ed., Harper & Row, Hagerstown, MD, 1977.

34. Hook, E.W., III and Holmes, K.K.: Gonococcal infections. Ann. Intern. Med. 102:229–243, 1985.

35. Hovelius, B., Mardh, P.A., and Bygren, P.: Urinary tract infections caused by Staphylococcus saprophyticus: Recurrences and complications. J. Urol. 122:645–647, 1979.

36. Hunter, G.W., Schwartzwelder, J.C., and Clyde, D.R.: Tropical Medicine, 5th Ed., W.B. Saunders, Philadelphia, 1976.

37. Jamieson, W.M.: Whooping cough. Br. Med. J. 1:223–225, 1973.

38. Johnson, R.T., Griffin, D.E., Hirsch, R.L., et al.: Measles encephalomyelitis—clinical and immunologic studies. N. Engl. J. Med. 310:137–141, 1984.

39. Jones, J.F., Ray, C.G., Minnich, L.L., et al.: Evidence for active Epstein-Barr virus infection in patients with persistent, unexplained illnesses: Elevated anti-early antigen antibodies. Ann. Intern. Med. 102:1–7, 1985.

40. Jordan, M.C., Rousseau, W.E., Stewart, J.A., et al.: Spontaneous cytomegalovirus mononucleosis. Ann. Intern. Med. 179:153–160, 1973.

41. Kaufmann, R.S. and Stone, G.: Osteomyelitis of frontal bone secondary to mucormycosis. N.Y.S.J. Med. 73:1325–1328, 1973.

42. Kaye, D.: Changes in the spectrum, diagnosis and management of bacterial and fungal endocarditis. Med. Clin. N. Am. 57: 941–957, 1973.

43. Kaye, D. (ed.): *Infective Endocarditis*, Univ. Park Press, Baltimore, 1976.

44. Latham, R.H., Running, K., and Stamm, W.E.: Urinary tract infections in young adult women caused by *Staphylococcus saprophyticus*. J.A.M.A. 250:3063–3066, 1983.

45. Lawrence, P.F., Tietjen, G.W., Gingrich, S., et al.: *Bacteroides* bacteremia. Ann. Surg. 186:559–563, 1977.

46. Leino, R. and Kalliomaki, J.L.: Yersiniosis as an internal disease. Ann. Intern. Med. 81:458–461, 1974.

47. Maegraith, B.G.: *Adams and Maegraith: Clinical Tropical Diseases*, 5th Ed., Blackwell Scientific Publications, Oxford and Edinburgh, 1980.

48. Meyers, B.R., Lawson, W., and Hirschman, S.Z.: Ludwig's angina, case report, with review of bacteriology and current therapy. Am. J. Med. 53:257–260, 1972.

49. Movsas, S.: Surgical treatment of amebic liver abscess. Am. J. Gastroenterol. 59:427–434, 1973.

50. Myerhoff, J.: Lyme disease. Am. J. Med. 75:663–670, 1983.

51. Neiderman, J.C.: Chronicity of Epstein-Barr virus infection. Ann. Intern. Med. 102:119–121, 1985.

52. Nishijimi, H., Weill, M.H., Shubin, H., and Cavanilles, J.: Hemodynamic and metabolic studies of shock associated with gram-negative bacteremia. Medicine 52:287–294, 1973.

53. Parenti, D.M. and Snydman, D.R.: *Capnocytophagus* species: Infections in non-immunocompromised and immunocompromised hosts. J. Infect. Dis. 151:140–147, 1985.

54. Petersdorf, R.G. and Bennett, I.L., Jr.: Factitious fever. Ann. Intern. Med. 46:1039–1062, 1957.

55. Rahimtoola, S.H.: *Infective Endocarditis*, Grune and Stratton, New York, 1978.

56. Robinson, H.M. (ed.): *The Diagnosis and Treatment of Fungal Infections*, Charles C. Thomas, Springfield, IL, 1974.

57. Romig, D.A., Voth, D.W., and Liu, C.: Facial sporotrichosis during pregnancy. A therapeutic dilemma. Arch. Intern. Med. 130:910–912, 1972.

58. Rose, H.D. and Varkey, B.: Deep mycotic infection in the hospitalized adult: A study of 123 patients. Medicine 54:499–507, 1975.

59. Ruebush, T.K., II, Weinstein, R.A., Baehner, R.L., et al.: An outbreak of *Pneumocystis* pneumonia in children with acute lymphocytic leukemia. Am. J. Dis. Child. 132:143–148, 1978.

60. Sarosi, G.A., Hammerman, K.J., Tosh, F.E., et al.: Clinical features of acute pulmonary blastomycosis. N. Engl. J. Med. 290:540–543, 1974.

61. Schumaker, J.D., Band, J.D., Lensmeyer, G.L., et al.: Thiabendazole treatment of severe strongyloidiasis in a hemodialyzed patient. Ann. Intern. Med. 89(part 1):644–645, 1978.

62. Southern, P.M. and Sanford, J.P.: Relapsing fever. Medicine 48:129–149, 1969.

63. Sparling, P.F.: Diagnosis and treatment of syphilis. N. Engl. J. Med. 284:642–653, 1971.

64. Stamm, W.E.: Guidelines for prevention of catheter-associated urinary tract infections Ann. Intern. Med. 82:386–390, 1975.

65. Steere, A.C., Bartenhagen, N.H., Craft, J.E., et al.: The early clinical manifestations of Lyme disease. Ann. Intern. Med. 99:76–82, 1983.

66. Steere, A.C., Grodzicki, R.L., Lornblatt, A.N., et al.: The spirochetal etiology of Lyme disease. N. Engl. J. Med. 308: 733–739, 1983.

67. Stover, D.E., White, D.A., Romano, P.A., et al.: Spectrum of pulmonary diseases associated with the acquired immune deficiency syndrome. Am. J. Med. 78:429–437, 1985.

68. Straus, S.E., Tosato, G., Armstrong, G., et al.: Persisting illness and fatigue in adults with evidence of Epstein-Barr virus infection. Ann. Intern Med. 102:7–16, 1985.

69. Sullivan, K.M., O'Toole, R.D., Fisher, R.H., et al.: Anaerobic empyema thoracis. The role of anaerobes in 226 cases of culture-proven empyemas. Arch. Intern. Med. 131:521–527, 1973.

70. Surakiatchanukul, S. and Ram, M.D.: Current patterns of subphrenic abscess. Am. J. Surg. 125:718–720, 1973.

71. Turner, L.H.: Leptospirosis. Br. Med. J. 1:231–233, 1969.

72. Van Dellen, R.G., Ottesen, E.A., Gocke, T.M., and Neafie, R.C.: *Loa loa*; An unusual cause of chronic urticaria and angioedema in the United States. J.A.M.A. 253:1924–1925, 1985.

73. Vartian, C., Lerner, P.I., Shlaes, D.M., and Gopalakrishna, K.V.: Infections due to Lancefield Group G streptococci. Medicine 64:75–88, 1985.

74. Watanakunakorn, C., Tan, J.S., and Phair, J.P.: Some salient features of *Staphylococcus aureus* endocarditis. Am. J. Med. 54:473–481, 1973.

75. Weiss, H. and Ottenberg, R.: Relation between bacteria and temperature in subacute bacterial endocarditis. J. Infect. Dis. 50:61, 1932.

76. Western, K.A., Benson, G.D., Gleason, N.N., et al.: Babesiosis in a Massachusetts resident. N. Engl. J. Med. 283:854–856, 1970.

77. Wilson, F.E. and Morse, S.R.: Therapy of acute meningococcal infections: Early volume expansion and prophylactic low-dose heparin. Am. J. Clin. Sci. 264:445–455, 1972.

78. Winberg, C.D., Rose, M.D., and Rappaport, H.: Whipple's disease of the lung. Am. J. Med. 65:873–880, 1978.

79. Winn, R.E., Chase, W.F., Lauderdale, P.W., et al.: Septic arthritis involving *Capnocytophaga ochracea*. J. Clin. Microbiol. 19:538–540, 1984.

12

Nephrology
Alvin E. Parrish, M.D., F.A.C.P.

DIRECTIONS: Each of the questions or incomplete statements below is followed by five suggested answers or completions. Select the **one** that is best in each case.

12.1. A patient is admitted with the following chemistries: $PCO_2 = 30$ mm Hg; $HCO_3^- = 20$ mEq/L. What is the pH?
  A. 7.44
  B. 7.61
  C. 7.34
  D. 7.21
  E. 7.00

12.2. A 69-year-old man has a history of asthma and chronic bronchitis. He is found to have:

Na^+	120 mEq/L
Cl^-	85 mEq/L
HCO_3^-	10 mEq/L
K^+	5 mEq/L
Creatinine	3.6 mg/dl

Which of the following does he most likely have?
  A. Respiratory acidosis
  B. Mixed respiratory and metabolic acidosis
  C. Metabolic acidosis
  D. Respiratory alkalosis and hyperchloremic acidosis
  E. Respiratory alkalosis

12.3. A 46-year-old man is admitted with a brief history of chills, fever, cough, and pain in his right chest. On examination he has a temperature of 40°C, marked shortness of breath, brownish colored sputum, dullness and rales in his right chest, and cyanosis. Which of the following sets of values would you expect?

	PO_2	PCO_2	HCO_3^-	Na^+	K^+
A.	50 mm Hg	70 mm Hg	25 mM/L	130 mEq/L	4.8 mEq/L
B.	20 mm Hg	50 mm Hg	12 mM/L	145 mEq/L	4.0 mEq/L
C.	50 mm Hg	40 mm Hg	25 mM/L	140 mEq/L	4.5 mEq/L
D.	100 mm Hg	80 mm Hg	45 mM/L	110 mEq/L	2.3 mEq/L

12.4. The following laboratory results are reported:

Creatinine   1.8 mg/dl
Na^+ 135 mEq/L
K^+ 2 mEq/L
Cl^- 110 mEq/L
HCO_3^- 15 mEq/L

You would do which of the following?
A. Measure his urinary $[H^+]$, NH_4^+, and β-2 microglobulin
B. Consider him for hemodialysis
C. Biopsy his kidney
D. Do a careful urinalysis to look for RBC
E. Measure urinary aldosterone levels

12.5. A 23-year-old diabetic is admitted with the following:

Blood sugar   450 mg/dl
Blood pH   7.16
Na^+ 120 mEq/L
K^+ 5.6 mEq/L

You would give him
A. insulin
B. insulin and sodium chloride or bicarbonate
C. sodium chloride and/or bicarbonate
D. insulin and sugar
E. glucose in water

12.6. Which of the following is NOT associated with acute post-streptococcal glomerulonephritis?
   A. Hematuria
   B. Fatty casts
   C. Red blood cell casts
   D. Edema
   E. Oliguria

12.7. Amyloidosis of the kidney may be associated with which of the following?
   A. Chronic pyelonephritis
   B. Chronic glomerulonephritis
   C. The aftereffects of acute renal failure
   D. Diabetic nephropathy
   E. Multiple myeloma

12.8. Which of the following drugs may produce nephrogenic diabetes insipidus?
   A. Declomycin
   B. Ampicillin
   C. Keflex
   D. Propranolol
   E. Chlorthalidone

12.9. Which of the following is useful in the treatment of the syndrome of inappropriate antidiuretic hormone secretion?
   A. Furosemide
   B. Cephalosporins
   C. 9-Fluorohydrocortisone
   D. Lithium chloride
   E. Streptomycin

12.10. The following values were obtained in a patient suspected of having renal disease: blood creatinine, 2.0 mg/dl; urine creatinine, 10 mg/dl; urine volume (24 hr), 993 ml. The creatinine clearance is
   A. 23.8 ml/min
   B. 51.2 ml/min
   C. 120.0 ml/min
   D. 5.8 ml/min
   E. 36.5 ml/min

12.11. A 24-year-old woman is admitted with a history of chronic renal failure. Her blood chemistries show:
$Na^+ = 125$ mEq/L; $K^+ = 5.6$ mEq/L; $Cl^- = 86$ mEq/L;
$HCO_2^- = 15$ mM/L
What is her approximate PCO_2?
A. 80 mm Hg
B. 70 mm Hg
C. 30 mm Hg
D. 22 mm Hg

12.12. In a patient with acute renal failure the PCO_2 is reported to be 46 mm Hg and the bicarbonate is 12 mM/L. Which of the following would you expect?
A. Respiratory alkalosis
B. Metabolic acidosis
C. Mixed respiratory and metabolic acidosis
D. Mixed respiratory alkalosis and metabolic acidosis

12.13. Which of the following will interfere with the determination of creatinine clearance?
A. Ingestion of a large amount of water
B. Azotemia
C. A collection of urine for less than 24 hr
D. Cefoxitin
E. Ingestion of leafy vegetables

12.14. In diabetic glomerulosclerosis which of the following is an uncommon finding?
A. Massive proteinuria (8+ g/24 hr)
B. Hematuria
C. Doubly refractile fat bodies (Maltese crosses) in the urine
D. Hypertension
E. Decreased insulin requirements

12.15. Interstitial nephritis may be caused by all of the following EXCEPT
   A. phenacetin
   B. streptomycin
   C. furosemide
   D. digoxin
   E. garamycin

12.16. The patient whose renal biopsy is shown in Figure 34 most likely has
   A. diabetes
   B. hypertension
   C. proteinuria
   D. a positive LE prep
   E. a positive throat culture for β-hemolytic streptococci

12.17. The determination of serum renin levels may in some instances be of value in the management of the hypertensive patient. Which of the following would NOT be associated with increased plasma renin activity (PRA)?
   A. Hypokalemia
   B. Diuretic therapy
   C. Propranolol therapy
   D. Low salt intake
   E. Birth control pills

12.18. The acidosis of renal failure is most likely associated with
   A. nonanion-gap acidosis
   B. metabolic alkalosis related to an abnormal K^+ metabolism
   C. a high blood chloride
   D. metabolic acidosis
   E. hypophosphatemia

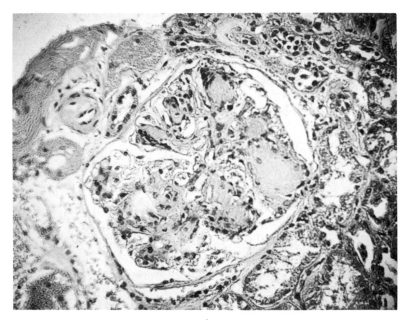

Figure 34

12.19. A 73-year-old man presents with a serum NA$^+$ of 170
mEq/L. He most likely is
   A.   eating excessive salt
   B.   uremic
   C.   dehydrated
   D.   suffering from the syndrome of inappropriate antidi-
        uretic hormone secretion (SIADH)
   E.   having the effects of an overdose of a diuretic

12.20. Which of the following would you NOT choose to determine
the suitability for surgical as opposed to medical (drug)
intervention in renovascular hypertension?
   A.   Single dose captopril test
   B.   Renal vein renin determinations
   C.   Renal artery angiography
   D.   Intravenous urogram
   E.   Radionuclide renal scan

12.21. Which of the following diseases would you expect to be consistent with these electrolytes:

Na^+ 138 mEq/L
K^+ 3 mEq/L
HCO_2^- 10mM/L
Cl^- 118 mEq/L

  A. Hyperchloremic alkalosis
  B. Renal tubular acidosis
  C. Diabetic ketoacidosis
  D. Pneumonia
  E. Chronic glomerulonephritis

12.22. The finding shown in Figure 35 can be found in the urine of all of the following EXCEPT
  A. Fabray's disease
  B. diabetic glomerulosclerosis
  C. interstitial nephritis
  D. lipoid nephrosis
  E. amyloidosis

12.23. The concentration of urine by the kidney is accompanied by the
  A. active reabsorption of NaCl by the thick ascending limb of Henle
  B. active transfer of urea across the epithelium of the collecting duct
  C. effect of ADH on the loop of Henle
  D. increased permeability of the ascending limb of Henle and decreased permeability of the descending limb
  E. active transfer of water across the epithelium of the distal nephron

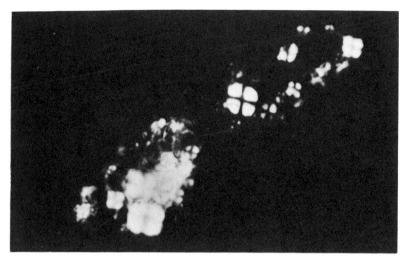

Figure 35

DIRECTIONS: Each group of questions below consists of several lettered headings followed by a list of numbered words or statements. For each numbered word or statement, select the **one** lettered heading that is most closely associated with it. Each lettered heading may be selected once, more than once, or not at all.

    A. Chloride reabsorption
    B. Sugar (glucose) reabsorption
    C. Hydrogen ion secretion
    D. Urine concentration (U_{max})
    E. Potassium reabsorption

12.24. Proximal convoluted tubule

12.25. Ascending loop of Henle

C **12.26.** Distal convoluted tubule

    A. Interstitial edema and lymphocyte infiltration
    B. Subepithelial immune complex deposits
    C. Subendothelial immune complex deposits
    D. Fusion of the podocyte foot processes
    E. Glomerular hyperplasia and polymorphonuclear leukocyte infiltration
    F. Onion-skin appearance of the arteriolar walls

C **12.27.** Lupus nephritis

B **12.28.** Membranous glomerulonephritis

F **12.29.** Malignant hypertension

DIRECTIONS: Each set of lettered headings below is followed by a list of numbered words or phrases. For each numbered word or phrase select

    (A) if the item is associated with A only
    (B) if the item is associated with B only
    (C) if the item is associated with both A and B
    (D) if the item is associated with neither A nor B

    A. Deposition of immune complexes in the glomerular basement membrane
    B. Proteinuria greater than 4 g/24 hr
    C. Both
    D. Neither

A **12.30.** Berger's disease

D **12.31.** Renal tubular acidosis of the distal type (type 1)

B **12.32.** Lipoid nephrosis

12.33. Membranous glomerulonephritis

    A. Hypokalemia
    B. Acts on luminal surface of cells in ascending loop of Henle
    C. Both
    D. Neither

12.34. Chlorthiazide

12.35. Furosemide

12.36. Allopurinol

12.37. Spironolactone

DIRECTIONS: For each of the questions or incomplete statements below, **one or more** of the answers or completions given is correct. Select
    (A) if only 1, 2, and 3 are correct
    (B) if only 1 and 3 are correct
    (C) if only 4 is correct
    (D) if all are correct

12.38. Type 2 renal tubular acidosis (proximal RTA) is associated with
    1. β-2 microglobulin in the urine
    2. inability to acidify the urine
    3. bicarbonate wasting by the kidney
    4. hyperkalemia

12.39. Acute glomerulonephritis is characterized by
    1. immune complex deposits on the subepithelial side of the glomerular basement membrane
    2. hematuria
    3. retinal edema
    4. massive proteinuria ($<$6g/24 hr)

12.40. Which of the following diseases is characterized by the nephrotic syndrome?
   1. Analgesic nephropathy
   2. Amyloidosis
   3. Nephrosclerosis
   4. Syphilitic nephropathy

12.41. Hypokalemia is often seen in
   1. diabetic nephropathy
   2. the syndrome of hyporeninemia and hypoaldosteronemia
   3. nonanion-gap acidosis
   4. Bartter's syndrome

12.42. Proteinuria of less than 3 g/24 hr is most often associated with
   1. nephrosclerosis
   2. diabetic glomerulosclerosis
   3. acute glomerulonephritis
   4. amyloidosis

12.43. Acute renal failure can result from which of the following?
   1. Acute glomerulonephritis
   2. Phenacetin
   3. Shock
   4. Goodpasture's syndrome

12.44. Hypochloremic acidosis is LEAST often associated with
   1. diabetic ketoacidosis
   2. chronic renal failure
   3. propionyl CoA carboxylase deficiency
   4. severe diarrhea

DIRECTIONS This section of the test consists of situations, each followed by a series of questions. Study each situation and select the **one** best answer to each question following it.

Questions 12.45–12.47: A 62-year-old woman presents with anasarca of 4 months duration. She has a blood pressure of 160—70 and a pulse of 78. Her urine shows 4+ protein which on electrophoresis consists of only albumin. The urine sediment contains many doubly refractile fat bodies and oval fat bodies and nothing else. Serum creatinine is 1.9 mg/dl, BUN is 72 mg/dl, and serum cholesterol is 550 mg/dl.

12.45. Which of the following would you expect to find on renal biopsy?
    A. Multiple small juxtamedullary cysts measuring several ml or more in diameter
    B. Thickening of the glomerular basement membrane with many subepithelial electron-dense deposits
    C. A normal-looking glomerulus on light microscopy but diffuse epithelial foot-process fusion on electron microscopy
    D. Linear deposits of IgG in the glomerular basement membrane
    E. Changes consistent with malignant hypertension

12.46. She is treated with intravenous furosemide (Lasix) without response. Which of the following might then be tried?
    A. Prednisone in large doses
    B. Ampicillin p. o. for 10 days
    C. Propranolol and oral lasix for her blood pressure
    D. Intravenous ethycrinic acid
    E. None of the above

12.47. The indications for hemodialysis in this patient would be
    A. anasarca
    B. a rising BUN
    C. progressive acidosis and hyperkalemia
    D. a rising blood pressure
    E. nausea and vomiting

Questions 12.48–12.50: A 54-year-old woman is admitted because of nausea and vomiting. Two years earlier she had had a duodeno-jejunal bypass for extreme obesity and had lost 100 lb during the succeeding 2 years. Approximately 6 months ago she developed hyperglycemia and was treated with insulin. On examination she appeared dehydrated and pale. BP 110/60, T 102°, pulse 90/min. The fundi could not be examined because of bilateral immature cataracts. There was a loud pericardial friction rub over the entire precordium. She had no edema. Laboratory studies showed a serum creatinine of 15.6 mg/dl, BUN 180 mg/dl, Na^+ 126 mEq/L, K^+ 6.3 mEq/L, Cl^- 92 mEq/L, CO_2 13 mM/L, cholesterol 180 mg/dl, serum albumin 6.2 gm/dl, blood sugar 240 mg/dl. Her urine output was 10 ml/hr.

12.48. She has
- **A.** respiratory acidosis
- **B.** anion gap
- **C.** hyperkalemia due to pulmonary congestion
- **D.** renal tubular acidosis
- **E.** evidence of obstructive uropathy (abnormal ratio of urea to creatinine)

12.49. She should be
- **A.** immediately started on dialysis
- **B.** treated for diabetic ketoacidosis
- **C.** given a liter of IV saline
- **D.** treated for impending alkalosis due to the persistent vomiting
- **E.** given a renal biopsy

12.50. Based on Figure 36, her most likely diagnosis is
- **A.** chronic glomerulonephritis
- **B.** amyloidosis
- **C.** chronic pyelonephritis
- **D.** oxalosis
- **E.** renal tubular acidosis

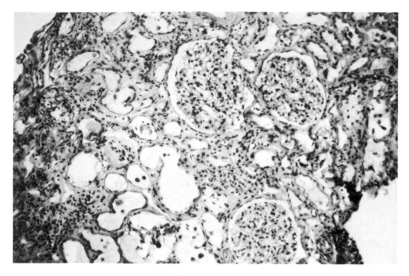

Figure 36

Answers and Comments

12.1. (A) With any of these three values the third may be estimated using the Henderson equation:

$[H^+] = k \times Pco_2/HCO_3$
$\quad k = 24$

$[H^+]$ may be estimated as follows:

$[H^+] = ph - 7.4 + 40 \qquad$ or $\qquad pH = (40 - [H^+]) + 40/100 +$
7 since the relationship is approximately as follows:

pH	$[H^\pm]$
7.50	30 nEq (nanoequivalents)
7.40	40 "
7.30	30 "
7.20	40 "

therefore:

$[H^+] = 24 \times 30/20$
$= 36 \text{ nEq}$

$pH = (40 - 36) + 40/100 + 7$
$= 7.44$

(Ref. 1, pp. 38–39).

12.2. (C) He has an anion gap and an elevated creatinine. If he had respiratory acidosis his HCO_3 would be expected to be higher although it rarely goes above 30 mEq/L. It usually rises at a rate of about 4 mEq/L for each 10 mm Hg rise in P_{CO_2}. Without either a P_{CO_2} or P_{O_2} one has to decide on the basis of the anion gap, low HCO_3, and, of course, elevated creatinine (Ref. 2, pp. 249–289).

12.3. (A) The values are internally inconsistent. A useful test is to use the Henderson equation:

$[H^+] = 24 \times P_{CO_2}/HCO_3$

An estimate of the relation between hydrogen ion concentration and pH is shown in the following table:

pH	H^+
7.50	30 (nanomol/L)
7.40	40 "
7.30	50 "
7.20	60 "

Calculating the equation:
$H^+ = 24 \times 50/25$ should give a H^+ of about 48 or a pH of about 7.48 rather 7.12 (Ref 8, pp. 295–298).

12.4. (A) The electrolyte pattern suggests renal tubular acidosis. Measurement of the 24 hr excretion of acid and NH_4^+ would help make the diagnosis. β-2-Microglobulin determinations in the urine in increased amounts might indicate tubular proteinuria such as that found in Fanconi's syndrome (Ref. 4, pp. 635–642).

12.5. (B) The laboratory results suggest diabetic ketoacidosis, and insulin with some sodium is probably the best treatment (Ref. 2, p. 260).

12.6. (B) Fatty casts usually are found in diseases associated with the nephrotic syndrome. The nephrotic syndrome is rare in acute glomerulonephritis (Ref. 4, p. 962).

12.7. (E) Multiple myeloma is the most likely of these to show amyloid in the kidney (Ref. 7, p. 315).

12.8. (A) Declomycin. In fact, this drug has been used because of this effect to treat the syndrome of inappropriate antidiuretic hormone secretion (SIADH) (Ref. 5, p. 22).

12.9. (D) Lithium chloride is another agent that will produce nephrogenic diabetes insipidus and is therefore useful in the treatment of SIADH. It is not as useful as declomycin because of its side effects (Ref. 5, p. 22).

12.10. (A) The basic formula for calculating clearance is:

Clearance of creatinine = urine creatinine × urine volume / serum creatinine

or

$$C_{cr} = U_{cr} \times V/S_{cr}$$

Each value must be first reduced to ml/min and mg/ml as appropriate
Therefore:

$$C_{cr} = 0.69 \times 0.69/0.02$$
$$= 23.8 \text{ ml/min}$$

(Ref. 4, p. 260).

12.11. (C) Using the equation developed by Albert et al.:

$$P_{CO_2} = HCO_3^- \times 1.5 + 8$$

the P_{CO_2} should be about 26 mm Hg (Ref. 11).

12.12. (C) Using the same equation as in Question 12.11 the measured P_{CO_2} is higher than one would expect suggesting that respiratory acidosis is also present or that this is an example of a mixed respiratory and metabolic acidosis (Ref. 11).

12.13. (D) Cephalosporins are among a group of substances which will interfere with the determination of creatinine. Incomplete collection of urine will interfere with the calculation of the creatinine clearance; however, there is nothing wrong with collecting urine over any period of time as long as all urine is collected and the time is known (Ref. 9).

12.14. (B) Hematuria is unusual and when it is present it is often associated with vascular disease (Ref. 4, p. 1264).

12.15. (D) Digoxin or other cardiac glycosides have not been associated with this (Ref. 5, p. 138).

12.16. (A) The biopsy shows diabetic glomerulosclerosis. There is diffuse and nodular mesangial sclerosis with thin-walled and dilated peripheral capillaries (Ref. 7, pp. 301–302).

12.17. (C) All of the remaining result in an increase in plasma renin activity (Ref. 4, pp. 482–484).

12.18. (D) Metabolic acidosis with an anion gap and low serum chloride is most often associated with uremia (Ref. 2, p. 257).

12.19. (C) Although there are several causes of hypernatremia, the most common is dehydration (Ref. 2, pp. 171–180).

12.20. (D) In the recent symposium on hypertension and the kidney sponsored by the National Kidney Foundation, Vaughan et al. suggest that the indications for intervention in patients with renovascular hypertension is best determined by the following: (1) the presence of a high PRA indexed against sodium excretion; (2) hypersecretion of renin following captopril administration; (3) absence of renin secretion from the contralateral kidney; and (4) an ipsilateral renal vein renin increment at least 50% greater than the matching inferior vena cava renin. These criteria are best met by performing A,B,C (Ref. 12).

12.21. (B) These electrolytes suggest renal tubular acidosis. A bicarbonate of 16 is in keeping with acidosis and a high chloride without an anion gap is consistent with RTA.

The estimation of anion gap is a useful way to approach an acid−base problem. In a normal person the sum of the cations $Na^+ + K^+$ should equal the sum of the anions $Cl^- + CO_2 + 17$. This is usually shortened to $Na^+ = Cl^- + CO_2 + 12$. In either case the 12 or 17 represent anions that are not usually measured. A number exceeding either of these two numbers represents an abnormal anion gap and is associated with acidosis. The presence of a normal anion gap with a low bicarbonate and a high chloride is consistent with renal tubular acidosis. It may also be associated with bicarbonate loss through the intestinal tract so that other findings are important in the differential diagnosis of such an electrolyte pattern (Ref. 10, pp. 223−257).

12.22. (C) Interstitial nephritis is not associated with doubly refractile fat (Maltese crosses) or usually with the nephrotic syndrome in which doubly refractile fat is commonly found in the urine. The rest of the entities are associated with the nephrotic syndrome (Ref. 4, pp. 994, 1003, 1012).

12.23. (A) It is thought that the reabsorption of NaCl by the ascending thick limb of Henle acts as the driving force to produce a hypertonic renal interstitium, and concentration of the urine as water is reabsorbed passively in the collecting ducts (Ref. 4, pp. 410−412).

12.24. (B) Sugar (glucose) is reabsorbed in the proximal tubule (Ref. 6, pp. 21−25).

12.25. (A) Chloride reabsorption takes place in the thick ascending limb of Henle (Ref. 8, pp. 90−93).

12.26. (C) Hydrogen ion secretion occurs in the distal convoluted tubule and first part of the collecting duct (Ref. 6, p. 35).

12.27. (C) Subendothelial deposits as well as subepithelial and basement membrane deposits (Ref. 7, pp. 158−199).

12.28. **(B)** Membranous glomerulonephritis is accompanied by multiple immune complex deposits on the epithelial side of the basement membrane often giving a "hair-on-end" appearance on light microscopy (Ref. 7, pp. 136−138).

12.29. **(F)** Malignant hypertension is associated with intimal hyperplasia of the arterioles and fibrinoid necrosis of the arterial walls (Ref. 7, p. 258).

12.30. **(A)** Deposits of IgG and IgA are present in the glomerular mesangium in Berger's syndrome (Ref. 7, pp. 86−89).

12.31. **(D)** Renal tubular acidosis has no histologic characteristics. Type 1 is not usually associated with proteinuria (type 2 may be) (Ref. 4, pp. 622−625).

12.32. **(B)** Lipoid nephrosis usually has massive proteinuria (>3.5 g/24 hr) (Ref. 4, pp. 994−996).

12.33. **(C)** Membranous glomerulonephritis has subepithelial immune complex deposits and proteinuria in excess of 3.5 g/24 hr (Ref. 7, pp. 136−138).

12.34. **(A)** Chlorthiazide is associated with low K^+ and acts mostly on the distal nephron (Ref. 4, pp. 747−750).

12.35. **(C)** Furosemide acts on the luminal surface of the thick ascending loop of Henle and is associated with low serum K^+ (Ref. 4, pp. 750−751).

12.36. **(D)** Allopurinol may produce an interstitial nephritis but has none of the effects listed (Ref. 5, p. 138).

12.37. **(D)** Spironolactone acts to inhibit the aldosterone effect on the distal nephron and promotes K^+ retention (Ref. 4, pp. 752−754).

12.38. **(B)** Patients with type 2 or proximal RTA can acidify their urine to below pH 6 and have associated hypokalemia, bicarbonate wasting, and sometimes tubular proteinuria (of which β-2 microglobulin is an example) (Ref. 5, pp. 52−54).

12.39. (A) Proteinuria (>3.5 g/24 hr) is not usually found in the urine in acute glomerulonephritis (Ref. 4, p. 962).

12.40. (C) Amyloidosis involving the kidney and syphilitic nephropathy are both characterized clinically by the nephrotic syndrome (Ref. 5, p. 122).

12.41. (D) All of the others are accompanied by a high serum potassium (Ref. 2, p. 257).

12.42. (B) Nephrosclerosis and acute glomerulonephritis usually have minimal proteinuria (<3.5 g/24 hr) (Ref. 2, pp. 25−33).

12.43. (E) Each of these can be accompanied by acute renal failure (Ref. 5, pp. 135−139).

12.44. (D) All but severe diarrhea are associated with an anion gap, hypochloremic acidosis. Severe diarrhea results in a bicarbonate loss in the stool, with a high serum chloride, nonanion gap acidosis, in which potassium may also be low. Propionyl CoA carboxylase deficiency is associated with episodes of ketoacidosis (Ref. 2, pp. 260−263).

12.45. (C) She most likely has lipoid nephrosis (minimal change disease) based on the selective proteinuria with only albumin being lost in the urine. This would be associated with a normal looking kidney biopsy on light microscopy but for the presence of foot process fusion on electron microscopy (Ref. 7, pp. 39−40).

12.46. (A) Steroid drugs are considered the treatment for this disease (Ref. 5, pp. 123−124).

12.47. (C) These patients rarely need dialysis. Occasionally, renal failure may occur and be associated with hyperkalemia and acidosis. This is more likely an indication that the diagnosis is really focal sclerosing glomerulonephritis, a more serious disease which initially may be mistaken for minimal change disease (Ref. 5, pp. 123−124).

12.48. (B) The concentration of Na^+ in the serum should approximately equal the sum of the Cl^- + HCO_3^- concentrations +12. If the Na^+ concentration is larger then an anion gap is present. In this case the difference is 11 (Ref. 5, p. 55).

12.49. (A) She is in renal failure with a high serum creatinine and BUN. She has acidosis as is indicated by her CO_2 of 13 mM/L and her urine output is low (Ref. 5, pp. 147–148).

12.50. (D) The intestinal bypass procedure is highly suspect as the cause of her problem and has been associated with oxalosis and renal failure (Ref. 4, pp. 1127–1130).

References

1. Brenner, B.M. and Stein, J.H.: *Acid–Base and Potassium Homeostasis*, Churchill Livingstone, New York, Edinburgh, London, 1978.

2. Klahr, S.: *Renal and Electrolyte Disorders*, Arco, New York, 1978.

3. Andreoli, T.E., Grantham, J.J., and Rector, F.C., Jr.: *Disturbances in Body Fluid Osmolality*, American Physiological Society, Bethesda, MD, 1977.

4. Brenner, B.M. and Rector, F.C., Jr.: *The Kidney*, W.B. Saunders, Philadelphia, London, Toronto, 1976.

5. Schrier, R.W.: *Manual of Nephrology*, Little, Brown, Boston, 1981.

6. Leaf, L. and Cotran, R.: *Renal Pathophysiology*, Oxford University Press, New York, 1976.

7. Antonovych, T.T. and Mostofi, F.K.: *Atlas of Kidney Biopsies*, Armed Forces Institute of Pathology, Washington, D.C., 1980.

8. Rose, B.D.: *Clinical Physiology of Acid−Base and Electrolyte Disorders*, McGraw-Hill, New York, 1977.

9. Saah, A.J., Koch, T.R., and Drusano, G.L.: Cefoxitin falsely elevates creatinine levels. J.A.M.A. 247:205−206, 1982.

10. Hruska, K.: Pathophysiology of acid-base metabolism. In *The Kidney and Body Fluids*, Klahr, S. (Ed.), Plenum, New York, London, 1983, pp. 223−257.

11. Albert, M.S., Dell, R.B., and Winters, R.W.: Quantitative displacement of acid−base equilibrium in metabolic acidosis. Ann. Int. Med. 66:312−322, 1967.

12. Vaughan, E.D., Jr., Case, D.B., Pickering, T.G., Sosa, R.E., Sos, T.A., and Laragh, J.H.: Indications for intervention in patients with renovascular hypertension. Am. J. Kid. Dis. 5: A136, 1985.

13

Neurology
William Pryse-Phillips, M.D., F.R.C.P., F.R.C.P.(C)

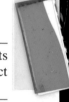

DIRECTIONS: Each of the questions or incomplete statements below is followed by five suggested answers or completions. Select the **one** that is best in each case.

13.1. The localizing value of diminished upward gaze is
   A. cerebellar vermis
   B. superior mesencephalon
   C. inferior occipital cortex
   D. midline pontomedullary junction
   E. lateral pons

13.2. Which of the following is NOT a sign of Parinaud's (dorsal midbrain) syndrome?
   A. Impaired vertical voluntary upward gaze
   B. Convergence nystagmus on upward gaze
   C. Impaired pupillary light response
   D. Preserved pupillary accommodation (near) response
   E. Rubral tremor

13.3. Regarding carotid endarterectomy for TIA/Stroke syndromes:
- **A.** the operation is seldom required because 50−75% of ischemic events occur in patients whose hearts may be a source of thromboembolism
- **B.** the acceptable risk in an institution for the combination of surgery and angiography is 2.9% mortality and morbidity
- **C.** recent U.S. overall morbidity and mortality is over 20%
- **D.** it is indicated in patients with asymptomatic carotid bruits
- **E.** this is the tenth most common operation performed in the U.S.

13.4. Drugs potentially able to cause malignant hyperpyrexia include both
- **A.** steroids and local anesthetics
- **B.** succinylcholine and tricyclic antidepressants
- **C.** succinylcholine and curare
- **D.** procainamide and local anesthetics
- **E.** none of the above

13.5. Multiple sclerosis
- **A.** has a prevalence of over 80/100,000 in high-risk areas
- **B.** occurs eventually in 95% of patients with preceding retrobulbar neuritis
- **C.** is made symptomatically worse by cold (cold bath test)
- **D.** tends to affect the spinal cord in younger and multiple sites in older patients
- **E.** is not a cause of V or VII cranial nerve palsies

13.6. The usual inheritance patterns in muscular dystrophy are which of the following?
- **A.** Facioscapulohumeral—autosomal recessive
- **B.** Limb girdle—autosomal dominant
- **C.** Facioscapulohumeral—autosomal dominant
- **D.** Duchenne—autosomal recessive
- **E.** Ocular—sex-linked recessive

13.7. Which of the following is NOT a feature of myotonic dystrophy?
A. Percussion myotonia of the tongue
B. Paradoxical hyperreflexia
C. Frontal baldness
D. Cataracts
E. Gonadal atrophy   *← Diagnostic*

13.8. Typical features of CT scan in dementias include
A. cerebral cortical atrophy in normal pressure hydrocephalus
B. temporal horn dilatation in Korsakoff's psychosis
C. scattered calcifications in hyperparathyroidism
D. caudate atrophy in Huntington's chorea   *a cortical atrophy*
E. cerebellar cortical atrophy in Pick's disease

13.9. A 23-year-old man complains of headache for 3 months and has noticed that he has not needed to shave for 6 months. The only neurologic signs are retractory nystagmus and lost upward gaze but his skin is greasy and his testes are atrophic. A cerebral tumor, which could present in this way, is
A. schwannoma of the cerebellopontine angle
B. pinealoma
C. colloid cyst of III ventricle
D. bifrontal glioma
E. infraclinoid meningioma

13.10 Raised intracranial pressure
A. always contraindicates lumbar puncture
B. indicates cerebral abscess rather than meningitis
C. is usually responsive to high-dosage dexamethasone therapy
D. is most profitably investigated with CT scanning
E. indicates lumbar intrathecal pressure greater than 20 mm H_2O

13.11. In syringomyelia the central cavity in the cord produces which of the following clinical findings?
  A. Proprioception and joint position lost in shawl distribution
  B. Sternomastoid atrophy
  C. Deep tendon reflexes in the arms diminished or absent
  D. Deep tendon reflexes in the arms and legs diminished or absent
  E. None of the above

13.12. Which of the following is NOT a member of the narcolepsy tetrad?
  A. Hypnogogic hallucinations
  B. Narcolepsy
  C. Ocular flutter
  D. Cataplexy
  E. Sleep paralysis

13.13. Which of the following is NOT characteristic of viral meningitis?
  A. Headache
  B. Vomiting
  C. Marked drowsiness
  D. Neck stiffness
  E. Fever

13.14. An acute labyrinthine insult is characterized by
  A. sensation of spinning of surroundings
  B. decreased hearing
  C. direction-changing nystagmus
  D. all of the above
  E. none of the above

13.15. Which of the following is NOT a typical feature of optic neuritis?
  A. Pain on movement of the eyeball
  B. Normal visual acuity
  C. Central scotoma
  D. Positive swinging flashlight test
  E. Close association with demyelinating disease of the nervous system

13.16. Initial management of a patient with myasthenia presenting with acute weakness should be
  A. IV edrophonium 2 + 8 mg with Ambu bag in room
  B. assessment of ventilatory capacity
  C. trial of neostigmine 15 mg p.o. until weakness is shown not to resolve
  D. atropine 0.6 mg IM
  E. EMG with repetitive stimulation

13.17. Neuralgic amyotrophy presents as a syndrome of (in order of appearance)
  A. pain, C7−8 sensory loss, and stiffness
  B. atrophy, paresthesiae, and fasciculations
  C. shoulder weakness, atrophy, and pain
  D. shoulder pain, weakness, and atrophy
  E. shoulder muscle atrophy and pain in the hand

13.18. A civil servant obtains a hunting license, a rifle, and a compass. After an 18-mile trek in the wilderness he returns home exhausted and without trophies. That night he complains of acute pains in the shins and back, and malaise. You examine him and find acute pain with swelling of the right anterior tibial muscles, and note that his urine is red and smoky in appearance. You would be justified in thinking
  A. this man is very unfit and probably has orthostatic hematuria
  B. people with porphyria should not hunt alone
  C. urine spectroscopy should be performed at once
  D. these symptoms are consistent with his having eaten beetroot sandwiches
  E. steroids should be prescribed at once

DIRECTIONS: Each group of questions below consists of five lettered headings followed by a list of numbered words or statements. For each numbered word or statement, select the **one** lettered heading that is most closely associated with it. Each lettered heading may be selected once, more than once, or not at all.

For each antiepileptic drug select the desirable blood level (therapeutic range)

  A. 1–5 mg/L (μg/ml)
  B. 5–10 mg/L (μg/ml)
  C. 10–20 mg/L (μg/ml)
  D. 50–150 mg/L (μg/ml)
  E. 100–200 mg/L (μg/ml)

13.19. Dilantin - Phenytoin

13.20. Sodium valproate

13.21. Carbamazepine

For each unwanted neurologic effect select the drug most likely to be responsible.

  A. Aminoglycoside antibiotics
  B. Phenobarbitone
  C. Aminophylline
  D. Birth control pill
  E. Ethambutol

13.22. Optic atrophy

13.23. Headache

13.24. Neuromuscular blockade

13.25. Seizures

DIRECTIONS: The set of lettered headings below is followed by a list of numbered words or phrases. For each numbered word or phrase select

(A) if the item is associated with A only
(B) if the item is associated with B only
(C) if the item is associated with both A and B
(D) if the item is associated with neither A nor B

A. Sensory neuropathy
B. Motor neuropathy
C. Both
D. Neither

13.26. Porphyria

13.27. Uremia

13.28. Charcot-Marie-Tooth disease

13.29. Vitamin B_{12} deficiency

DIRECTIONS: For each of the questions or incomplete statements below, **one or more** of the answers or completions given is correct. Select

(A) if only 1, 2, and 3 are correct
(B) if only 1 and 3 are correct
(C) if only 2 and 4 are correct
(D) if only 4 is correct
(E) if all are correct

13.30. Parkinsonism may result from
1. prior exposure to vinyl chloride fumes
2. propranolol toxicity
3. multiple sclerosis
4. medications for hypertension

13.31. In a patient with subacute sclerosing panencephalitis, which of the following statements hold(s) true?
  1. Brain biopsy will show arrays of papova virus
  2. The EEG shows a characteristic pattern
  3. Myoclonus, dementia, and fasciculations are likely clinical features
  4. Measles antibody titers in CSF are abnormally high

13.32. Factors increasing cerebral blood flow include
  1. raised PaO_2
  2. severe anemia
  3. barbiturate anesthesia
  4. halothane anesthesia

13.33. The abnormal movements of dystonia musculorum deformans resemble those of
  1. postencephalitic parkinsonism
  2. haloperidol toxicity
  3. Wilson's disease
  4. rheumatic fever

13.34. Migraine sufferers should be advised to refuse
  1. sweet and sour pork balls with soy sauce
  2. Chianti Classico '73
  3. hot dogs with pickled gherkins
  4. smoked salmon and mushroom soufflé

13.35. Concerning multiple sclerosis (MS) arising after the age of 50:
  1. it usually has a relapsing/remitting rather than a chronic/progressive course
  2. it may be diagnosed with the help of CSF oligoclonal banding and evoked potential studies
  3. it seldom affects the eyes
  4. it occurs in about 10% of all MS cases

13.36. Alcoholic peripheral neuropathy
1. accounts for up to a third of all cases of generalized peripheral neuropathy
2. paresthesias and burning dysesthesias are the main presenting symptoms
3. is associated with substantial weight loss in the recent past
4. is an acutely evolving demyelinating neuropathy with mainly motor signs

13.37. Factors favoring a diagnosis of multiinfarct dementia over dementia of the Alzheimer type include
1. stepwise deterioration
2. emotional incontinence
3. presence of focal neurologic signs
4. evidence of generalized atherosclerosis

13.38. A febrile child with headache and bilateral cerebellar signs may be suffering from
1. acute viral cerebellitis
2. cholesteatoma in the CP angle
3. cerebellar abscess secondary to otitis
4. carbamazepine toxicity

DIRECTIONS: This section of the test consists of situations, each followed by a series of questions. Study each situation and select the **one** best answer to each question following it.

Questions 13.39–13.42: A 24-year-old woman complains of 2 months of increasing headache and right facial numbness. Examination confirms a right V nerve subjective hypoesthesia and shows right VIII nerve deafness and minimal intention tremor of the right arm in the finger–nose test only.

13.39. Possible sites of the lesion include
  A. right lateral lobe of cerebellum
  B. cerebellar vermis, mainly right-sided
  C. left foramen magnum lesion with IV ventricle compression
  D. cerebellopontine angle
  E. pons

13.40. Which of the following investigations would be irrelevant in this case?
  A. Brainstem (auditory) evoked potentials
  B. Carotid angiography
  C. Blink reflexes
  D. Audiometry
  E. CT scan with intrathecal air

13.41. The corneal reflex
  A. is polysynaptic
  B. tests only homolateral V and VII cranial nerves
  C. is not affected by cortical lesions
  D. is a sensitive indicator of cerebellar pathology
  E. is usually reduced with CP angle masses

13.42. Isolated facial numbness may occur in
  A. stilbamidine toxicity
  B. motor neuron disease
  C. pontine glioma
  D. syringobulbia
  E. Arnold-Chiari malformation

Questions 13.43–13.45: A 16-year-old man is admitted in a drowsy state complaining of mild headache and fever. His parents have noticed progressive irritability in the last 4 days. Six months ago he was involved in a road traffic accident and sustained a fractured skull base with CSF rhinorrhea which ceased spontaneously. Examination reveals meningism, temperature 38.5°C, and loss of retinal venous pulsations.

13.43. Lumbar puncture in this circumstance
  A. is potentially dangerous and not indicated here
  B. is essential and must be done at once
  C. is preferably delayed until CT/isotope scan or EEG have ruled out a cerebral abscess
  D. is safe if only a small volume of fluid is removed
  E. must be accompanied by a Queckenstedt maneuver

13.44. The organisms to be expected here would include
  A. *Staphylococcus* or *Hemophilus*
  B. *Escherichia coli* or group B streptococcus
  C. pneumococcus, *Streptococcus* sp, or *Bacteroides*
  D. *Listeria monocytogenes*
  E. viral agents

13.45. Which statement about chloramphenicol in the treatment of meningitis is NOT correct?
  A. It is the drug of choice in patients allergic to penicillin with *Hemophilus influenzae* meningitis
  B. It is the drug of choice in patients with β-lactamase producing *H. influenzae* meningitis
  C. Its safe therapeutic range is between 25 and 50 μg/ml serum
  D. It is preferred in all patients with pneumococcal meningitis
  E. It is preferred in patients with meningococcal meningitis who are penicillin-sensitive

Answers and Comments

13.1. (B) The center is at the level of the superior colliculus; for downward gaze, it is the pons (Ref. 1, p. 516).

13.2. (E) In Parinaud's syndrome, a mesodiencephalic lesion, such as a pineal tumor, encephalitis, or MS, produces any or all of the first four signs. A rubral tremor is thought to be due to a more ventral lesion affecting the red nucleus and is not part of the syndrome (Ref. 3, pp. 54−60).

13.3. (B) The intense controversy over the indications for carotid endarterectomy will only be quenched by a prospective study but it is reasonable to analyze surgical procedures in the same way as we analyze drug treatments and if the morbidity/mortality of angiography and surgery is over 3%, then the best current evidence is that medical treatment is superior. Nevertheless, the operation is the third most commonly performed in the U.S. It has not been shown to be of any benefit in asymptomatic carotid bruits, and only 15–25% of ischemic events are probably cardiogenic (Ref. 4, pp. 941–943).

13.4. (B) Local anesthetics, muscle relaxants, and tricyclics have all been incriminated. Procainamide is part of the therapy (Ref. 1, p. 569).

13.5. (A) Retrobulbar neuritis leads to MS in about two-thirds of cases. Heat, not cold, worsens symptoms. The sites in choice D are reversed for the age groups. Brainstem involvement is well recognized (Ref. 1, pp. 654–658).

13.6. (C) Limb girdle dystrophy is usually autosomal recessive; Duchenne dystrophy, sex-linked; and ocular dystrophy, autosomal dominant or recessive (Ref. 1, pp. 605–614).

13.7. (B) All of the others are features of myotonic dystrophy. Arm reflexes are depressed early, those in the legs later (Ref. 1, pp. 614–615).

13.8. (D) The CT scan picture is almost diagnostic in this condition. Apart from the caudate atrophy, cortical atrophy would also be seen (Ref. 1, p. 640).

13.9. (B) This is usually seen in young men. None of the other conditions present in this way. CP-angle tumors should produce V, VII, VIII cranial nerve and cerebellar features. III ventricle cysts commonly are asymptomatic or cause raised intracranial pressure (Ref. 1, p. 516).

13.10. (D) It may be necessary to do LP if CNS infection is suspected; any such infection could raise intracranial pressure. Raised ICP indicates pressure over 180 mm of water (Ref. 1, pp. 234–237).

13.11. (C) This is almost essential for diagnosis. Spinothalamic, not posterior, column sensation may be lost in shawl distribution. Reflexes in the legs will be increased. Sternomastoid atrophy is possible but highly unusual (Ref. 1, p. 684).

13.12. (C) The other four are, in any combination. Narcolepsy alone is the most common single presentation (Ref. 1, p. 265).

13.13. (C) Drowsiness denotes generalized depression of cortical function and thus encephalitis. Viral illnesses are, of course, causes of encephalitis but with viral meningitis only, marked drowsiness should not occur (Ref. 1, p. 469).

13.14. (A) Hearing loss and tinnitus both indicate cochlear, not labyrinthine, damage. A spinning sensation (true vertigo) is characteristic. Nystagmus in this condition will be direction-fixed, i.e., always with the fast component in the same direction, whichever way the eyes are looking (Ref. 1, p. 320).

13.15. (B) Optic neuritis produces scotomas, usually central, so that macular vision may be 20/200 but peripheral vision almost intact. All the other features are characteristic although such causes as cranial arteritis, nonarteritic ischemia, and infectious and toxic agents are also important (Ref. 1, p. 276).

13.16. (B) Ventilatory failure may be killing this patient and the first thing to do is to determine its extent. Tensilon, if used, must wait until this is done. All other choices are irrelevant or useless (Ref. 1, p. 627).

13.17. (D) Pain is the first symptom, preceding weakness and atrophy by a day or two and clearing in weeks or months The pain is felt in C5–6 dermatomes (Ref. 1, p. 385).

13.18. (C) You are looking for myoglobinuria with the anterior tibial syndrome due to unaccustomed use of the anterior compartment muscles. This has led to swelling of those muscles in their enclosed space, with secondary nerve and muscle damage and myoglobin release from the muscles. Myoglobin may damage the renal tubules. Steroids are not valuable treatment. Decompression of the swollen muscles is essential and a careful watch on renal function is necessary because diuresis or dialysis may be needed (Ref. 1, p. 630).

13.19. (C)
13.20. (D)
13.21. (B) Constant drug-level monitoring is the key to successful therapy and permits the avoidance of polypharmacy. It is the greatest single advance in antiepileptic therapy in recent years (Ref. 1, p. 224).

13.22. (E)
13.23. (D)
13.24. (A)
13.25. (C) Numerous neurologic syndromes follow drug therapy especially in the elderly and subjects with any type of brain damage. These are the common examples. No drug should be prescribed without awareness of its potential unwanted effects (Ref. 1, pp. 560, 564, 568).

13.26. (B)
13.27. (C)
13.28. (C)
13.29. (A) The classification of neuropathy (sensory/motor/mixed: proximal/distal:genetics/acquired:neuronal/demyelinating, etc.) allows a likely clinical recognition diagnosis in over half the cases seen (Ref. 1, p. 583).

13.30. (D) Methyldopa, in particular, may cause parkinsonism. MS almost never produces parkinsonism and propranolol may be therapeutic at least against the tremor (Ref. 1, pp. 562, 632).

13.31. (E) The condition is considered to be a slow virus infection and the clinical and diagnostic test findings are as in the question (Ref. 1, p. 494).

13.32. (C) An increase in PaO_2 will lower cerebral blood flow as will barbiturate anesthesia. CBF is, however, much more dependent upon $PaCO_2$ and blood pressure than these factors (Ref. 1, p. 396).

13.33. (A) Rheumatic fever produces Sydenham's chorea. All of the other choices may induce abnormal dystonic movements resembling dystonia musculorum deformans (Ref. 1, p. 642).

13.34. (E) Soy sauce, nitrites, red wine, and many other foods can precipitate vascular headaches (Ref. 1, p. 255).

13.35. (C) When MS occurs after the age of 50, cord and brainstem involvement are most common. The course is seldom of a relapsing/ remitting kind and diagnostic tests are more often positive than in patients with onset at a younger age (Ref. 5, pp. 1537–1544).

13.36. (A) This neuropathy is indeed common but usually develops insidiously. Axonal damage with both sensory and motor deficits (paresthesias, pain, blunted pinprick and light touch, hyper reflexia, distal atrophy, and weakness) is characteristic. Any demyelination of peripheral neurones is secondary to the axonal damage. Nutritional deficiency is the cause rather than a direct toxic effect of alcohol (Ref. 6, pp. 183–187).

13.37. (B) Features most helpful in differentiating MID from DAT are abrupt onset, stepwise deterioration, history of stroke, focal neurologic signs, and focal neurologic symptoms. Hypertension is of secondary importance, whereas somatic complaints and emotional incontinence are questionably of any value. Because these two are the most common kinds of dementia seen in the older population, differentiation by clinical means is of great value (Ref. 7, pp. 486–588).

13.38. **(B)** Fever is uncommon in choices 2 and 4, although carbamazepine has very rarely caused serious neutropenia (Ref. 1, p. 667).

13.39. **(D)** None of the other choices can explain V and VII cranial nerve and unilateral cerebellar signs. The lateral lobes are too far away, a vermis lesions should extend forward and damage the brainstem bilaterally; the foramen magnum is too low and the pons is too high for VIII nerve involvement (Ref. 1, pp. 511−512).

13.40. **(B)** This would not demonstrate a posterior fossa lesion. All of the other choices may do so and are part of the diagnostic workup (Ref. 1, pp. 102, 511).

13.41. **(E)** It is oligosynaptic, tests both of the VII nerves, is reduced in stroke, and is uninfluenced by cerebellar disease (Ref. 1, p. 25).

13.42. **(A)** In all of the other disorders multiple signs may be expected. Trichlorethylene inhalation may also cause facial numbness in isolation. This is a sign that always demands careful investigation (Ref. 1, p. 305).

13.43. **(C)** Abscess is a real possibility and some investigation is wise prior to doing the LP. This is potentially dangerous but may be necessary because meningitis is the alternative diagnosis and the organism must be identified. The Queckenstedt test is extremely hazardous in this situation (Ref. 1, pp. 88−90).

13.44. **(C)** These are most likely because of the history of prior skull fracture (Ref. 2, p. 313).

13.45. **(D)** This agent should be used in patients with pneumococcal meningitis when they are allergic to penicillins, which are otherwise the drugs of choice. The other statements are correct (Ref. 2, p. 320).

References

1. Pryse-Phillips, W., Murray, T.J.: *Essential Neurology*, 3rd Ed., Medical Examination Publishing Co., New York, 1982.

2. Bell, W.E.: Treatment of bacterial infections of the nervous system. Ann. Neurol. 9:313–327, 1981.

3. Baloh, R.W., et al.: Neurol. 35:54–60, 1985.

4. Barnett, H.J.M., et al.: Stroke 15:941–943, 1984.

5. Noseworthy, J., et al.: Neurol. 33:1537–1544, 1983.

6. Shields, R.W.: Muscle Nerve 8:183–187, 1985.

7. Rosen, W.G., et al.: Ann. Neurol. 7:486–588, 1980.

14

Oncology

Michael A. Baker, M.D., F.R.C.P.(C), F.A.C.P.

DIRECTIONS: Each of the questions or incomplete statements below is followed by five suggested answers or completions. Select the **one** that is best in each case.

14.1. High-dose methotrexate infusions require "rescue" of normal tissues by
  A. *cis*-platinum
  B. intrinsic factor
  C. leucovorin
  D. hypoxanthine
  E. hypothermia

14.2. Which of the following factors implicates a high risk of recurrence in resected carcinoma of the breast?
  A. One positive axillary node
  B. Clinical stage I
  C. Primary tumor 1.5 cm
  D. Age over 65
  E. Vascular invasion

14.3. A stage I malignant melanoma of the skin that is invasive into the papillary zone of the dermis, but does not expand to fill the papillary dermis, would be classified in the Clark level system as level
A. I
B. II
C. III
D. IV
E. V

14.4. Which of the following clinical presentations is most characteristic of the clinical onset of ovarian cancer?
A. Sudden back pain
B. Gradual anemia
C. Fever of unknown origin
D. Gradual abdominal bloating
E. Menorrhagia

14.5. Which of the following markers is most useful for following patients with gestational trophoblastic neoplasms?
A. β subunit of hCG in serum
B. Serum levels of CEA
C. Urine levels of luteinizing hormone
D. Serum levels of growth hormone
E. Urine levels of progesterone

14.6. Children with common acute lymphoblastic leukemia achieving complete remission
A. must receive central nervous system prophylaxis
B. require no further therapy
C. should receive a bone marrow transplantation if a donor is available
D. have a mean survival of 3 years
E. should receive prophylactic penicillin for 2 years

14.7. Which of the following forms of Hodgkin's disease carries the best prognosis?
  A. Stage II B, lymphocyte-depleted
  B. Stage III A, nodular-sclerosing
  C. Stage III A, mixed cellularity
  D. Stage III B, nodular-sclerosing
  E. Stage II A, lymphocyte-predominant

14.8. All of the following diseases are associated with blastic lesions of the bone EXCEPT
  A. breast cancer
  B. multiple myeloma
  C. hypernephroma
  D. Hodgkin's disease
  E. prostate cancer

DIRECTIONS: Each group of questions below consists of five lettered headings followed by a list of numbered words or statements. For each numbered word or statement, select the **one** lettered heading that is most closely associated with it. Each lettered heading may be selected once, more than once, or not at all.

  A. Cyclophosphamide
  B. Vincristine
  C. Tamoxifen
  D. Doxorubicin
  E. Bleomycin

14.9. Cumulative dose limited by cardiac toxicity

14.10. Dose limited by neurotoxicity

14.11. Hydration necessary to prevent hemorrhagic cystitis

DIRECTIONS: The set of lettered headings below is followed by a list of numbered words or phrases. For each numbered word or phrase select

(A) if the item is associated with A only
(B) if the item is associated with B only
(C) if the item is associated with both A and B
(D) if the item is associated with neither A nor B

A. Acute lymphoblastic leukemia
B. Chronic lymphocytic leukemia
C. Both
D. Neither

14.12. Equal frequency in children and adults

14.13. No treatment given when asymptomatic

14.14. Hemolytic anemia and hypogammaglobulinemia

DIRECTIONS: For each of the questions or incomplete statements below, **one or more** of the answers or completions given is correct. Select

(A) if only 1, 2, and 3 are correct
(B) if only 1 and 3 are correct
(C) if only 2 and 4 are correct
(D) if only 4 is correct
(E) if all are correct

14.15. Small-cell anaplastic carcinoma of the lung metastasizes to the
1. mediastinal lymph nodes
2. brain
3. bone
4. liver

14.16. Tissue obtained from a 60-year-old woman suspected of having breast cancer should be studied for
   1. testosterone receptors
   2. progesterone receptors
   3. carcinoembryonic antigen
   4. estrogen receptors

14.17. The main prognostic indicators in malignant melanoma are
   1. level of invasion of the primary
   2. sex and age of the patient
   3. anatomic site of the primary
   4. presence of a preexisting benign mole

DIRECTIONS: This section of the test consists of a situation followed by a series of questions. Study the situation and select the **one** best answer to each question following it.

Questions 14.18–14.20: A 60-year-old man develops sudden onset of pain in the right lateral chest while playing golf. He has a history of progressive weakness over the past 6 months. On examination he is pale and has joint tenderness over the right lateral eighth rib. His hemoglobin is 9.0 g/100 ml with marked rouleaux seen on the blood film and an ESR of 110 mm/hr. Total serum proteins are elevated. The chest x-rays are shown in Figure 37.

14.18. The most likely diagnosis is
   A. metastatic lung cancer
   B. pulmonary embolism secondary to carcinoma of the prostate
   C. multiple myeloma
   D. carcinoma of the male breast
   E. acute myeloblastic leukemia

14.19. Further investigations should include all of the following EXCEPT
   A. bone marrow aspiration
   B. intravenous pyelogram
   C. serum immunoelectrophoresis
   D. 24-hr urine protein
   E. serum calcium

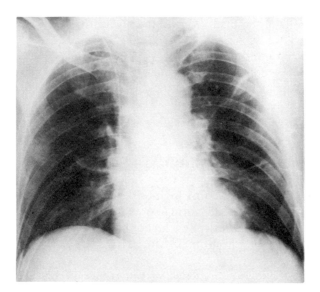

Figure 37A

Figure 37B

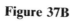

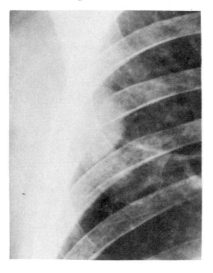

14.20. Initial attempts to control the severe rib pain will probably
require
   -**A.** radiotherapy
   B. prednisone
   C. bleomycin
   D. rhyzotomy
   E. acyclovir

Answers and Comments

14.1. (C) The technique of high-dose methotrexate infusion requires "rescue" with leucovorin to prevent lethal damage to normal
tissues. There is theoretically a higher methotrexate-to-leucovorin
ratio in tumor than in normal tissues (Ref. 1, pp. 106–107).

14.2. (E) There is a high risk of recurrence of resected breast
cancer if vascular invasion is seen on pathologic examination. Other
high-risk factors include over four positive axillary nodes, clinical
stage II or III, and primary tumor greater than 5 cm (Ref. 1, pp.
148–149).

14.3. (B) Clark's level II invasion goes through the epidermis to
the papillary zone of the dermis. If the reticular dermis is invaded, it
is level IV, and subcutaneous fat is invaded in level V (Ref. 1, pp.
316–317).

14.4. (D) The clinical onset of ovarian cancer is characterized by
insidious abdominal bloating and weight gain. These symptoms
usually progress to subacute intestinal obstruction (Ref. 1, p. 244).

14.5. (A) Measurement of β subunit of human chorionic gonado-
tropin (hCG) is the most effective method of following trophoblastic tumors. Urine levels are much less accurate. A radioimmunoassay is the technique of choice (Ref. 1, p. 424).

14.6. (A) Children with common acute lymphoblastic leukemia
achieving complete remission must receive central nervous system
treatment with intrathecal methotrexate and cranial irradiation. If
this is not given, the nervous system is the most likely site of relapse.

There is a high potential cure rate with chemotherapy therefore marrow transplants are not indicated (Ref. 2, pp. 1518–1520).

14.7. **(E)** Clinical stage II indicates two lymph-node bearing areas on the same side of the diaphragm, and A refers to the absence of systemic symptoms. The lymphocyte-predominant histology carries the best prognosis and the lymphocyte-depleted type has the worst (Ref. 2, pp. 1648–1653).

14.8. **(B)** Multiple myeloma produces generalized osteoporosis or lytic bone lesion but is not associated with blastic lesions of bone. As a corollary, the alkaline phosphatase is not a useful test in evaluating myeloma bone damage, nor is the bone scan (Ref. 2, pp. 1739–1744).

14.9. **(D)** Doxorubicin is limited in dose to a total of about 450 mg/m^2. Cumulative doses beyond this level may cause myocardial damage that leads to irreversible cardiac failure. Monitoring of cardiac output is necessary before exceeding this dose (Ref. 2, p. 1874).

14.10. **(B)** Vincristine will cause peripheral neuropathy in doses over 1.5 mg/m^2 but the total single dose in adults must be kept below 2 mg, with the usual weekly schedule. Excessive doses will cause peripheral neuropathy in the toes and fingers but if continued will cause loss of motor innervation as well (Ref. 2, p. 1873).

14.11. **(A)** Cyclophosphamide is metabolized in the liver. Metabolic breakdown products are excreted by the kidney and if allowed to remain in high concentration in the bladder will cause hemorrhagic cystitis (Ref. 2, p. 1869).

14.12. **(D)** Acute lymphoblastic leukemia is most common in childhood and chronic lymphocytic leukemia is most common after the fifth decade. Acute lymphoblastic leukemia is rare over age 45 and chronic lymphocyte leukemia is very rare under age 20 (Ref. 2, p. 1457).

14.13. **(B)** Chronic lymphocytic leukemia is not treated in asymptomatic patients. The disease may persist for several months or years without requiring therapy. Indications for treatment include weight loss, weakness, and bleeding (Ref. 2, pp. 1642–1644).

14.14. (B) Chronic lymphocytic leukemia may be associated with hemolytic anemia with a positive antiglobulin (Coombs' test). Hypogammaglobulinemia occurs frequently and may contribute to susceptibility to bacterial infection (Ref. 2, p. 1642).

14.15. (E) Small-cell anaplastic carcinoma commonly metastasizes to lymph nodes, brain, bone, and liver. Investigation of a new patient includes chest x-ray, brain scan, bone scan, liver scan, alkaline phosphatase, and bone marrow biopsy (Ref. 3, pp. 1721–1723).

14.16. (C) Breast cancer tissue obtained at initial biopsy must be studied for content of hormonal receptors. Patients demonstrating cytoplasmic receptors for estrogens and progesterone have a significantly greater response to hormonal manipulation (Ref. 3, pp. 964, 2397).

14.17. (A) The single most important prognostic indicator is the depth of invasion of the primary lesion through the layers of the epidermis and subcutaneous tissues. Women have a better outlook than men, an advantage that disappears after menopause. Lesions on the back, neck, and scalp have a better prognosis for the same depth of invasion compared to lesions in areas of thinner skin (Ref. 3, pp. 2123–2127).

14.18. (C) Anemia and bone pain in a 60-year-old patient should alert the clinician to the diagnosis of multiple myeloma. The sudden onset of pain and the point tenderness are clues to the pathologic fracture with extraosseous myeloma seen in the figure. The elevated serum protein and high ESR are further supportive of the diagnosis (Ref. 3, pp. 1558–1559).

14.19. (B) An intravenous pyelogram should not usually be done in a patient with multiple myeloma because the accompanying dehydration may cause hyperviscosity. In addition, acute renal failure has been reported and interaction of abnormal proteins with radiopaque dyes has been postulated (Ref. 3, p. 1564).

14.20. **(A)** Bone pain in myeloma may respond dramatically to radiotherapy. Prednisone is useful in the reduction of protein excess by catabolism but does not relieve the bone pain. Chemotherapy with alkylating agents should control the lesion over the longer term (Ref. 3, p. 1570).

References

1. Greenspan, E.M.: *Clinical Interpretation and Practice of Cancer Chemotherapy*, 1st Ed., Raven Press, New York, 1982.

2. Wintrobe, M.M., Lee, G.R., Boggs, D.R., Bithell, T.C., Foerster, J., Athens, J.W., and Lukens, J.W.: *Clinical Hematology*, 8th Ed., Lea & Febiger, Philadelphia, 1981.

3. Holland, J.F. and Frei, E.: *Cancer Medicine*, 2nd Ed., Lea & Febiger, Philadelphia, 1982.

Pulmonary

15

Pulmonary Medicine

**N. LeRoy Lapp, M.D.,
Edward L. Petsonk, M.D.,
and Joseph Renn, M.D.**

DIRECTIONS: Each of the questions or incomplete statements below is followed by five suggested answers or completions. Select the **one** that is best in each case.

15.1. A homogeneous shadow that obscures the lateral portion of the left hemidiaphragm, but not the left cardiac border, represents abnormality in the
   A. lingula
   B. left upper lobe
   C. superior segment of left lower lobe
   D. basilar segment of left lower lobe
   E. left middle lobe

15.2. All of the following are suggestive of sleep disordered breathing (sleep apnea syndrome) EXCEPT
   A. snoring plus violent movements during sleep
   B. findings consistent with cor pulmonale without lung disease
   C. inappropriate daytime somnolence
   D. bilateral hilar adenopathy
   E. severe morning headaches

15.3. All of the following are accepted criteria for the ECG diagnosis of chronic cor pulmonale EXCEPT
  A. increased (greater than 3 mV) P-wave amplitude in leads II, III, and AVF
  B. incomplete right bundle branch block
  C. QRS axis of greater than 110°
  D. R/S amplitude ratio in V_1 of greater than 1
  E. marked counterclockwise rotation of the QRS axis

15.4. Which of the following best characterizes the pleural fluid exudate from a patient with pneumonia?
  A. pH 7.5, glucose 70 mg/dl, WBC 950 mm^3
  B. pH 7.10, pleural fluid:serum protein ratio 0.7, pleural fluid: serum protein ratio 0.3
  C. pH 7.10, pleural fluid:serum protein ratio 0.3, pleural fluid:serum LDH ratio 0.4
  D. pH 7.10, specific gravity 1.011, LDH 185 IU/L
  E. pH 7.5, glucose 75 mg/dl, WBC 2400 mm^3

15.5. A 19-year-old female foreign exchange student from East India presents to you with breathlessness and radiographic evidence of a massive right pleural effusion. Thoracentesis reveals a fluid with exudative characteristics and a glucose of 25 mg/dl. Cultures of the fluid for acid-fast organisms, fungi, and bacteria are negative. Intermediate PPD-S skin test is negative and the mumps control is positive. Radiographic follow-up shows that the effusion gradually and completely resolves. You suspect the likely diagnosis and start treatment with which of the following?
  A. Penicillin
  B. Bleomycin, vincristine
  C. INH, rifampin
  D. Prednisone
  E. Gold

15.6. A 57-year-old woman is discovered on physical examination to have dullness, absent tactile fremitus and egophony, and diminished breath sounds at the right base. Pelvic examination reveals a right ovarian mass. You would expect to find all of the following on thoracentesis EXCEPT
   A. pleural fluid:serum protein ratio 0.4
   B. pleural fluid glucose 80 mg/dl
   C. WBC 450 mm^3
   D. pleural fluid LDH 1110 IU/L
   E. pleural fluid:serum LDH ratio 0.4

15.7. All of the following connective tissue diseases may cause pleuritic involvement EXCEPT
   A. systemic lupus erythematosus
   B. progressive systemic sclerosis (scleroderma)
   C. rheumatoid arthritis
   D. ankylosing spondylitis
   E. dermatomyositis

15.8. Initial therapy of the mild-to-moderate asthmatic in the outpatient setting is best achieved with which of the following?
   A. Inhaled β-2 selective agonist
   B. Corticosteroids
   C. Oral β-2 selective agonist
   D. Inhaled racemic epinephrine
   E. Oral fixed combination of theophylline and ephedrine

15.9. Sarcoidosis is characterized by all of the following features EXCEPT
   A. intrathoracic hilar lymph node or pulmonary parenchymal involvement at some point in the disease in greater than 90% of cases
   B. worsening of the disease during pregnancy
   C. impaired cellular immunity
   D. elevated serum levels of angiotensin-converting enzyme
   E. eventual resolution in thhe majority of stage I cases (bilateral hilar lymphadenopathy)

15.10. Therapy with corticosteroid drugs is usually recommended in sarcoidosis when any of the following manifestations are present EXCEPT
A. facial palsy and papilledema
B. single breath DLCO of 60% and vital capacity of 80% predicted
C. left bundle branch block and intrathoracic lymphadenopathy
D. erythema nodosum and bilateral hilar lymphadenopathy
E. persistent hypercalciuria

15.11. A 24-year-old man is 5'6" tall and weighs 268 lb. He is otherwise healthy and does not smoke. All of the following might be found in this patient EXCEPT
A. polycythemia
B. hypoxemia
C. decreased expiratory reserve volume
D. impaired perfusion of the lung bases
E. impaired ventilation of the lung bases

15.12. All of the following are known to result from ventilation with positive end-expiratory pressures (PEEP) EXCEPT
A. opening of collapsed airways and reduction of intrapulmonary shunt
B. misleading pulmonary artery pressure readings (Swan-Ganz catheter)
C. tension pneumothorax
D. pneumomediastinum
E. increased cardiac output

15.13. All of the following are indications for endotracheal intubation via an oral or nasotracheal tube EXCEPT

A. a patient with asthma who has been sitting up for the past three nights because of dyspnea and wheezing. Arterial blood gases show pH 7.29, PO_2 48 mm Hg, and PCO_2 57 mm Hg on room air

B. a patient involved in an automobile accident who presents in the emergency room with a depressed fracture of the mandible, marked dyspnea, and noisy breathing. Arterial blood gases on room air show pH 7.34, PO_2 58 mm Hg, and PCO_2 47 mm Hg

C. a patient is admitted to the emergency room with crushing substernal chest pain of 2 hr duration, whose blood pressure rose to 70/30 mm Hg on a dopamine drip and whose arterial blood gases on 100% O_2 showed pH 7.24, PO_2 45 mm Hg, and PCO_2 28 mm Hg

D. a patient undergoing chemotherapy in an attempt to induce a remission from acute leukemia and who has 300 neutrophils/mm^3 suddenly develops a fever to 41°C, hypotension, and somnolence. Arterial blood gases while breathing oxygen via face mask reveal pH 7.24, PO_2 38 mmHg, and PCO_2 24 mm Hg

E. a patient involved in an automobile accident sustaining a midshaft fracture of the left femur and comminuted fractures of the right distal tibia and fibula. Shortly after admission and stabilization of the fractures, the patient became tachypneic to 40 breaths/min, had a fever of 39°C, and a tachycardia of 140 beats/min. Petechiae were evident in the axillary folds. While breathing oxygen by face mask, the arterial blood gases showed pH 7.57, PO_2 45 mm Hg, and PCO_2 23 mm Hg

15.14. In an acute asthmatic attack, all of the following may indicate impending respiratory failure EXCEPT

A. heart rate over 130

B. normal arterial carbon dioxide tension (PCO_2)

C. decreased wheezing in the chest

D. arterial oxygen on room air (PO_2) less than 60 mm Hg

E. decreased pulsus paradoxus

15.15. Of the following, the feature that most clearly separates the emphysematous (type A) from the bronchitic (type B) patient with chronic, irreversible obstructive airway disease is
  A. dyspnea on exertion
  B. residual volume elevation
  C. hyperinflation on chest radiograph
  D. arterial oxygen tension (PO_2) at rest
  E. static lung compliance and lung recoil pressure

15.16. Which of the following is correct concerning the α-1-antitrypsin deficiency disorder?
  A. Familial emphysema is associated with the MM phenotype
  B. a heterozygous state (phenotype MZ) occurs in about 20% of the population
  C. Population studies have clearly demonstrated that subjects with MZ phenotype develop an excess of respiratory disorders
  D. The emphysema associated with homozygous deficiency occurs in middle age rather than in the fifth to sixth decade
  E. Cigarette smoking plays little role in influencing the development of emphysema in subjects with homozygous deficiency

15.17. A 46-year-old obese woman who is recuperating from a cholecystectomy suddenly develops left chest pain of a pleuritic nature and marked tachypnea. Which of the following would give you the greatest degree of confidence that you were dealing with a pulmonary embolus?
  A. Pulmonary angiogram demonstrating a vascular defect
  B. Elevated bilirubin and LDH with a normal SGOT
  C. PaO_2 of 60 mm Hg on room air
  D. A perfusion lung scan with multiple nonsegmental defects
  E. ECG evidence of right axis deviation

15.18. All of the following are manifestations of acute massive pulmonary embolism EXCEPT

    A. syncope
    B. central chest pain
    C. dyspnea
    D. pleuritic chest pain
    E. accentuated P_2

15.19. Essential steps in the management of massive, life-threatening hemoptysis include all of the following EXCEPT

    A. emergency bronchoscopy to localize the site of bleeding
    B. notification of thoracic surgeon to prepare for possible lung resection
    C. maintaining the affected lung in the nondependent (up) position
    D. type and cross-match blood
    E. immediate chest radiograph

15.20. Examination of the chest in pulmonary fibrosis is likely to show

    A. medium and high pitched wheezes in expiration
    B. fine crackles (crepitations) at the lung bases heard throughout inspiration
    C. coarse crackles heard only during expiration
    D. hyperresonance to percussion
    E. medium crackles at the right base only

15.21. Fiberoptic bronchoscopy is useful in all of the following settings EXCEPT

    A. hemoptysis in a patient with rheumatoid cervical spondylitis
    B. removal of large foreign bodies
    C. biopsy of pulmonary nodules
    D. treatment of atelectasis due to secretions
    E. biopsy in chronic interstitial lung disease

15.22. You would advise a 40-year-old 50 pack-year male smoker to have surgical removal of a solitary pulmonary nodule if all of the following were present EXCEPT
- **A.** eccentric flecks of calcium
- **B.** negative sputum cytology
- **C.** negative transthoracic needle aspiration of the nodule
- **D.** negative fiberbronchoscopy with brushings under fluoroscopic control
- **E.** chest radiograph of 2 years previous showing no change in the size of the nodule

15.23. Chemoprophylaxis with isoniazid in a dosage of 300 mg once daily for a period of 1 year is recommended for which one of the following clinical situations?
- **A.** A 3-year-old child with low-grade fever, anorexia, and general lassitude given a skin test with intermediate strength PPD shows a 12-mm area of induration
- **B.** An 18-year-old high school student who underwent a college entrance physical examination and was given a skin test with intermediate strength PPD, the reaction to which was 15 mm of induration
- **C.** A 54-year-old alcoholic admitted to hospital for recent onset of melena is given skin test with intermediate strength PPD which results in 5 mm of induration. Repeat testing with 250 TU of PPD results in 12 mm of induration
- **D.** A 60-year-old man is admitted to hospital because of a 15-lb weight loss, anorexia, and general malaise. His admission chest radiograph shows some haziness in the right upper zone, just beneath the clavicles
- **E.** A 5-year-old boy is seen by his family physician because of 10 days of fever, lack of energy, a brassy cough, and several painful, raised, purple-red lumps on his legs. Among other investigations a skin test with intermediate strength PPD was performed; the result was 11 mm of induration

15.24. A 61-year-old man, heavy smoker, presents in your office with complaints of shortness of breath. He worked in the Newport News, Virginia, shipyards during World War II. All of the following conditions might be related to his former occupation EXCEPT
   A. pleural mesothelioma
   B. emphysema
   C. interstitial pulmonary fibrosis
   D. bronchogenic carcinoma
   E. diffuse pleural thickening

15.25. A 42-year-old woman smoked half a pack of cigarettes per day since age 21. She notes a cough productive of scant amounts of clear sputum, and progressive dyspnea on mild exercise for 3 months. Examination reveals fine inspiratory crackles at both lung bases. She has had a chronic bladder infection for 2 months, and has taken nitrofurantoin for this. The most likely explanation of the symptoms is
   A. chronic renal failure and "uremic lung"
   B. drug-induced lung disease
   C. chronic bronchitis and emphysema due to cigarettes
   D. viral (walking) pneumonia
   E. the findings are probably normal for a person this age and physical condition

15.26. A 60-year-old man 75 pack-year smoking pipefitter is referred to you for evaluation of an abnormal chest roentgenogram showing a right infrahilar mass and a bilateral lower zone reticular pattern. You discover clubbing and expect to find all the following EXCEPT
   A. proliferating subperiosteal osteitis of the distal long bones of the extremities
   B. asymmetric subperiosteal new bone formation
   C. chronic synovitis
   D. pannus formation in joints
   E. joint effusions of ankles, knees, and wrists

15.27. A 68-year-old man is receiving radiotherapy to the left hilar area for an unresectable squamous cell carcinoma of the lung. The radiotherapist asks you to reassess the clinical situation because of an interim change in the chest radiograph showing elevation of the left hemidiaphragm. You expect to find all of the following EXCEPT
  A. fluoroscopic movement of the diaphragm superiorly with sniffing
  B. recent onset of dyspnea on exertion
  C. fluoroscopic movement of the diaphragm inferiorly with cough
  D. forced vital capacity approximately equivalent to that done when the chest radiograph was normal
  E. movement of the mediastinal structures on inspiration to the right

15.28. A 65-year-old jaundiced female 60 pack-year smoker is referred for preoperative evaluation of a left hilar mass and a left pleural effusion. Physical examination reveals dilated jugular veins and fullness of the face. Fiberbronchoscopy reveals the lesion to be almost totally occluding the left mainstem bronchus approximately 4.5 cm from the carina and not involving the carina. Pleural biopsy is performed. All of the following are evidence that the tumor is unresectable EXCEPT
  A. a positive sniff test after evacuating the pleural effusion
  B. pleural biopsy positive for carcinoma
  C. hepatic involvement
  D. superior vena cava syndrome
  E. a mass 4.5 cm in diameter

15.29. When a compliant asthmatic patient is not responding to the usual therapy, all of the following should be considered EXCEPT
  A. theophylline level less than 6 μg/ml
  B. employment in a plastics factory
  C. concurrent therapy with an aspirin-containing drug
  D. elevated serum IgE level
  E. concurrent therapy with erythromycin

DIRECTIONS: Each group of questions below consists of five lettered headings followed by a list of numbered words or statements. For each numbered word or statement, select the **one** lettered heading that is most closely associated with it. Each lettered heading may be selected once, more than once, or not at all.

Match the lung neoplasm with the paramalignant syndrome most closely associated with it.

    A. Epidermoid (squamous) carcinoma
    B. Small-cell anaplastic carcinoma
    C. Adenocarcinoma
    D. Large-cell carcinoma
    E. Mesothelioma

15.30. Cushing's syndrome

15.31. Hypercalcemia

15.32. Inappropriate antidiuretic hormone

15.33. Hypertrophic pulmonary osteoarthropathy

15.34. Nonbacterial thrombotic endocarditis

For each of the arterial blood gas results, indicate the most likely clinical situation.

    A. P_{CO_2} 80 mm Hg, pH 7.17, P_{O_2} 60 mm Hg
    B. P_{CO_2} 20 mm Hg, pH 7.58, P_{O_2} 108 mm Hg
    C. P_{CO_2} 20 mm Hg, pH 7.60, P_{O_2} 50 mm Hg
    D. P_{CO_2} 20 mm Hg, pH 7.19, P_{O_2} 88 mm Hg
    E. P_{CO_2} 70 mm Hg, pH 7.22, P_{O_2} 40 mm Hg

15.35. Thirty-year-old man who is semicomatose with Kussmaul's respiration, fruity breath odor, glycosuria, and ketonuria

15.36. Twenty-five-year-old male asthmatic who is semicomatose and combative, with diminished but normal breath sounds, brought in by the emergency medical squad, receiving oxygen by mask

15.37. A 19-year-old woman, auto accident victim, intubated on continuous mandatory ventilation and oxygen concentration of 30% for "flail" chest, 3 hours following the accident

15.38. A 60-year-old woman with a temperature of 39°C, radiographic evidence of pneumonia, and a white blood count of 25,000/mm³

15.39. A 27-year-old resident from the southeast coastal plains of Kenya, attempting his first climb of the Himalayas

---

DIRECTIONS: Each set of lettered headings below is followed by a list of numbered words or phrases. For each numbered word or phrase select

    (A) if the item is associated with A only
    (B) if the item is associated with B only
    (C) if the item is associated with both A and B
    (D) if the item is associated with neither A nor B

    A. Air-space consolidation (acinus-filling pattern)
    B. Interstitial pattern
    C. Both
    D. Neither

15.40. Acute pulmonary hemorrhage

15.41. Asbestos exposure, long term

15.42. Asthma

    A. Obstructive pattern of pulmonary function
    B. Restrictive pattern of pulmonary function
    C. Both
    D. Neither

15.43. Centrilobular emphysema

15.44. Idiopathic pulmonary fibrosis

15.45. Acute hypersensitivity pneumonitis (allergic alveolitis)

DIRECTIONS: For each of the questions or incomplete statements below, **one or more** of the answers or completions given is correct. Select

(A) if only 1, 2, and 3 are correct
(B) if only 1 and 3 are correct
(C) if only 2 and 4 are correct
(D) if only 4 is correct
(E) if all are correct

15.46. Which of the following are commonly reported causes of pulmonary infiltrates in patients with acquired immune deficiency syndrome (AIDS)?
 1. *Pneumocystis carinii*
 2. Atypical mycobacteria
 3. Cytomegalic virus
 4. *Mycoplasma pneumoniae*

15.47. Which of the following are characteristics of Legionnaire's disease?
 1. Chest radiographs show patchy infiltates early, that often progress to segmental or lobar consolidations bilaterally
 2. The mortality rate from infection is often greater than 50%
 3. Microscopic hematuria, often accompanied by cylindruria and proteinuria, occurs in about one-third of patients
 4. Pleural effusions, nearly always exudates, are seen in the majority of patients

15.48. Infection by *Mycoplasma pneumoniae* is characterized by which of the following?
 1. Tracheobronchitis without clinical or radiographic evidence of pneumonia is distinctly uncommon
 2. Infection without evidence of pneumonia is common in preschool children
 3. The characteristic radiographic finding is a segmental infiltrate
 4. Physical examination of the chest often demonstrates rhonchi and wheezes, as well as fine-to-medium rales over the affected areas

15.49. Progressive hematogenous tuberculosis (miliary tuberculosis) is characterized by which of the following?
1. A diffuse small nodular pattern on chest x-ray in all cases
2. Tuberculous meningitis is frequently present
3. Intermediate-strength tuberculin skin tests are virtually always positive
4. It may mimic sepsis with fever and rigors, or present as a chronic wasting illness

15.50. A 2-year-old child of a recent immigrant from Southeast Asia is seen in a clinic because of fever and lassitude. A tine test produced a confluent reaction. Which of the following would be expected on a chest radiograph?
1. Bilateral widely disseminated irregular nodular opacities
2. Lower zone parenchymal infiltrate
3. Apical cavity
4. Ipsilateral hilar adenopathy

15.51. A 47-year-old alcoholic woman is diagnosed as having chronic cavitary tuberculosis. Expected findings include
1. persistent cough productive of sputum containing large numbers of acid-fast bacilli
2. chest x-ray abnormality predominantly in the apical and posterior segments of the upper lobes
3. a high rate of tuberculin reactivity in household contacts
4. normochromic anemia

15.52. Histoplasmosis is the most common respiratory fungal infection in the United States. Clinical syndromes resulting from this fungus include
1. primary histoplasmosis: a common, self-limited, flulike illness with cough, fever, and myalgia
2. chronic histoplasmosis: chronic cough and fever arising from fungal growth in preexisting emphysematous blebs
3. disseminated histoplasmosis: a progressive, multiorgan infection with hepatosplenomegaly
4. epidemic histoplasmosis: high rates of infection due to crowding and person-to-person spread

A	B	C	D	E
DIRECTIONS SUMMARIZED				
1,2,3	1,3	2,4	4	All are
only	only	only	only	correct

15.53. Nocardiosis is characterized by
  1. more commonly infecting immunosuppressed patients
  2. presenting, in most cases, as a pneumonic process
  3. hematogenous spread
  4. its susceptibility to amphotericin B

15.54. Pneumocystosis is a pulmonary disease caused by *Pneumocystis carinii*. It is characterized by
  1. progressive pulmonary symptoms in an immunocompromised host
  2. being easily found in transtracheal aspirates stained with methenamine silver
  3. cysts with sporozoites stained with methenamine silver
  4. its susceptibility to the therapy of choice, pentamidine

15.55. Viral pneumonia can be differentiated from bacterial pneumonia by
  1. low-grade fever of 38°C or less
  2. normal-to-low white blood count
  3. typical radiographic signs
  4. appropriate culture of respiratory secretions or tissue

DIRECTIONS: This section of the test consists of situations, each followed by a series of questions. Study each situation and select the **one** best answer to each question following it.

Question 15.56: A 52-year-old woman requests a check-up. She has little change in her chronic productive cough, but a recent onset of "feeling tired all the time" and numbness in the left hand. She has smoked 1−2 packs of cigarettes per day for 31 years. Physical examination reveals a well-developed female, with a few coarse crackles and low-pitched wheezes in the chest. There is an ill-defined decrease in pin sensation in the left upper extremity. There are no abnormal lymph nodes palpable. The chest x-ray is shown in Figure 38. No old films are available.

15.56. Initial workup in this case should include all of the following EXCEPT
    A. sputum cytologies and cultures
    B. liver enzymes, alkaline phosphatase, and serum calcium
    C. serum electrolytes and urea nitrogen
    D. mediastinoscopy with biopsies
    E. fiberoptic bronchoscopy with biopsy

Question 15.57: Serum electrolytes and urea nitrogen showed the following:
    Sodium 120 mEq/L   Chloride 86 mEq/L   BUN 9
    Potassium 4.3 mEq/L   Bicarbonate 24 mEq/L

15.57. The most likely explanation of these findings is
    A. the patient has the coincidental development of Cushing's disease
    B. the patient has Cushing's syndrome secondary to the lung lesion
    C. the patient has widespread disease which has caused this, and is preterminal
    D. the low BUN indicates a primary kidney problem
    E. the urinary osmolarity is inappropriately high compared to the serum osmolarity

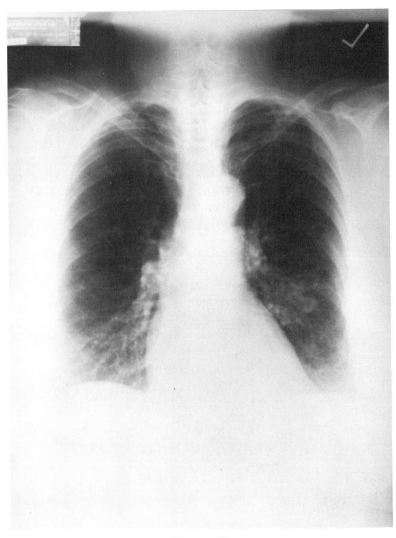

Figure 38

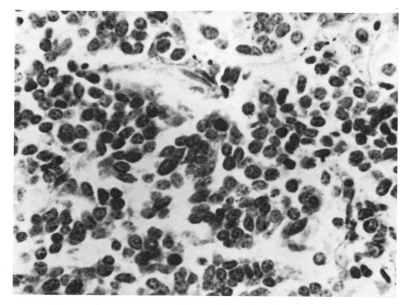

Figure 39

Question 15.58: Biopsy of a mass lesion, seen during bronchoscopy, is shown in Figure 39.

15.58. The best approach regarding treatment of this problem is to
  A. prepare immediately for resectional surgery, because any delay will reduce the chances of prolonged survival
  B. begin treatment with isoniazid and rifampin and repeat the chest x-ray at monthly intervals. If the lesion enlarges, proceed to surgery
  C. perform computerized tomogram of the head to pursue the neurologic abnormality on physical examination
  D. perform a thorough workup, including radionucleotide scans of the bones, liver, and spleen, and computerized tomogram of the brain, and if these are all normal, refer for surgery
  E. begin treatment with intravenous penicillin G, then switch to oral penicillin after 2 weeks .

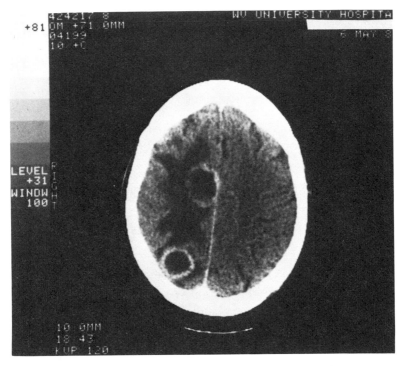

Figure 40

Question 15.59: The results of a computerized tomogram of the head are shown in Figure 40.

15.59. The next step in management in this patient is
- **A.** consult a neurosurgeon to remove the brain lesions prior to lung resection
- **B.** administer dexamethasone to reduce brain edema, and then proceed to resection of the lung lesion
- **C.** advise patient that no further therapy could be helpful
- **D.** refer for cancer chemotherapy, since surgical therapy would be ineffective
- **E.** perform mediastinoscopy, and if negative proceed to remove the pulmonary lesion

Questions 15.60–15.61: A 52-year-old male office worker complains of 2 weeks of fever, night sweats, and cough productive of dark, foul-smelling sputum. He smokes half a pack of cigarettes per day, and had two teeth extracted several weeks ago, but has no other known medical problems. Examination reveals an ill-appearing male, temperature 38.7°C, pulse 108, respirations 26. There is dullness to percussion and diminished breath sounds in the right midlung field posteriorly with a few persistent coarse inspiratory crackles. The chest x-ray is shown in Figure 41.

Figure 41

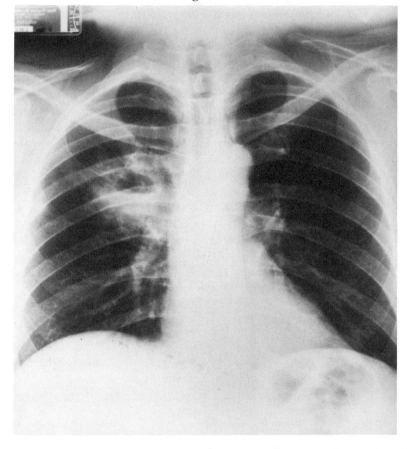

15.60. Appropriate specimens for diagnosis include all of the following EXCEPT
   A. sputum for anaerobic culture
   B. routine blood cultures
   C. transtracheal aspirate for smears and cultures
   D. bronchoscopic brushings for quantitative cultures
   E. anaerobic blood culture

15.61. The most appropriate therapy at this time would be
   A. a cephalosporin and aminoglycoside parenterally
   B. isoniazid and rifampin
   C. preparation for surgical drainage or resection of the lesion
   D. high-dose intravenous penicillin G
   E. tetracycline orally for 2–3 months

Question 15.62: Several days later, a right pleural effusion is noted. A thick brown pleural fluid was cultured and reported as growing three different organisms.

15.62. True statements at this time include all of the following EXCEPT
   A. the thoracentesis should be repeated because the culture was likely to have been contaminated
   B. a chest-tube drainage of the pleura is necessary at this time
   C. bronchopleura fistula is an expected complication of this condition
   D. brain abscess is an expected complication of this condition
   E. the organism(s) causing this condition is/are found normally in the mouth

Question 15.63: A 72-year-old man presents with a 2-day history of cough, fever, and prostration. He felt as if he were getting a cold while driving home to West Virginia from Florida. The cough was initially nonproductive, but within 12 hours he experienced a chill associated with rigors, pain in the right upper anterior chest, myalgia, and profound weakness. The cough became productive of phlegm that was blood-streaked and looked like prune juice. He had had a cardiac pacemaker implanted several years earlier for complete heart block. Physical examination revealed an acutely ill elderly man with hot skin. The temperature was 40°C rectally. The heart rate was 84 and regular. The respiratory rate was 35/min with use of accessory inspiratory muscles, and there was audible grunting with each expiration. The chest radiograph is shown in Figure 42.

15.63. The most likely diagnostic impression in this case is
  - **A.** infected pulmonary embolism with infarction
  - **B.** *Klebsiella pneumonia*
  - **C.** lung abscess
  - **D.** pneumococcal pneumonia
  - **E.** bronchogenic carcinoma

Questions 15.64–15.65: A deep-cough specimen of sputum was obtained in the emergency room. Gram stains of this material showed the presence of more than 25 polymorphonuclear neutrophils per low-power field. Organisms were identified as shown in Figure 43.

15.64. Based upon this and the the clinical information, the most appropriate initial treatment is
  - **A.** lung scan, pulmonary angiogram, and intravenous heparin
  - **B.** intravenous penicillin, 4,000,000 U/day
  - **C.** intravenous penicillin, 20,000,000 U/day
  - **D.** cephalothin and gentamicin in full dosage
  - **E.** fiberoptic bronchoscopy before treatment is initiated

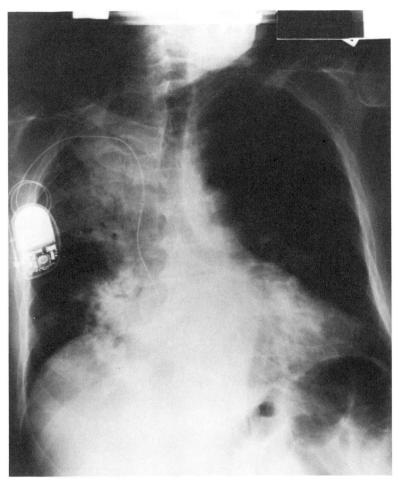

Figure 42

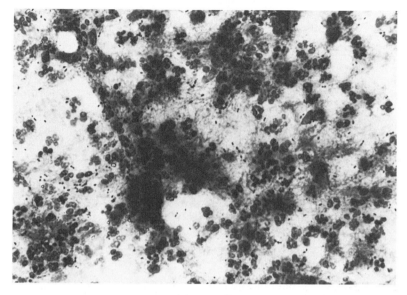

Figure 43

15.65. If after the appropriate therapy were given for 72 hours, the patient's fever recurred, it would be appropriate to assume that a complication of the original disease had occurred. All of the following are complications that might be expected to occur *at this time* EXCEPT
   A. empyema
   B. pericarditis
   C. peritonitis
   D. meningitis
   E. bronchopleura fistula

Answers and Comments

15.1. (D) When the air-containing lung is adjacent to another structure, a sharp margin is usually seen on the chest radiograph. Loss of this margin indicates consolidation, collapse, or fluid in the adjacent lobe or segment. On a routine posteroanterior chest film, the left heart border is adjacent to the lingular division of the left upper lobe. The fact that the left cardiac border is well seen, indicates that the lesion in this case cannot be in the lingula. The basilar segments of the lower lobe are adjacent to the diaphragm and disease in these will obscure the diaphragm contour. There is no left middle lobe (Ref. 3, p. 487).

15.2. (D) Virtually all persons decrease their arterial oxygen tension during sleep. Snoring is common and alone is not necessarily suggestive of sleep apnea. Severe nocturnal hypoxemia is associated with morning headaches, and in time with pulmonary hypertension. Recognition of this syndrome is important because life-threatening cardiac arrhythmias may occur (Ref. 1, p. 1934).

15.3. (E) Marked clockwise rotation, rather than counterclockwise rotation, occurs with right ventricular hypertrophy. Other criteria are an S_1Q_3 or S_1, S_2, S_3 pattern, and R/S amplitude ratio in V_2 less than 1 (Ref. 4, p. 1674).

15.4. (B) A parapneumonic effusion may have an acid, alkaline, or neutral pH; however, as it progresses toward empyema stage, it becomes progressively more acidic. A pleural fluid:serum protein ratio of greater than 0.5 and a pleural fluid:serum LDH ratio of greater than 0.6 are the most reliable parameters of a pleural exudate, of which pneumonia is one etiology (Ref. 3, pp. 314–318).

15.5. (C) A young person from a country with a high incidence of tuberculosis and little reason to suspect other etiologies of a low pleural-fluid glucose (such as malignancy, rheumatoid pleuritis, or pneumonia) should be suspect of having tuberculosis. The PPD skin test is usually negative, and culture is also rarely positive. A pleural biopsy is the most rewarding procedure and, if negative initially, should be repeated. A tuberculous pleural effusion will spontaneously disappear without treatment, but within 5 years approximately 66% of patients will develop clinically-manifest tuberculosis. Steroids may hasten resolution of the effusion, but should not be used without appropriate concomitant chemotherapy (Ref. 1, pp. 423, 1548).

15.6. (D) The patient has Meig's syndrome, usually a benign ovarian tumor associated with a pleural effusion, usually a transudate. Any pleural effusion, which is of long duration, may become an exudate, but the separation of effusions into transudate and exudate helps to narrow the diagnostic possibilities. One of the characteristics of a transudate is an LDH less than 200 IU/L. (Ref. 1, pp. 422–424).

15.7. (D) Systemic lupus erythematosus and rheumatoid arthritis are the connective tissue diseases that are most frequently associated with pleuritis and pleural effusions. The effusions are generally an exudate. In SLE effusions, complement is decreased, and LE cells may be found; in rheumatoid effusions the glucose is low. Pleural effusions are uncommonly encountered in progressive systemic sclerosis or dermatomyositis. Ankylosing spondylitis is no longer considered to be a variant of rheumatoid arthritis, and pleural involvement has not been reported (Ref. 1, pp. 380, 424, 1824, 1878).

15.8. (A) In mild-to-moderate asthmatics, recent studies have shown that inhaled β-2 agonists are effective and better tolerated than other therapy. Long-acting oral theophylline preparations are also useful in this setting. Fixed combinations of theophylline with other agents are to be avoided because they result in increased adverse reactions and ineffective control of the bronchospasm (Ref. 2, pp. 1518, 1519).

15.9. (B) Many patients with sarcoidosis improve and are able to discontinue steroid therapy from the second trimester on. Cellular immunity is impaired, but there is evidence of increased humoral immunity with increased B-cell activity and raised immunoglobulin levels. Serum angiotensin-converting enzyme levels are raised in about 60% of active cases. Stage I disease resolves spontaneously in around 65% of cases (Ref. 1, pp. 1891–1895).

15.10. (D) Erythema nodosum with bilateral hilar adenopathy and iritis (Lofgren's syndrome) has an excellent prognosis for spontaneous resolution. Neurologic, cardiac, and significant pulmonary functional impairments are indications for treatment, as well as a persistently abnormal calcium metabolism, uveitis, and hypersplenism (Ref. 1, pp. 1892–1896).

15.11. (D) Morbid obesity frequently affects lung function, even when the lungs are histologically normal. Hypoxemia is due to impaired ventilation of the lung bases, particularly in the supine position, with normal perfusion. Polycythemia is occasionally seen. Certain individuals may have hypoventilation and/or sleep apnea (Ref. 3, pp. 1924–1925).

15.12. **(E)** Positive end-expiratory pressures (PEEP) can improve arterial blood oxygenation in patients with reduced lung compliance and hypoxemia. Shunting of venous blood through collapsed lung regions is decreased, but cardiac output usually falls. Thus, oxygen delivery may improve at low PEEP but decrease at higher levels, even with high arterial oxygen tension. A pulmonary artery (Swan-Ganz) catheter helps to quantify this effect, but the effects of PEEP on pressure measurements must be taken into account. Particularly in patients with increased lung compliance (chronic bronchitis and emphysema), PEEP frequently results in barotrauma, which can be rapidly fatal if not recognized. It should be used with caution, if at all, in these individuals (Ref. 2, pp. 1593–1594).

15.13. **(B)** Endotracheal intubation for respiratory failure manifested by either arterial hypoxemia, hypercapnea, or both is proper management. The preferred method of establishing an airway in most emergencies is via either a nasal or oral endotracheal tube. The one exception is acute obstruction of the upper airways from foreign bodies, inflammation due to infection or burns in the area, or as in this case, a fracture of the larynx (Ref. 1, p. 4331).

15.14. **(E)** Increased pulsus paradoxus is a useful finding indicating the severity of an asthmatic attack. A decrease in wheezing occurs in severe asthma, when air-flow is very low. The $PaCO_2$ is usually low; an increase, even to normal, suggests fatigue and that mechanical ventilation may soon be required. Arterial PO_2 does not correlate well with the severity of asthma, but is usually less than 60 mm Hg in severe attacks (Ref. 3, pp. 1344–1351).

15.15. **(E)** The destruction of lung parenchyma characteristic of emphysema is reflected very accurately by an increased static lung compliance with a shift of the pressure-volume curve upward and to the left of normal. Thus, at comparable lung volumes there is reduced lung recoil pressure. There is considerable overlap or variability in the result of arterial blood oxygen tension. The radiograph and residual volume elevation reflect widespread air trapping. Dyspnea is a nonspecific symptom, with little discriminating value (Ref. 1, p. 368).

15.16. (D) The normal phenotype is MM. The homozygous deficiency (phenotype ZZ) is associated with the development of emphysema by age 40 if the patient smokes, and about age 60 if he does not. In contrast, "ordinary" emphysema develops between 55 and 65 years. While some family studies have shown an increased tendency to COPD, population studies have failed to show any overall tendency for heterozygous (phenotype MZ) subjects to develop an excess of respiratory disease or for respiratory disorders to be related to the level of serum-trypsin inhibitor capacity. The heterozygous state (phenotype MZ) occurs in about 3−5% of the population (Ref. 1, p. 367).

15.17. (A) Pulmonary angiography is the standard by which all other methods of detecting pulmonary emboli are measured. CPK, SGOT, LDH, and bilirubin are of no real benefit. While it is true that the PaO_2 is less than 80 mm Hg in 85% of patients with pulmonary embolism, it is also true that many of the disorders with which pulmonary embolism is associated also produce hypoxemia. Electrocardiographic evidence may be suggestive but not confirmatory; it is also usually transient and only found in large emboli. Perfusion lung scans are affected by anything that causes a radiographic density or obstruction to ventilation, thus limiting their diagnostic specificity. A normal perfusion lung scan virtually eliminates the possibility of pulmonary embolus but an abnormal scan does not necessarily mean the presence of emboli. Multiple *segmental* defects are the finding most associated with a high incidence of pulmonary emboli confirmed by pulmonary angiography. The appropriate clinical situation and a high probability perfusion lung scan are generally enough to decide that pulmonary emboli are present. If either is not present, then pulmonary angiography should be the standard by which one decides to use or continue heparin anticoagulation (Ref. 1, pp. 389, 393).

15.18. (D) Pleuritic chest pain is more likely to be found in a medium-sized pulmonary embolism involving primarily the segmental and subsegmental pulmonary artery branches. Hypotension and many signs of right ventricular overload may be found in addition to an accentuation of P_2 (Ref. 1, p. 390).

15.19. (C) Massive hemoptysis is defined as bleeding of 600 cc or more in 48 hours and is a medical emergency. To prevent flooding in the *normal* lung, the affected lung should be kept in the dependent (down) position. Bronchoscopy is most safely performed with a rigid bronchoscope, and should be done as soon as possible to localize the site of bleeding. Early surgical intervention is often required, although the postoperative course is frequently complicated (Ref. 1, pp. 336−337).

15.20. (B) Fine crackles, so-called velcro rales, late in inspiration are heard in many diffuse fibrosing lung diseases. Wheezes are occasionally heard on inspiration. Medium crackles are more suggestive of pulmonary edema, and hyperresonance suggests emphysema. Of note is the frequent absence of crackles in granulomatous lung diseases, such as sarcoidosis and eosinophilic granuloma (Ref. 3, pp. 288−289, 1678, 1690−1695, 1731−1740).

15.21. (B) Fiberoptic bronchoscopy has become the procedure of choice for investigation of a variety of pulmonary disorders, due to the ease and low complication rate of the technique in experienced hands. It is also useful in treatment of secretions and atelectasis, and is preferred in patients with reduced mobility of the cervical spine. In the presence of active life-threatening hemoptysis, or in the removal of large foreign bodies, the rigid bronchoscope is preferable (Ref. 2, p. 1510).

15.22. (E) The age and smoking history require that you suspect malignancy. The sex of a patient is no longer a consideration in lung cancer. A malignancy may incorporate flecks of calcium as it grows; concentric rings or a central nidus of calcium are reliable indicators of the presence of a granuloma. Sputum cytology and fiberbronchoscopy have a very low yield in this type of lesion, even if malignant. Transthoracic needle aspiration has a good yield, but you cannot be certain the lesion is not malignant if cytology is negative. If a solitary nodule can be documented by previous chest radiograph to be unchanged in size over 2 years, it is almost always benign (Ref. 1, pp. 410−421).

15.23. (B) Chemoprophylaxis with INH (isoniazid) is recommended in all known recent tuberculin convertors regardless of age, and in all household contacts of newly diagnosed active cases regardless of tuberculin status. Persons with a positive tuberculin reaction (greater than 10 mm induration to 5 TU, intermediate strength) of unknown duration or history are generally treated if under the age of 20 and some extend this to age 35. Persons with symptoms or radiographic changes consistent with *active* tuberculosis are not candidates for chemoprophylaxis. Similarly, positive reactions to large doses (250 TU) of tuberculin are not considered indications for chemoprophylaxis (Ref. 1, p. 1542).

15.24. (B) Exposure to asbestos was common in the shipyards during World War II. All of the above manifestations are related to exposure to asbestos except pulmonary emphysema. Cigarette smoking plus asbestos exposure increases the risk of bronchogenic carcinoma (Ref. 1, pp. 400–402).

15.25. (B) A large number of drugs have been reported to cause lung reactions. An acute reaction with fever, infiltrates, and eosinophilia can be seen after several days of treatment. Chronic insidious reactions can arise after months or years of therapy. The findings are nonspecific. Nitrofurantoin can cause either acute or insidious disease. Withdrawal of the offending agent is essential (Ref. 1, pp. 380–381).

15.26. (B) Subperiosteal new bone formation occurs *symmetrically* in hypertrophic pulmonary osteoarthropathy. Clubbing is almost always found in association with pulmonary osteoarthropathy, but the reverse is not true, and clubbing may occur in association with other disorders. Hypertrophic osteoarthropathy may be associated with various neoplasms, but is most commonly associated with bronchogenic carcinoma. Bronchogenic carcinoma is 60–90 times more likely to occur in the smoking worker exposed to asbestos than it is in the general population. Resection of the lesion, vagotomy, or just thoracotomy may cause the osteoarthropathy to regress (Ref. 1, p. 416).

15.27. (B) Unilateral diaphragmatic paralysis is frequently found with interruption of the phrenic nerve by tumor. Metastatic or local extension of bronchogenic tumor is one of the more common tumors causing unilateral paralysis. Unilateral paralysis does not significantly affect lung function and it is usually clinically asymptomatic; dyspnea on exertion would not be expected. The paralyzed hemidiaphragm moves paradoxically on sniffing or coughing (Ref. 1, pp. 350, 427–428).

15.28. **(E)** The size of a lesion does not determine whether or not it is resectable. The positive sniff test indicative of diaphragmatic paralysis and invasion of the phrenic nerve, jaundice suggesting liver metastases, SVC syndrome, and a positive pleural biopsy are indicative of mediastinal and distant metastases; therefore, surgery would be an exercise in futility. In this case, the presence of an SVC syndrome indicates extensive mediastinal involvement because the superior vena cava is on the right side in the mediastinum. Pleural biopsies are performed only on the parietal pleura and are, therefore, indicative of chest-wall invasion. Other signs of unresectability are mediastinal lymph-node invasion, Horner's syndrome, and other evidence of distant metastases, such as CNS and bone, and paralysis of the recurrent laryngeal nerve (Ref. 1, p. 418).

15.29. **(E)** The therapeutic plasma concentrations of theophylline lie between 10 and 20 μg/ml but the dosage required to achieve this level varies widely from patient to patient due to differences in disposition (excretion) of the drug. Aspirin and related compounds ingested by susceptible patients make asthma worse. A variety of compounds used in industry can cause asthma in susceptible people, these include metal salts, vegetable and wood dusts, industrial chemicals and plastics, pharmaceutical agents, biological enzymes, and animal and insect dusts, serum, and secretions. Allergic bronchopulmonary aspergillosis often presents with wheezing associated with transient pulmonary infiltrates. Such flares are usually preceded by elevations of the total IgE levels (Ref. 2, pp. 1513, 1514).

15.30. **(B)** Small-cell anaplastic tumors arise from cells derived from the neural crest, and thus give rise to a variety of endocrine syndromes, including Cushing's syndrome (Ref. 1, pp. 414, 416).

15.31. **(A)** Hypercalcemia most commonly is caused by epidermoid tumors, but is also seen with bone metastasis and small-cell cancers (Ref. 1, pp. 414–416).

15.32. **(B)** The syndrome of inappropriate antidiuretic hormone is most commonly seen with small-cell cancers (Ref. 1, pp. 414–416).

15.33. **(E)** Digital clubbing is common in bronchogenic carcinoma, but the syndrome of hypertrophic pulmonary osteoarthropathy, including joint effusions and subperiosteal new bone formation, is unusual. It is often associated with bulky tumors involving the pleura such as mesothelioma (Ref. 1, pp. 414–416).

15.34. **(C)** Sterile vegetations, usually involving the mitral and/or aortic valves, are seen with adenocarcinomas. Systemic embolization is often the clue to their presence (Ref. 1, pp. 414–416).

15.35. **(D)** Kussmaul's respiration is a severe form of hyperventilation, a singular manifestation of metabolic acidosis. There are many causes of metabolic acidosis and thus of Kussmaul's respiration, but the concomitant occurrence of both glycosuria and ketonuria almost certainly makes the diagnosis diabetic ketoacidosis (Ref. 1, p. 491).

15.36. **(A)** An increase in PCO_2 and a decrease in pH in asthma indicate fatigue and impending cardiorespiratory arrest. The adequate oxygenation seen here is misleading because of supplemental administration of oxygen (Ref. 3, pp. 1344–1351).

15.37. **(B)** This auto accident victim is being hyperventilated and has an acute respiratory alkalosis. She is also being overoxygenated for her needs, and the oxygen concentration should be decreased to keep her PaO_2 between 60 and 100 mm Hg. The increased $A\text{-}aDO_2$ gradient suggests parenchymal as well as chest-wall injury (Ref. 1, pp. 2192, 2194–2195, 2198).

15.38. **(C)** Pneumonia leads to hyperventilation manifested by uncompensated respiratory alkalosis. It also produces a large intrapulmonary shunt through the involved unventilated but perfused lung (Ref. 4, p. 695).

15.39. **(C)** Unacclimated persons who ascend to high altitude may develop acute mountain sickness; this usually occurs in those in poor physical condition, and during a rapid ascent requiring strenuous physical activity. The mechanism is thought to be hyperventilation stimulated by hypoxia with a resultant acute respiratory alkalosis (Ref. 1, p. 406).

15.40. **(A)** Alveolar edema, bleeding into the acini (idiopathic pulmonary hemorrhage), aspiration of blood or lipid, alveolar-cell carcinoma, and certain idiopathic conditions, such as alveolar proteinosis, are all capable of producing acinar shadows (Ref. 3, p. 345).

15.41. **(B)** Early asbestosis may produce an extremely fine reticulation. A transition from this early form through all stages of fine, medium, and coarse reticulation to honeycombing has been described in asbestosis, rheumatoid lung, and idiopathic interstitial fibrosis (Ref. 3, p. 429).

15.42. **(D)** Uncomplicated spasmodic asthma may demonstrate overinflation on the chest radiograph, but there are no air-space consolidations or interstitial infiltrations of consequence (Ref. 3, pp. 543–544).

15.43. **(A)** Chronic bronchitis and centrilobular emphysema are caused by prolonged exposure to inhaled toxins (e.g., cigarette smoke) and give rise to air-flow obstruction. As the condition progresses, air trapping may result in a reduction in vital capacity as well (Ref. 2, p. 1549).

15.44. **(B)** Idiopathic pulmonary fibrosis results in reduced lung volumes and diffusing capacity, a typical restrictive pattern (Ref. 2, p. 1557).

15.45. **(B)** Hypersensitivity pneumonitis can result in acute reversible or chronic restrictive lung impairment. Wheezes and obstruction are occasionally seen, but they are not typical (Ref. 2, pp. 1521–1522).

15.46. **(B)** *Pneumocystis carinii* is the pneumonia classically associated with either congenital or acquired immunodeficiency. Oral and anal mucosal lesions, from which *Candida albicans*, herpes simplex type 2, and cytomegalovirus have been isolated alone or in combination should be studied. Cytomegalovirus has been isolated also from the lungs and is presumed to be the cause of pulmonary infiltrates in the absence of *Pneumocystis carinii* (Ref. 2, p. 361).

15.47. **(B)** The mortality rate, while high, is about 15–20%, *not* greater than 50%. Renal involvement occurs in about one-third of cases, azotemia in about half of these, and occasionally requires dialysis. Pleural effusions occur in only about one-third of patients. Analysis of the pleural effusion indicates that about half are exudates, the other half transudates (Ref. 1, p. 1440).

15.48. (C) Tracheobronchitis without pneumonia is more common than pneumonia. In infants and preschool children asymptomatic infection is endemic. No chest radiographic pattern is either typical or diagnostic of mycoplasma pneumonia. Since tracheobronchitis is common, the physical signs of airways obstruction may be quite prominent even in the presence of pneumonic infiltrations (Ref. 1, pp. 1427−1428).

15.49. (C) Miliary tuberculosis may present as an acute or chronic illness, especially in adults. A biopsy is often required to establish the diagnosis; transbronchial lung biopsy, bone marrow, and liver biopsies are most productive. The chest radiograph may be normal, even late in the illness. Anergy is common and thus skin tests are unreliable. Meningeal involvement is frequent and may be seen with normal clinical and laboratory findings, although this is unusual (Ref. 1, pp. 1549−1550).

15.50. (C) Tuberculosis is a common chronic pulmonary disease occurring in immigrants from Southeast Asia. A 2-year-old would be expected to have primary, symptomatic tuberculosis. Symptoms would be a brassy cough, fever, and lassitude. Hilar adenopathy is a distinguishing characteristic of primary tuberculosis and is not found in melioidosis, which also is an endemic chronic pulmonary infection found in Southeast Asia (Ref. 1, p. 1542; 3, p. 711).

15.51. (E) This picture of chronic cough and sputum, hemoptysis, anemia, fatigue, and weight loss, with an apical cavity on chest x-ray, suggests chronic pulmonary tuberculosis. The sputum has large numbers of organisms, and household contacts are at high risk of infection. Treatment with two or three active drugs reduces risk of infection within 1−2 weeks (Ref. 1, pp. 1543−1545).

15.52. (A) Histoplasma infection results from inhalation of fungal spores, found in high numbers in bird or bat feces. Person-to-person spread is not reported. Reexposure to the spores may result in acute symptoms, so-called reinfection histoplasmosis. Intestinal ulcerations or painful ulcers of the tongue suggest disseminated disease, which is confirmed by serum antibodies and identification of the fungus in sputum, tissue, and by culture (Ref. 1, p. 1698).

15.53. (A) *Nocardia asteroides* is a gram-positive, weakly acid-fast aerobe found worldwide in soil. Nocardiosis can occur in normal persons and patients with chronic obstructive pulmonary disease but most commonly infects those who are immunocompromised. Seventy-five percent of cases present as the pneumonic form but if the pulmonary involvement is subclinical or transient, the hematogenous spread to other organ systems, especially the CNS, may be the presenting manifestation. Sulfonamides are the treatment of choice (Ref. 1, pp. 1533–1535).

15.54. (B) Pneumocystis only rarely occurs outside of the lungs. It is one of the opportunistic infections and, in the adult, attacks mostly those who have received chemotherapy for hematologic malignancies or organ transplantation. Sputum or transtracheal aspirates are diagnostic in less than 15% of patients; bronchoscopic washings and brushings, percutaneous needle or transbronchial biopsy of the lung, and open-lung biopsy are the preferred procedures with the highest diagnostic yield. Trimethoprim with sulfamethoxazole has supplanted pentamidine as the therapy of choice (Ref. 1, pp. 1742–1744).

15.55. (D) Viral pneumonia cannot be differentiated from bacterial pneumonia by clinical or radiographic signs. Fever in viral pneumonia can range as high as 41°C and the white blood count is normal-to-markedly elevated in most. Although viral pneumonic radiographic signs may be more widespread, there is actually no typical radiographic appearance. With viral pneumonia there is more likely to be a paucity of physical findings when radiographic signs are abundant and vice versa (Ref. 1, pp. 1627–1633).

15.56. (D) In the initial workup of bronchogenic carcinoma, history, physical examination, chest radiographs, sputum examination, routine biochemistries, and bronchoscopy are nearly always indicated. Further staging should be directed by these results; routine scans are not productive, but biopsy of an abnormal lymph node, liver, bone, or pleura is often helpful. If no metastatic lesions are found, mediastinoscopy may be indicated in order to help determine resectability (Ref. 1, pp. 414–415).

15.57. **(E)** Hyponatremia is often due to tumor secretion of antidiuretic hormone, resulting in an inappropriate urine osmolarity. Treatment consists of fluid restriction (Ref. 1, pp. 477–479).

15.58. **(C)** This patient has anaplastic small-cell carcinoma. Surgery has not been effective in improving survival in small-cell cancers, as they are invariably metastatic when discovered. It is the treatment of choice in all other bronchogenic carcinomas that prove resectable. Other tumor-related disorders occur in this setting, such as hypercalcemia and Cushing's syndrome, as well as nonmetastatic neurologic syndromes and brain metastases (as found in this patient) (Ref. 1, pp. 414–415).

15.59. **(D)** While surgery remains the most effective therapy for most bronchogenic carcinomas, one exception is the patient with small-cell anaplastic carcinoma. This tumor has an extremely poor prognosis, and for limited disease radiation therapy is superior to surgery. For metastatic disease, a combination of radiation and chemotherapy has produced encouraging results (Ref. 1, pp. 417–719).

15.60. **(A)** This patient has a lung abscess. The etiologic organisms are mainly the normal flora of the mouth, and arise from aspiration during altered consciousness (seizures, alcohol intoxication) or after oral anesthesia. Expectorated sputum specimens are invariably contaminated with anaerobes, and thus a more invasive procedure is required for a reliable culture (Ref. 1, pp. 383–386).

15.61. **(D)** Most lung abscesses will heal on high-dose intravenous penicillin (over 10,000,000 U/day) followed by prolonged oral treatment (Ref. 1, pp. 383–386).

15.62. **(A)** Multiple organisms, including both anaerobes and aerobes, are expected. Empyema is a frequent complication and requires tube drainage. Other recognized complications of lung abscess include bronchopleural fistula, brain abscess, hemoptysis, and lung flooding from sudden, spontaneous drainage of the abscess contents (Ref. 1, pp. 383–386).

15.63. **(D)** The clinical presentation, with a preceding upper respiratory infection, sudden onset of chill, rigor, myalgia, profound weakness, blood-streaked or prune-juice sputum, associated with high fever, tachypnea, use of accessory inspiratory muscles and grunting, is charactertistic. The lack of tachycardia is due to the fixed rate pacemaker. The radiograph showing lobar consolidation and air bronchograms is also typical of pneumococcal pneumonia (Ref. 1, pp. 1422–1424).

15.64. (B) When presented with a typical clinical presentation and chest radiograph, an adequate sputum specimen (defined as showing greater than 25 polymorphonuclear leukocytes/low-power field and no epithelial cells) showing gram-positive, bullet-shaped diplococci provides good evidence of pneumococcal infection. Appropriate initial treatment in this setting is low-dose penicillin (Ref. 1, p. 1425).

15.65. (E) Bronchopleural fistula tends to occur in association with bacterial infection with anaerobes, staphylococci, and gram-negative organisms. The remaining choices are all recognized complications of pneumococcal pneumonia (Ref. 1, pp. 423–424, 1426).

References

1. Wyngaarden, J.P. and Smith, L.H., Jr.: *Cecil's Textbook of Medicine*, 16th Ed., W.B. Saunders, Philadelphia, 1982.

2. Petersdorf, R.G., et al.: *Harrison's Principles of Internal Medicine*, 10th Ed., McGraw-Hill, New York, 1983.

3. Fraser, R.G. and Pare, J.A.P.: *Diagnosis of Diseases of the Chest*, 2nd Ed., W.B. Saunders, Philadelphia, 1977–1979.

4. Braunwald, E.: *Heart Disease*, W.B. Saunders, Philadelphia, 1980.

16

Rheumatology
Steven J. Wees, M.D.

DIRECTIONS: Each of the questions or incomplete statements below is followed by five suggested answers or completions. Select the **one** that is best in each case.

16.1. Which of the following laboratory tests is most crucial in the assessment of acute monarticular arthritis?
  A. Mucin clot test
  B. Synovial fluid glucose
  C. Synovial fluid complement
  D. Synovial fluid cell count and differential
  E. Microscopic examination of synovial fluid

16.2. Which of the following is NOT characteristic of the fibrositis syndrome?
  A. Generalized pain
  B. Morning stiffness
  C. Insomnia
  D. Joint swelling
  E. Exhaustion

16.3. Common clinical characteristics of scleroderma include all of the following EXCEPT
   A. Raynaud's phenomenon
   B. pleural effusions
   C. arthralgias and arthritis
   D. restrictive lung disease
   E. esophageal dysfunction

16.4. The most common cause of acute pyogenic arthritis in adults is
   A. *Staphylococcus aureus*
   B. *Hemophilus influenzae*
   C. *Escherichia coli*
   D. *Neisseria gonorrhoeae*
   E. *Proteus mirabilis*

16.5. Classic historical features of back pain in ankylosing spondylitis include all of the following EXCEPT
   A. duration over 3 months
   B. worsening with rest
   C. onset over 40 years of age
   D. prolonged morning stiffness
   E. insidious onset

16.6. The presence of which of the following antibodies is generally considered a sine qua non for the diagnosis of mixed connective tissue disease (MCTD)?
   A. SS-A
   B. SS-B
   C. Sm
   D. DNA
   E. RNP

16.7. Acute attacks of gout rarely affect the
   A. first metatarsophalangeal joint
   B. shoulder
   C. ankle
   D. wrist
   E. elbow

16.8. Clinical manifestations of Sjögren's syndrome include all of the following EXCEPT
   A. salivary gland enlargement
   B. dental caries
 - **C.** subcutaneous calcifications
   D. Raynaud's phenomenon
   E. lower extremity purpura

16.9. Which of the following is NOT indicated in the treatment of acute pyogenic arthritis?
   A. Passive range of motion exercises
   B. Analgesics
   C. Joint splinting
   D. Open surgical drainage
 - **E.** Intraarticular instillation of antibiotics

16.10. Symptoms suggesting osteoarthritis rather than inflammatory arthritis include all of the following EXCEPT
   A. 15 minutes of morning stiffness
   B. slowly worsening course
   C. absence of pain at rest
 - **D.** fatigue
   E. relative absence of acute flares

DIRECTIONS: Each group of questions below consists of five lettered headings followed by a list of numbered words or statements. For each numbered word or statement, select the **one** lettered heading that is most closely associated with it. Each lettered heading may be selected once, more than once, or not at all.

   A. Prednisone
   B. Hydroxychloroquine
   C. Cyclophosphamide
   D. Methotrexate
   E. Azathioprine

16.11. Relapsing polychondritis

ᴅ **16.12.** Discoid lupus

ᴀ **16.13.** Giant-cell arteritis

ᴄ **16.14.** Wegener's granulomatosis

DIRECTIONS: Each set of lettered headings below is followed by a list of numbered words or phrases. For each numbered word or phrase select

    (A) if the item is associated with A only
    (B) if the item is associated with B only
    (C) if the item is associated with both A and B
    (D) if the item is associated with neither A nor B

    A. Speckled antinuclear antibody pattern
    B. Peripheral antinuclear antibody pattern
    C. Both
    D. Neither

ᴄ **16.15.** Systemic lupus erythematosus (SLE)

ᴀ **16.16.** Rheumatoid arthritis

ᴀ **16.17.** Mixed connective tissue disease

DIRECTIONS: For each of the questions or incomplete statements below, **one or more** of the answers or completions given is correct. Select
    (A) if only 1, 2, and 3 are correct
    (B) if only 1 and 3 are correct
    (C) if only 2 and 4 are correct
    (D) if only 4 is correct
    (E) if all are correct

16.18. Mucocutaneous lesions characteristically seen in Reiter's syndrome include
    1. erythema chronicum migrans
    2. Gottron's papules
    3. erythema elevatum diutinum
    4. circinate balanitis

16.19. Complications of giant-cell arteritis include
    1. myocardial infarction
    2. dissecting aortic aneurysm
    3. congestive heart failure
    4. blindness

16.20. Typical joint changes of osteoarthritis include
    1. Bouchard's node
    2. hallux valgus
    3. genu varus
    4. boutonniere deformity

16.21. The arthritis of SLE is typically
    1. asymmetric
    2. polyarticular
    3. erosive
    4. nondeforming

DIRECTIONS: This section of the test consists of situations, each followed by a series of questions. Study each situation and select the **one** best answer to each question following it.

Question 16.22: A 45-year-old white man complains of gradually worsening fatigue and muscle weakness over a 4-month period of time. On physical examination he has difficulty raising both arms over his head as well as lifting both feet to step onto the examining table.

16.22. Which of the following is LEAST likely in the differential diagnosis of this patient's problem?
  A. Polymyositis
  B. Trichinosis
  C. Hypothyroidism
  D. Polymyalgia rheumatica
  E. Myasthenia gravis

Question 16.23: A 30-year-old woman with rheumatoid arthritis of 5 years duration complains of pain in the first three fingers of her right hand over the past 6 weeks. The pain seems especially severe at night, often awakening her from her sleep.

16.23. The more likely cause of this patient's complaint is
  A. atlantoaxial subluxation of the cervical spine
  B. sensory peripheral neuropathy
  C. carpal tunnel syndrome
  D. DeQuervain's tenosynovitis
  E. rheumatoid vasculitis

Question 16.24: A healthy 50-year-old white man awakens suddenly from sleep with painful swelling of the first right metatarsophalangeal joint. Physical examination reveals the joint to be hot, swollen, and very tender.

16.24. The most useful diagnostic test or maneuver is
  A. radiograph of the involved joint
  B. joint aspiration
  C. CBC with peripheral smear
  D. serum uric acid level
  E. blood cultures

16.25. A 24-year-old white woman presents to her physician's office with a 3-week history of painful swelling of the knees and ankles. She has been previously healthy and denies the use of any medications except acetaminophen for her recent joint pain. Examination reveals small knee and ankle effusions and slightly raised, very tender, purplish nodules on the anterior legs. The most likely diagnosis of this patient's condition is

    A. rheumatoid arthritis
    B. acute rheumatic fever
    C. Lofgren's syndrome
    D. acute gouty arthritis
    E. viral arthritis

Answers and Comments

16.1. **(E)** Two of the major causes of acute monarticular arthritis are crystal disease (gout and pseudogout) and bacterial arthritis. Even a single drop of synovial fluid can be examined first for crystals as a wet mount and then allowed to dry for Gram staining. The Gram stain is essential to begin appropriate antibiotic treatment in bacterial arthritis. Clearly, early treatment of bacterial arthritis is essential to guarantee the best long-term results; failure to institute antibiotic treatment early may lead to irreversible destruction of the joint (Ref. 1, pp. 388−391).

16.2. **(D)** The fibrositis syndrome is characterized by widespread pain or aching of more than 3 months duration, disturbed sleep with significant complaints of morning stiffness and fatigue, and localized areas of tenderness in the cervical and upper scapular region. Soft tissue joint swelling is not seen in this syndrome, and when encountered must make one consider the various forms of inflammatory arthritis (Ref. 1, pp. 488−490).

16.3. **(B)** Pleural effusions are unusual in scleroderma. Pulmonary function abnormalities occur in at least two-thirds of these patients with restrictive ventilatory defects being most common. Esophageal dysfunction occurs in 90% of patients, and 95% of scleroderma patients have Raynaud's phenomenon. Articular complaints are common, and synovitis mimicking rheumatoid arthritis is often the first manifestation of the disease (Ref. 3, pp. 994—1036).

16.4. **(D)** *Neisseria gonorrhoeae* is responsible for the overwhelming proportion of septic arthritis in adults (Ref. 1, p. 1560).

16.5. **(C)** Ankylosing spondylitis classically affects adolescent or young adult males. Careful study has made it clear that this disease has its onset before age 40 (Ref. 2, pp. 621—622).

16.6. **(E)** Patients with MCTD have high titer antibody levels to the antigen ribonucleoprotein (RNP). Antibodies to SS-A, SS-B, Sm, and DNA are usually not seen in these patients (Ref. 4, p. 1117).

16.7. **(B)** Acute attacks of gout most commonly involve the first metatarsophalangeal joint. Other frequent sites of initial attack are the ankle, wrist, and elbow. Acute attacks very rarely involve the shoulder (Ref. 2, p. 1197).

16.8. **(C)** Subcutaneous calcifications are noted in scleroderma and polymyositis, but not in Sjögren's syndrome (Ref. 2, pp. 797, 811—813).

16.9. **(E)** Parenterally administered antibiotics achieve concentrations in synovial fluid that are many times greater than the minimal inhibitory concentration necessary for most bacteria invading joints. Intraarticular administration of antibiotics is therefore unnecessary. More importantly this practice may produce a chemical synovitis and introduces the risk of another infecting organism (Ref. 1, pp. 1564—1567).

16.10. **(D)** Malaise and fatigue are characteristic of inflammatory joint disease (i.e., rheumatoid arthritis) but not of osteoarthritis. Joint stiffness in osteoarthritis is short lived (30 min) and is better referred to as gelling. Osteoarthritic joint pain worsens with use and disappears with rest; pain that occurs at rest indicates far advanced osteoarthritis. Inflammatory joint pain subsides somewhat with rest but does not resolve. The course of osteoarthritis is one of very gradual worsening over time (Ref. 1, pp. 393—395).

16.11. (A) An acute inflammatory attack of cartilage may be brought under complete control with prednisone in daily dosages ranging from 20 to 60 mg (Ref. 2, p. 877).

16.12. (B) Antimalarial drugs are very effective treatment for discoid skin lesions. Systemic corticosteroids can be effective, but they usually require such large doses that it is impractical to treat these lesions in this fashion (Ref. 1, p. 1136).

16.13. (A) High dose corticosteroids are very effective treatment for giant cell arteritis. It is customary to use 60 mg of prednisone daily for 1 month, and then taper the dose while following the erythrocyte sedimentation rate (Ref. 2, p. 683).

16.14. (C) The most extensive experience with cytotoxic agents in the treatment of Wegener's granulomatosis has been with cyclophosphamide, and the majority of patients can undergo clinical remission with this agent. Treatment with corticosteroids is rarely beneficial, though they may help to control the systemic features of this disease. Hydroxychloroquine has not been used to treat this disease (Ref. 1, pp. 1176–1177).

16.15. (C)
16.16. (A)
16.17. (A) The peripheral antinuclear antibody (ANA) pattern has been shown to be produced by antibodies to native (or double-stranded) DNA, and is almost exclusively seen in patients with SLE. The speckled pattern results from the interaction of antibody with nuclear material which can be extracted with saline. This nuclear material consists of a number of antigens, collectively referred to as extractable nuclear antigens (ENA). The speckled antinuclear antibody pattern is seen in many chronic rheumatic diseases including SLE, rheumatoid arthritis, scleroderma, mixed connective tissue disease, and polymyositis (Ref. 1, pp. 691–706).

16.18. (D) Painless, superficial erosions on the glans penis in patients with Reiter's syndrome are referred to as circinate balanitis. Gottron's papules are characteristic skin lesions of dermatomyositis. Erythema chronicum migrans is the classic skin lesion of Lyme arthritis. Erythema elevatum diutinum is characterized by reddened papules and nodules, but is not seen in Reiter's syndrome (Ref. 1, pp. 543, 1038–1039, 1596).

16.19. **(E)** Blindness is usually caused by ischemia of the optic nerve secondary to arteritis of the ophthalmic or posterior ciliary arteries. Myocardial infarction and congestive heart failure may rarely occur secondary to coronary arteritis. Large artery involvement may result in aortic dissection and rupture (Ref. 1, pp. 1191– 1192).

16.20. **(A)** The boutonniere deformity is seen in rheumatoid arthritis and is characterized by flexion of the proximal interphalangeal joint and hyperextension of the distal interphalangeal joint. Bony enlargement of the proximal interphalangeal joint (Bouchard's node), lateral deviation of the first metatarsophalangeal joint (hallux valgus), and predominant cartilage loss in the medial compartment of the knee (genu varus) are cardinal clinical findings of osteoarthritis (Ref. 1, pp. 946, 1479).

16.21. **(C)** One typically sees a symmetric polyarticular arthritis in SLE. Deformities, however, are unusual. Approximately 10% of patients develop swan neck deformities and ulnar deviation of the metacarpophalangeal joints. Radiographs of hands and feet reveal absence of bony erosions (Ref. 2, pp. 696–699).

16.22. **(D)** The patient's primary clinical manifestation is muscle weakness. Polymyositis merits strong consideration and must be differentiated from trichinosis, hypothyroid myopathy, and myasthenia gravis by appropriate examinations. Muscle strength is generally unimpaired in polymyalgia rheumatica, but pain with movement may make objective assessment of muscle strength difficult. Polymyalgia rheumatica only rarely presents before age 50 (Ref. 1, pp. 1192, 1263–1264).

16.23. **(C)** The patient's complaints are classic for carpal tunnel syndrome. Tenosynovitis in the enclosed flexor compartment of the wrist may result in compression of the nearby median nerve as illustrated in Figures 44 and 45. Symptoms may be reproduced by percussion at the volar surface of the wrist (Ref. 2, p. 995).

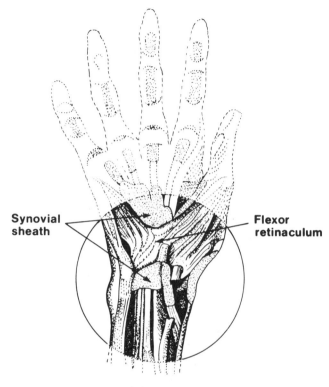

Synovial sheath

Flexor retinaculum

Figure 44

16.24. **(B)** The patient suffers from a classic attack of acute gouty arthritis. Joint aspiration is mandatory. Inspection of synovial fluid under polarized microscopy will reveal the strongly negatively birefringent crystals of monosodium urate and establish the diagnosis of gout with absolute certainty (Ref. 1, pp. 388–391).

16.25. **(C)** The leg nodules described are erythema nodosum. The presence of these lesions in combination with inflammation in the knees and ankles is typical of acute sarcoid arthritis. A chest x-ray would likely reveal bilateral hilar adenopathy. Lofgren's syndrome is the triad of erythema nodosum, bilateral hilar adenopathy, and arthritis.

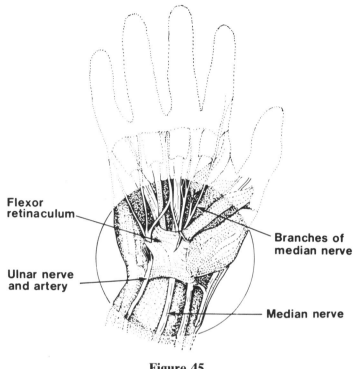

Flexor retinaculum

Ulnar nerve and artery

Branches of median nerve

Median nerve

Figure 45

The nodules, which appear in rheumatoid arthritis, acute rheumatic fever, and gouty arthritis, are nontender. Though one might suspect rheumatoid arthritis in a young woman with 3 weeks of joint inflammation, a minimum of 6 weeks is necessary before this diagnosis can be made. Acute gouty arthritis occurs only rarely in premenopausal women. One must always consider the possibility of viral arthritis in patients presenting with joint inflammation of less than 4 weeks' duration, however, other types of skin lesions than that described are found (Ref. 3, p. 1128).

References

1. Kelley, W.N., Harris E.D., Ruddy, S., and Sledge, C.B.: *Textbook of Rheumatology*, W.B. Saunders, Philadelphia, 1981.

2. McCarty, D.J.: *Arthritis and Allied Conditions*, 9th Ed., Lea & Febiger, Philadelphia, 1979.

3. McCarty, D.J.: *Arthritis and Allied Conditions*, 10th Ed., Lea and Febiger, Philadelphia, 1985.

4. Kelley, W.N., Harris, E.D., Ruddy, S., and Sledge, C.B.: *Textbook of Rheumatology*, 2nd Ed., W.B. Saunders, Philadelphia, 1985.

PEDIATRICS

17

Pediatric Allergy and Immunology

R. Michael Sly, M.D.

DIRECTIONS: Each of the questions or incomplete statements below is followed by five suggested answers or completions. Select the **one** that is best in each case.

17.1. Digital clubbing is LEAST likely to be found in a child with which of the following?

    A. Asthma
    B. Bronchiectasis
    C. Cyanotic congenital heart disease
    D. Cystic fibrosis (mucoviscidosis)
    E. Lung abscess

17.2. Appropriate management of a 10-year-old child who had generalized urticaria 4 days ago after having been stung by a honey bee should include
  A. immediate allergy skin testing with bee venom
  B. immunotherapy
  C. hydroxyzine for immediate administration after any subsequent stings
  D. epinephrine for subcutaneous injection for any life-threatening reaction that may follow subsequent stings
  E. prescription for albuterol metered dose inhaler for emergency use

17.3. Optimal response to treatment with theophylline without signs or symptoms of toxicity is most likely at serum concentrations of
  A. 10−20 mg/ml
  B. 2−5 μg/ml
  C. 10−15 μg/ml
  D. 20−30 μg/ml
  E. 30−40 μg/ml

DIRECTIONS: The group of questions below consists of five lettered headings followed by a list of numbered words or statements. For each numbered word or statement, select the **one** lettered heading that is most closely associated with it. Each lettered heading may be selected once, more than once, or not at all.

  A. Vascular ring
  B. Bronchiectasis
  C. Atelectasis of the right middle lobe
  D. Asthma
  E. Foreign body in left mainstem bronchus

17.4. Shift of mediastinum to right on expiration

17.5. Generalized hyperinflation

17.6. Obliteration of right cardiac border

DIRECTIONS: For each of the questions or incomplete statements below, **one or more** of the answers or completions given is correct. Select
(A) if only 1, 2, and 3 are correct
(B) if only 1 and 3 are correct
(C) if only 2 and 4 are correct
(D) if only 4 is correct
(E) if all are correct

17.7. Common causes of airway obstruction in asthmatics include
  1. running
  2. inhalation of cold air
  3. viral respiratory infections
  4. bacterial infections

17.8. Drugs of well-established efficacy in the treatment of asthma include
  1. β-agonists
  2. methyl xanthines
  3. adrenal corticosteroids
  4. antihistamines

DIRECTIONS: This section of the test consists of a situation followed by a series of questions. Study the situation and select the **one** best answer to each question following it.

Questions 17.9–17.10: The 6-year-old boy in Figure 46 has a 3-year history of perennial clear, watery nasal discharge with frequent paroxysmal sneezing and persistent nasal itching. He sleeps on a feather pillow and shares his bed with his dog, acquired 4 years ago. There is a large oak tree outside his bedroom window, and a vacant lot next door is overgrown with weeds. He drinks approximately 1 quart of chocolate milk each day. He has always resided in New York. Allergy skin testing discloses 4+ reactions to feathers, dog dander, and house dust and negative reactions to pollen extracts, including oak and ragweed.

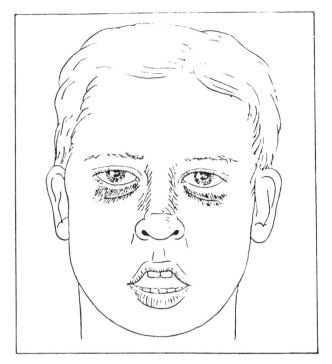

Figure 46

17.9. The measures most likely to be beneficial include
  A. elimination of milk and chocolate from the diet
  B. adenoidectomy and tonsillectomy
  C. elimination of the dog and feather pillow from the house
  D. moving to Arizona
  E. allergy injections with dog dander and feather extract

17.10. Common complications of this disorder include
  A. cor pulmonale
  B. nasal polyposis
  C. hyperimmunoglobulin E syndrome
  D. epistaxis
  E. none of the above

Answers and Comments

17.1. (A) The disease most commonly associated with digital clubbing in children in the U.S. is probably cyanotic congenital heart disease. The most common pulmonary cause is bronchiectasis, usually due to cystic fibrosis in white children. Other pulmonary causes include empyema and lung abscesses. Even minimal digital clubbing occurs only very rarely in children with uncomplicated asthma (Ref. 1, pp. 58–60).

17.2. (D) Immunotherapy is indicated for patients who have had life-threatening systemic reactions to *Hymenoptera* venom and who also have positive skin tests to venom. Patients whose only manifestation of allergy has been generalized urticaria do not frequently have life-threatening reactions after subsequent stings. Because of the refractory period that may follow systemic anaphylaxis, allergy skin testing should be deferred 2–4 weeks to avoid false-negative reactions to testing. Patients who have had systemic reactions should keep 1:1000 aqueous epinephrine on hand for subcutaneous injection in case a life-threatening systemic reaction should follow a subsequent sting. Hydroxyzine is effective for treating urticaria, but much less important than epinephrine for the treatment of more serious reactions. Inhaled β-agonist drugs are much less effective than 1:1000 aqueous epinephrine by subcutaneous injection in the treatment of systemic anaphylaxis (Ref. 1, pp. 286, 287; 2, p. 687).

17.3. (C) Both toxic symptoms and therapeutic response correlate closely with serum concentrations of theophylline. Most patients require concentrations of at least 10 µg/ml for optimal bronchodilation and most experience toxic symptoms at concentrations that exceed 20 µg/ml (Ref. 1, p. 111).

17.4. (E) When a bronchial foreign body forms a check valve, permitting inflation but preventing deflation of a lung or lobe, comparison of inspiratory and expiratory roentgenograms of the chest is helpful in identifying the location of the obstruction. The obstructed lung or lobe remains hyperinflated after expiration, causing shift of the mediastinum to the opposite side (Ref. 1, p. 86).

17.5. **(D)** Chest roentgenograms during acute asthma typically disclose evidence of hyperinflation: hyperlucency, depression of the diaphragm, increase in the anteroposterior diameter of the chest, and an increase in the size of the retrosternal radiolucency evident on the lateral view (Ref. 1, p. 78).

17.6. **(C)** Roentgenographic evidence of atelectasis of the right middle lobe includes obliteration of the right cardiac border on the PA view, inferior displacement of the right hilum, and inferior displacement of the horizontal fissure (Ref. 1, p. 81).

17.7. **(A)** Vigorous exercise for several minutes while inhaling cold, dry air through the mouth can cause airway obstruction in most asthmatics. Inhalation of cold air can cause bronchoconstriction in many asthmatics even without exercise. Viral respiratory infections are among the most common triggers of bronchoconstriction in children with asthma, but bacterial infection rarely if ever causes bronchoconstriction in asthmatics (Ref. 1, pp. 48–52).

17.8. **(A)** Beta agonists, methyl xanthines such as theophylline, and adrenal corticosteroids are all of established efficacy in the treatment of asthma. Antihistamines have not been found helpful in the treatment of most asthmatics despite their effectiveness in the treatment of allergic rhinitis (Ref. 1, pp. 98–116, 119, 128).

17.9. **(C)** The history and physical findings of allergic "shiners," transverse nasal crease, Dennie's lines, and mouth breathing are typical of perennial allergic rhinitis. The history and results of allergy skin testing indicate allergy to feathers and dog dander, for which elimination of exposure is the most effective treatment. Immunotherapy with neither dog dander nor feather extract has been shown to be effective. Although food allergy can cause allergic rhinitis, this is not a likely cause after the first few years of life, and with the correlation between the positive skin tests to inhalants and the history, further testing with food extracts would not be indicated. Tonsillectomy and adenoidectomy might provide some temporary partial relief of obstruction, but regression of these tissues is likely, and avoidance of the offending allergens may relieve most of the symptoms (Refs. 1, pp. 169–174, 178, 249; 2, p. 524).

17.10. **(D)** Epistaxis is a common complication of allergic rhinitis, probably because of frequent rubbing and scratching of the congested nasal mucosa. Cor pulmonale and nasal polyposis are rare complications of allergic rhinitis. Nasal polyposis occurs in children more often as a complication of cystic fibrosis. Some increase in the total serum IgE concentration occurs in some patients with allergic rhinitis, but the hyperimmunoglobulinemia E syndrome is characterized by chronic dermatitis and recurrent staphylococcal abscesses. Although some of these patients also have allergic rhinitis, there is no evidence that the hyperimmunoglobulin E syndrome occurs as a complication of allergic rhinitis (Refs. 1, p. 178; 2, p. 111).

References

1. Sly, R.M.: *Textbook of Pediatric Allergy*, Medical Examination Publishing, New York, 1985.

2. Bierman, C.W. and Pearlman, D.S. (eds.): *Allergic Diseases of Infancy, Childhood and Adolescence*, W.B. Saunders, Philadelphia, 1980.

18

Pediatric Cardiology
John W. Downing, Jr., M.D., F.A.C.C.

DIRECTIONS: Each of the questions or incomplete statements below is followed by five suggested answers or completions. Select the **one** that is best in each case.

18.1. Which of the following vessels carries highly oxygenated blood from the placenta toward the heart?
  A. Coronary artery
  B. Umbilical artery
  C. Inferior vena cava
  D. Umbilical vein
  E. Ductus arteriosus

18.2. Which of the following closes first after birth?
  A. Ductus arteriosus
  B. Foramen ovale
  C. Ductus venosus
  D. Foramen magnum
  E. Azygous vein

18.3. Cyanotic congenital heart lesions include all of the following EXCEPT
   A. transposition of the great vessels
   B. tetralogy of Fallot
   C. isolated ventricular septal defect
   D. tricuspid atresia
   E. pulmonary atresia with intact ventricular septum

DIRECTIONS: The group of questions below consists of five lettered headings followed by a list of numbered words or statements. For each numbered word or statement, select the **one** lettered heading that is most closely associated with it. Each lettered heading may be selected once, more than once, or not at all.

   A. Atrial septal defect
   B. Innocent murmur
   C. Pulmonary valvular stenosis
   D. Mitral stenosis
   E. Patent ductus arteriosus

18.4. Harsh ejection systolic murmur preceded by an ejection click which varies with respiration and is associated with a thrill

18.5. Fixed splitting of the second heart sound

18.6. Low-pitched, vibratory systolic murmur

DIRECTIONS: For each of the questions or incomplete statements below, **one or more** of the answers or completions given is correct. Select
- **(A)** if only 1, 2, and 3 are correct
- **(B)** if only 1 and 3 are correct
- **(C)** if only 2 and 4 are correct
- **(D)** if only 4 is correct
- **(E)** if all are correct

18.7. An innocent murmur is best described as
1. low-pitched, vibratory
2. diastolic
3. grade 3/6 or less in intensity
4. associated with fixed splitting of the second heart sound

18.8. Patent ductus arteriosus is associated with which of the following?
1. Bounding peripheral pulses
2. Commonly seen in premature infants
3. Continuous murmur at pulmonary area
4. May be managed medically by the use of indomethacin

DIRECTIONS: This section of the test consists of a situation followed by a series of questions. Study the situation and select the **one** best answer to each question following it.

Questions 18.9–18.10: A 2-month-old male infant, born full term without complications, was well until 4 weeks of age when he became tachypneic, had difficulty in feeding, and a loud pansystolic murmur was noted at the lower left sternal border. Also, an apical middiastolic rumble was heard. The chest x-ray taken at that time is shown in Figure 47 and the electrocardiogram is seen in Figure 48.

18.9. The congenital heart lesion that is most likely present in this patient is
- **A.** atrial septal defect
- **B.** hypoplastic left heart syndrome
- **C.** transposition of the great vessels
- **D.** pulmonary valvular stenosis
- **E.** ventricular septal defect

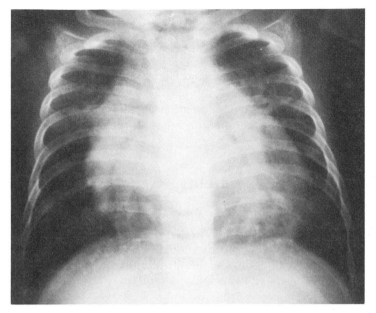

Figure 47

Figure 48

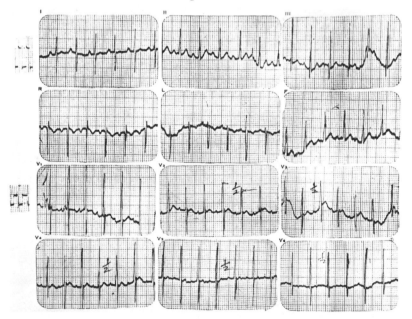

18.10. The best explanation for the change in the status of this patient since birth is
  A. the congenital heart defect has enlarged
  B. he developed pneumonia
  C. there was a significant fall in pulmonary vascular resistance
  D. he has developed acute bronchiolitis
  E. he is shunting right to left through an atrial septal defect

Answers and Comments

18.1. **(D)** The placenta is the major route of gas exchange in the fetus. Highly oxygenated blood leaves the placenta via the umbilical vein and subsequently joins the blood of low saturation returning from the lower half of the body in the inferior vena cava (Ref. 1, p. 11).

18.2. **(B)** Immediately after delivery as the infant takes his first breath, there is a rapid fall in pulmonary vascular resistance and an increase in pulmonary blood flow. This increases pulmonary venous return to the left atrium, which raises left atrial pressure and closes the foramen ovale (Ref. 1, pp. 13–14).

18.3. **(C)** Isolated ventricular septal defect is not normally a cause of cyanosis because it results in a left-to-right shunt, which increases pulmonary blood flow, and the systemic oxygen saturation is normal. In the other lesions, cyanosis results from right to left shunting with blood of decreased oxygen saturation in the systemic arterial circulation (Ref. 2, pp. 29, 154, 166, 212, 342).

18.4. **(C)** The striking feature of valvular pulmonary stenosis is a harsh, loud ejection systolic murmur with maximal intensity at the second and third left intercostal spaces. It is usually associated with a systolic thrill at the same area where the murmur is best noted. In mild to moderate valvular stenosis, the murmur is preceded by an ejection click at the upper left sternal border, where it is louder on expiration (Ref. 1, pp. 235–236).

18.5. (A) Persistent splitting of the second heart sound is a hallmark of atrial septal defect. This results from the delayed pulmonary valve closure due to the prolonged emptying time of the volume-overloaded right ventricle (Ref. 2, p. 8).

18.6. (B) Several phonocardiographic studies of murmurs in normal children have shown that most fall in the frequency range of 90–250 cycles/sec. The majority were located at the pulmonary area, with less incidence at the lower left sternal border and apex (Ref. 3, pp. 107–108).

18.7. (B) Innocent murmurs generally are not loud, usually less than grade 3 (of 6). They are also low pitched. Those best heard at the midprecordium generally are of a characteristic vibratory or buzzing acoustic quality. Those at the pulmonary area are usually more humming or blowing in quality (Ref. 3, pp. 88–100).

18.8. (E) The presence of a patent ductus arteriosus usually results in a run-off of blood from the aorta into the pulmonary artery during systole and diastole. Thus, a continuous murmur generally is heard at the pulmonary area. The pattern of blood flow in this condition causes a widening of the pulse pressure, resulting in bounding peripheral pulses. In addition to surgical closure, the ductus arteriosus may be closed pharmacologically in premature infants by either oral or parenteral indomethacin, a prostaglandin inhibitor (Refs. 4, pp. 177–178; 5, pp. 307–308).

18.9. (E) The chest x-ray demonstrates cardiomegaly and increased pulmonary vascularity indicative of a left-to-right shunt, and the electrocardiogram shows biventricular hypertrophy. These are associated with the pansystolic murmur at the lower left sternal border and apical middiastolic murmur, which are typical of a moderate to large ventricular septal defect. These findings are not usually noted in any of the other lesions listed (Ref. 1, pp. 147–153).

18.10. (C) The tachypnea in this patient is indicative of congestive heart failure. The onset of tachypnea and tiring on feeding usually begins during the latter part of the first month of life as pulmonary vascular resistance falls substantially, resulting in a marked increase in pulmonary blood flow and overloading of the left heart, leading to congestive heart failure (Ref. 1, pp. 146–147).

References

1. Moss, A.J., Adams, F.H., and Emmanouilides, G.C.: *Heart Disease in Infants, Children and Adolescents*, 2nd Ed., Williams and Wilkins, Baltimore, 1977.

2. Downing, J.W., Jr. and James, F.W.: *Pediatric Cardiology Case Studies*, Medical Examination Publishing, New York, 1981.

3. Cacares, C.A. and Perry, L.W.: *The Innocent Murmur*, Little, Brown, Boston, 1967.

4. Rudolph, A.M.: *Congenital Diseases of the Heart*, Year Book Medical Publishers, Chicago, 1974.

5. Heymann, M.A. and Rudolph, A.M.: Neonatal manipulation: Patent ductus arteriosus. In *Pediatric Cardiovascular Disease*, Engle, M.A., (Ed.), F.A. Davis, Philadelphia, 1981.

19

Pediatric Dermatology
William P. Coleman III, M.D.

DIRECTIONS: Each of the questions or incomplete statements below is followed by five suggested answers or completions. Select the **one** that is best in each case.

19.1. Which of the following treatments is NOT appropriate for verruca plantaris (plantar wart)?
  A. Cryosurgery
  B. Keratolytic agents
  C. Excision and repair
  D. Cantharidin
  E. Laser photocoagulation

19.2. Often found in children, which of the following diseases is characterized by myalgia, calcinosis, poikilodermatous skin rashes, and periorbital edema (Figure 49)?
  A. Dermatomyositis
  B. Lupus erythematosus
  C. Scleroderma
  D. Mixed connective tissue disease
  E. Still's disease

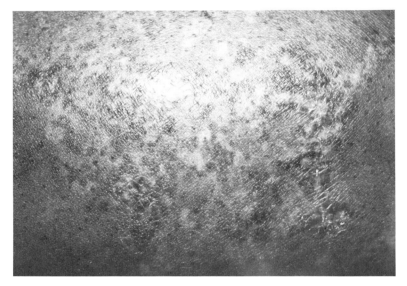

Figure 49

19.3. Which of the following is NOT a precusor of melanoma?
   A. Blue nevus
   B. Halo nevus
   C. Congenital compound nevus
   D. Hutchinson's freckle
   E. None of the above

DIRECTIONS: For each of the questions or incomplete statements below, **one or more** of the answers or completions given is correct. Select
- **(A)** if only 1, 2, and 3 are correct
- **(B)** if only 1 and 3 are correct
- **(C)** if only 2 and 4 are correct
- **(D)** if only 4 is correct
- **(E)** if all are correct

19.4. Which of the following drugs is useful for treating tinea versicolor?
1. Miconazole
2. Selenium sulfide
3. Clotrimazole
4. Griseofulvin

19.5. Which of the following skin parasites are too small to be visible to the human eye?
1. *Pediculus humanis capitis*
2. *Pediculus humanis corporis*
3. *Phthirus pubis*
4. *Sarcoptes scabiei*

Answers and Comments

19.1. (C) Verrucae (warts) are viral infections. Various destructive modalities may be used to effectively treat these lesions. These include the application of keratolytic agents, liquid nitrogen (cryosurgery), superficial electrosurgery, caustic agents (trichloroacetic acid), cantharidin (a cytotoxic substance), immunotherapy, and laser photocoagulation. All of these treatments must be used carefully to avoid the production of scars. Excision and repair provides a poorer cure rate for warts than any of the previously mentioned treatments and *always* produces a scar. Scars on the plantar surfaces of the feet may be painful and are permanent (Ref. 1, pp. 148–160).

19.2. (A) Dermatomyositis is the collagen disease seen most commonly in children. Calcinosis especially dominates the clinical picture in patients under 15. The prognosis is extremely poor (Ref. 2, pp. 188–190).

19.3. (E) All of the listed lesions can develop into malignant melanoma. The blue nevus is a black or dark blue mole which either appears at birth or is acquired. The halo nevus is a mole which suddenly develops a hyperpigmented ring around it. The congenital nevi, especially larger ones, have an increased risk of developing melanoma. The Hutchinson's freckle or lentigo maligna is a slow-growing, flat pigmented lesion which gradually develops into melanoma (Refs. 1, pp. 431–437; 2, pp. 862–880).

19.4. (A) Tinea versicolor, unlike other superficial fungal infections, is not responsive to oral griseofulvin. A wide variety of topical antifungal agents are effective (Ref. 1, pp. 126–127).

19.5. (D) Choices 1, 2, and 3 are head, body, and pubic lice, respectively. These mobile parasites are easily visible (1–3 mm in size). The scabies mite is microscopic (0.2–0.4 mm) (Ref. 2, pp. 554–557, 566–570).

References

1. Coleman, W.P., III and McBurney, E.I.: *Pediatric Dermatology: New Directions in Therapy*, Medical Examination Publishing, New York, 1981.

2. Domonkos, A.N., Arnold, H.L., and Odom, R.B.: *Andrew's Diseases of the Skin*, W.B. Saunders, Philadelphia, 1982.

20

Developmental and Behavioral Pediatrics

John E. Williams, M.D.

DIRECTIONS: Each of the questions or incomplete statements below is followed by five suggested answers or completions. Select the **one** that is best in each case.

20.1. When a full-term newborn is compared to a healthy infant who was born at 30 weeks' gestation but is now 10 weeks old (i.e., 40 weeks postconception), the premature infant should
  A. have more muscle tone
  B. be more active
  C. lie more flexed when prone
  D. have more head control
  E. have a more coordinated walking reflex

20.2. It has been found that psychogenic vomiting
  A. can be an aspect of school phobia
  B. is associated with enuresis and fire setting
  C. is a symptom of a pervasive developmental disorder
  D. is preceded by pica in infancy
  E. is related to a failure in the development of basic trust

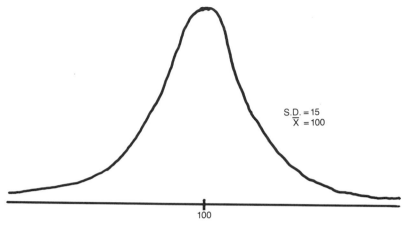

S.D. = 15
$\overline{X}$ = 100

100

Figure 50

20.3. Figure 50 illustrates the distribution of WISC-R Full Scale IQ scores for a random sample of 8-year-olds. What is the lowest score in the range of normal if 2.3% of the population is classified as mentally retarded?
   A. 55
   B. 60
   C. 65
   D. 70
   E. 75

DIRECTIONS: The group of questions below consists of five lettered headings followed by a list of numbered words or statements. For each numbered word or statement, select the **one** lettered heading that is most closely associated with it. Each lettered heading may be selected once, more than once, or not at all.

   A. 3 months
   B. 4 months
   C. 5 months
   D. 6 months
   E. 7 months

20.4. Passes cube from hand to hand

20.5. Follows objects through a 180° arc

20.6. Voluntarily grasps objects with a bidextrous approach and takes them to the mouth

---

DIRECTIONS: For each of the questions or incomplete statements below, **one or more** of the answers or completions given is correct. Select

   (A) if only 1, 2, and 3 are correct
   (B) if only 1 and 3 are correct
   (C) if only 2 and 4 are correct
   (D) if only 4 is correct
   (E) if all are correct

20.7. Late sequelae of the congenital rubella syndrome include
   1. progressive panencephalitis
   2. diabetes mellitus
   3. chronic renal disease
   4. thyroid disease

20.8. According to Erikson, the stages of psychosocial development include
   1. initiative versus guilt
   2. autonomy versus shame and doubt
   3. industry versus inferiority
   4. sensorimotor versus concrete operations

DIRECTIONS: This section of the test consists of a situation followed by a series of questions. Study the situation and select the **one** best answer to each question following it.

Questions 20.9–20.10: A 2-year, 11-month-old girl is brought to you by her mother with a complaint of poor speech. The perinatal history is significant in that the birth weight was 2450 g (36 weeks AGA), and an ABO incompatibility with jaundice was present. She walked at 11 months and began using words at 23 months. Presently she does not make sentences and people other than her immediate family members have difficulty understanding her. The physical and neurologic examinations are completely normal. You administer the Denver Developmental Screening Test and find several delays and no passes through the age line in the language area. As a part of your evaluation of children with speech language disorders, you refer this child to an audiologist who obtains the audiogram shown in Figure 51.

20.9. This audiogram indicates a/an
  A. conductive hearing loss
  B. sensorineural hearing loss
  C. cholesteatoma
  D. perinatal injury to the middle ear
  E. otosclerosis

Figure 51

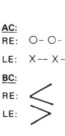

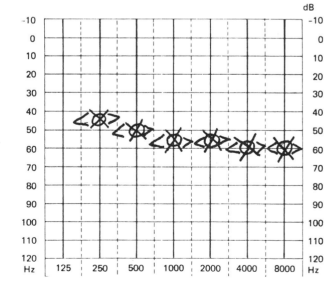

20.10. All of the following could be etiologies for this type of audiogram EXCEPT
  A. subclinical congenital cytomegalovirus infection
  B. otitis media
  C. ototoxicity
  D. hyperbilirubinemia
  E. genetic

Answers and Comments

20.1. (B) The prematurely born baby who has reached term is different from the term newborn infant in that the former has less muscle tone, less head control, a less rhythmic and coordinated walking reflex, lies with the extremities more extended when prone, and is more active (Ref. 1, pp. 104–105).

20.2. (A) Psychogenic vomiting may be a part of the school phobia picture. Although it can be a symptom of serious conflicts in the child or family, it is not a part of the enuresis/fire-setting syndrome or a symptom of pervasive developmental disorders (Ref. 2, p. 68).

20.3. (D) IQ scores follow a gaussian distribution in random populations. The standard deviation of the Wechsler Intelligence Scale for Children-Revised is 15. The 2.3 percentile (2.3% of the population) marks 2 S.D. below the mean of 100 and the threshold of the categories of mental subnormality, 70 (Ref. 2, p. 61).

20.4. (E)
20.5. (A)
20.6. (C) The development of binocular coordination and interest in objects in the visual field precedes manual coordination. The ability to track objects through a 180° arc occurs by 3 months. Bidextrous manipulation develops at 5 months and the ability to transfer a cube from hand to hand comes later, at 7 months (Ref. 1, pp. 150–152).

20.7. (E) The congenital rubella syndrome represents a chronic viral infection in utero. Viremia can persist long after birth with shedding of the virus in oral secretions and urine. Direct effects of the infection and antigenemia include progressive rubella panencephalitis, pancreatic infection with hypoinsulinism, chronic renal damage, and hypo- or hyperthyroidism (Ref. 2, pp. 631–636).

20.8. (A) According to Erikson, the stages of psychosocial development are: infancy—basic trust versus mistrust; toddler stage— autonomy versus shame and doubt; preschool stage—initiative versus guilt; school age—industry versus inferiority; adolescence— identity versus identity confusion; young adulthood—intimacy versus isolation; middle adulthood—generativity versus stagnation; late adulthood—integrity versus despair. Operational and sensorimotor cognitive processes are concepts in Piaget's theories of development (Ref. 2, pp. 51–52).

20.9. (B) The pattern on the audiogram indicates a moderate bilateral sensorineural hearing loss. A perinatal injury to the middle ear, cholesteatoma, and otosclerosis would cause a conductive hearing loss (Ref. 4, pp. 1–15).

20.10. (B) Frequently the etiology of sensorineural hearing loss is obscure and the true cause is determined by exclusion. Sensorineural hearing loss can be caused by all of those agents listed except otitis media (Ref. 4, pp. 43–75).

References

1. Illingworth, R.S.: *The Development of the Infant and Young Child, Normal and Abnormal*, 5th Ed., Churchill Livingstone, Edinburgh, London, and New York, 1976.

2. Rudolf, A.M. and Hoffman, J.I.E.: *Pediatrics*, 17th Ed., Appleton-Century-Crofts, New York, 1982.

3. The American Psychiatric Association: *Diagnostic and Statistical Manual of Mental Disorders*, 3rd Ed., American Psychiatric Association, Washington, D.C., 1980.

4. Northern, J.L. and Downs, M.P.: *Hearing in Children*, 2nd Ed., Williams and Wilkins, Baltimore, 1978.

21

Pediatric Drug Therapy
Raymond M. Russo, M.D., F.A.A.P.

DIRECTIONS: Each of the questions or incomplete statements below is followed by five suggested answers or completions. Select the **one** that is best in each case.

21.1. Which of the following are the only currently available antiasthmatic agents that can reverse the bronchodilator-unresponsive component of asthmatic airway obstruction?
- **A.** Intermittent positive-pressure breathing devices, metered-dose inhalers, or air-driven nebulizers
- **B.** Subcutaneous epinephrine
- **C.** β_2 agonists, such as terbutaline
- **D.** Round-the-clock maintenance of serum theophylline concentrations at levels within the $10-20$ mg/ml range
- **E.** Corticosteroids

21.2. Which of the following relaxes smooth muscle, inhibits insulin secretion, and has *no* diuretic activity?
- **A.** Hydralazine (Apresoline)
- **B.** Diazoxide (Hypostat)
- **C.** Sodium nitroprusside (Nipride)
- **D.** Minoxidil (Loniten)
- **E.** Prazosin (Minipress)

21.3. Which of the following may produce these symptoms: "gray syndrome," reversible bone marrow suppression, and "idiosyncratic" aplastic anemia?

    A. 1000 mg/day quinidine in conjunction with 100% normal digoxin dose

    B. 1000 mg/day quinidine in conjunction with 50% normal digoxin dose

    C. 25 mg/kg/day chloramphenicol

    D. 100−200 mg/kg/day chloramphenicol

    E. 16−20 mg/kg phenobarbital

DIRECTIONS: The group of questions below consists of five lettered headings followed by a list of numbered words or statements. For each numbered word or statement, select the **one** lettered heading that is most closely associated with it. Each lettered heading may be selected once, more than once, or not at all.

For questions 21.4−21.6, refer to Figure 52.

    A. Treatment by chemotherapy alone

    B. Treatment by laser therapy

    C. Treatment by radiation alone

    D. Treatment by a combination of chemotherapy and irradiation

    E. Treatment by radical surgery

21.4. Stages I and II Hodgkin's disease

21.5. Stage III Hodgkin's disease

21.6. Stage IV Hodgkin's disease

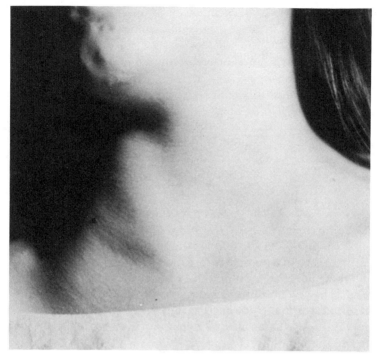

Figure 52

DIRECTIONS: For each of the questions or incomplete statements below, **one or more** of the answers or completions given is correct. Select
  (A) if only 1, 2, and 3 are correct
  (B) if only 1 and 3 are correct
  (C) if only 2 and 4 are correct
  (D) if only 4 is correct
  (E) if all are correct

21.7. Rifampin has been recommended as a prophylactic antibiotic to intimate contacts of patients diagnosed to have the following illnesses:
   1. tuberculous meningitis
   2. meningococcal meningitis
   3. pneumococcal meningitis
   4. *Hemophilus influenzae* meningitis

21.8. Which specific binding antibodies can reverse or prevent toxicity produced by digoxin or digitoxin overdose?
1. Furosemide
2. Gamma globulin or specific immunoglobulin (IgG)
3. Fc elements
4. F(ab') 2 fragments

DIRECTIONS: This section of the test consists of a situation followed by a series of questions. Study the situation and select the **one** best answer to each question following it.

Questions 21.9−21.10: A 6-month-old infant is brought to your office for his first well-baby visit. The child was noted to have a cleft lip at birth and to be small for gestational age. Your office nurse's measurements of length indicate that the baby's growth rate is below normal. The mother tells you that the child has not yet smiled, and you note that he does not follow light with his eyes. Other features make you increasingly concerned. He has a short nose with a low nasal bridge, hypertelorism, ptosis, and a heart murmur (Figure 53).

Figure 53

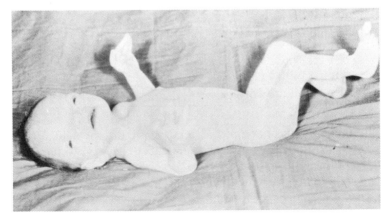

21.9. In making a diagnosis, further questioning is most likely to be helpful in which of the following areas?
  A. The infant's nutritional history
  B. Maternal medication history
  C. The history of present illness
  D. The history of past illness
  E. The social history

21.10. The most likely diagnosis is
  A. fetal hydantoin syndrome
  B. mitral valve prolapse
  C. trisomy 13−15
  D. Torch syndrome
  E. Waardenburg's syndrome

Answers and Comments

21.1. (E) Intermittent positive-pressure machines (bird or Bennet) are about as effective as metered-dose inhalers or air-driven nebulizers. None of these methods, used alone, are likely to be effective in the bronchodilator-resistant asthmatic. Subcutaneous epinephrine is an excellent bronchodilator for initial therapy. However, it is useless to continue treatment with epinephrine if prompt bronchodilation does not occur after three subcutaneous injections. In the bronchodilator-resistant patient, epinephrine cannot be relied upon to work. Terbutaline, theophylline, and other β_2 agonists are bronchodilators. An asthmatic who is bronchodilator-resistant to one of these drugs is likely to be resistant to the others. The corticosteroid drugs are the treatment of choice for reversing the unresponsive asthmatic's bronchoconstriction (Ref. 1, pp. 47−75).

21.2. (B) Diazoxide relaxes smooth muscle and inhibits insulin secretion. It has no diuretic effect whatsoever, unlike older antihypertensive agents. Diazoxide relaxes vascular, uterine, and urethral smooth muscle as well. Hydralazine is a smooth muscle relaxant affecting arteriolar muscle primarily. Sodium nitroprusside affects venules and arterioles, minoxidil causes arteriolar vasodilation, and prazosin reduces peripheral vascular tone. None of these have significant insulin inhibiting effects (Ref. 2, pp. 135−144).

21.3. (D) The only drug listed that has been known to cause all the effects listed is the antibiotic chloramphenicol. Quinidine has cardiac effects but will not cause gray syndrome, nor will phenobarbital or digoxin. Chloramphenicol is a bacteriostatic antibiotic with bacteriocidal action against *H. influenzae* and *N. meningitidis* and has been known to cause fatal aplastic anemia in children and adults. It can produce a more benign reversible bone marrow suppression as well. The gray syndrome primarily occurs in newborns who are given an older child's dosage of 100 mg/kg/day or more. Doses in the 25 mg/kg/day range are still effective and are not known to cause the gray syndrome (Ref. 3, pp. 195−202).

21.4. (C) Stages I and II Hodgkin's disease are routinely treated with radiation therapy only. Radiation is directed to clinically evident lesions (involved field) and/or contiguous lymphatics (extended field). This therapy is very effective, providing the staging has been accurate (by laparoscopy); some 96−98% survive 3 or more years (Ref. 4, pp. 145−160).

21.5. (D) Stage III Hodgkin's disease, defined as involvement of lymph nodes on both sides of the diaphragm, is treated with both chemotherapy and radiation. The outcome, if complete remission is achieved, is good; the 5-year survival rate is close to 90% (Ref. 4, pp. 145−160).

21.6. (A) Stage IV Hodgkin's disease, when the illness involves one or more extralymphatic organs (liver, lung, etc.), is managed with chemotherapy alone. Combination therapy with vincristine, prednisone, nitrogen mustard, and procarbazine is used initially. The cure rate approaches 40% (Ref. 4, pp. 145−160).

21.7. (C) Although rifampin has been used in the treatment of tuberculosis, it is not recommended as a prophylactic agent in this illness. It does serve as a prophylactic agent in both meningococcal and *H. influenzae* meningitis (Ref. 5, pp. 159 and 174).

21.8. (C) It seems odd to use a binding antibody in treating drug intoxication; yet gamma globulin, specific immunoglobulin (IgG), or F(ab')2 fragments derived from IgG all have the effect of reversing or preventing digoxin or digitoxin toxicity. The antibody apparently binds itself to the steroid portion of the digoxin or digitoxin molecule where myocardial receptors are also attached. In effect, then, the antibody performs as a blocking antibody (Ref. 6, pp. 203–216).

21.9. (B) Of course, all areas of the medical history may reveal important information useful in diagnosing or advising patients on health care. However, the most likely area to be of diagnostic help in this instance is a history of maternal medication. The findings here are indicative of an adverse prenatal influence affecting fetal development. Adverse influences are likely to be genetic, infections, interference with growth support mechanisms, or maternal medications. The description of present, past, nutritional, and social histories is not likely to explain the cleft lip, facial anomalies, and small size for gestational age (Ref. 7, pp. 179–194).

21.10. (A) The diagnosis that fits the clinical findings best is the fetal hydantoin syndrome. This condition can cause all of the findings described, in addition to cleft palate. Your suspicions would strengthened if the mother indicated she was receiving phenytoin (Dilantin) for a seizure disorder during the child's pregnancy. Mitral valve prolapse would not cause any but the cardiac findings described. The Torch syndrome causes small size for gestational age but not cleft lip or facial anomalies. Waardenburg's syndrome causes hypertelorism with a broad nasal root but not ptosis, cleft lip, or palate. Trisomy 13–15 can cause cleft lip or palate but not hypertelorism or ptosis (Ref. 7, pp. 179–194).

References

1. Weinberger, M., Hendeles, L., and Aherns, R.: Clinical pharmacology of drugs used for asthma. Pediatr. Cl. N. Am., 28, 1981.

2. Pruitt, A.W.: Pharmacologic approach to the management of childhood hypertension. Pediatr. Cl. N. Am., 28, 1981.

3. Dajani, A.S. and Kauffman, R.E.: The renaissance of chloramphenicol. Pediatr. Cl. N. Am., 28, 1981.

4. Smith, S.D.: Advances in the pharmacology of cancer chemotherapy. Pediatr. Cl. N. Am., 28, 1981.

5. Russo, R.M., Gururaj, V.J., and Freis, P.: *Practical Points in Pediatrics*, 4th Ed., Medical Examination Publishing Co., New York, 1986.

22

Pediatric Emergencies and Accidental Poisoning
Shirley K. Osterhout, M.D.

DIRECTIONS: Each of the questions or incomplete statements below is followed by five suggested answers or completions. Select the **one** that is best in each case.

22.1. The venom of which animal results in tissue ischemia progressing to a large area of necrosis and eschar formation?
  A. Black widow spider
  B. Southeastern tarantula
  C. Woolly slug
  D. Brown recluse spider
  E. Saddleback caterpillar

22.2. The approved antidote for toxicity of acetaminophen, which is primarily hepatotoxic, is acetylcysteine. The dose to treat toxicity is a

A. loading dose of 140 mg/kg p.o. within the first 24 hr followed by a maintenance dose of 70 mg/kg p.o. every 4 hours for a total of 17 doses

B. loading dose of 140 mg/kg IV within the first 24 hr followed by a maintenance dose of 70 mg/kg IV every 4 hr for a total of 17 doses

C. loading dose of 140 mg/kg p.o. no later than within the first 14 hr followed by a maintenance dose of 70 mg/kg p.o. every 4 hr for a total of 17 doses

D. loading dose of 140 mg/kg IV no later than with the first 14 hr followed by a maintenance dose of 70 mg/kg IV every 4 hr for a total of 17 doses

E. loading dose of 140 mg/kg IV within the first 24 hr followed by a maintenance dose of 70 mg/kg p.o. every 4 hr for a total of 17 doses

22.3. Repeated doses of activated charcoal orally can be highly effective in lowering the blood level in all EXCEPT the following

A. phenobarbital
B. diazepam
C. amitriptyline
D. theophylline
E. propranolol

DIRECTIONS: Each group of questions below consists of five lettered headings followed by a list of numbered words or statements. For each numbered word or statement, select the **one** lettered heading that is most closely associated with it. Each lettered heading may be selected once, more than once, or not at all.

    A. Naloxone
    B. Atropine
    C. Ethyl alcohol
    D. Physostigmine
    E. Deferoxamine

22.4. Ferrous sulfate

22.5. Ethylene glycol

22.6. Jimson weed

For each abnormality, indicate the most appropriate toxin.

    A. Methyl alcohol
    B. Phenytoin
    C. Tricyclic antidepressants
    D. Butyl nitrite
    E. Carbon monoxide

22.7. Abnormal electrocardiogram

22.8. Severe acidosis

22.9. Methemoglobinemia

For each toxin, indicate the most appropriate set of physical findings.

    A. Phenytoin
    B. Clonidine
    C. Hydrochloric acid
    D. Propanolol
    E. Sodium hydroxide

22.10. Miosis, decreased deep tendon reflexes, bradycardia

22.11. Edematous, soapy-appearing lips

22.12. Ataxia, nystagmus, mydriasis

DIRECTIONS: For each of the questions or incomplete statements below, **one or more** of the answers or completions given is correct. Select
(A) if only 1, 2, and 3 are correct
(B) if only 1 and 3 are correct
(C) if only 2 and 4 are correct
(D) if only 4 is correct
(E) if all are correct

22.13. Naloxone is indicated in poisoning with
1. narcotics
2. propoxyphene
3. pentazocine
4. glutethimide

22.14. Which of the following toxins cause pinpoint pupils?
1. Phenothiazine
2. Lithium
3. Carbamate insecticides
4. Camphorated oil

DIRECTIONS: This section of the test consists of situations, each followed by a series of questions. Study each situation and select the **one** best answer to each question following it.

Questions 22.15–22.17: A 16-year-old high school student is brought into the emergency room by the police, who found him wandering aimlessly after his parents had reported him missing. He had to be restrained with difficulty, as he was markedly agitated. Vigorous efforts were made to quiet him to obtain a history and physical. His parents stated his health was excellent. On physical examination: BP 165/110, P 130, R 36, T 102°F. Skin color normal. Neurologically he was normal except for fine tremors and dilated pupils. The most prominent physical finding was marked sweating with dryness of mouth. He was able to void for urine specimen. No needle holes or tracks were found. Odor of breath was noted.

22.15. Although anxiety and hyperactive states can occur from a variety of disease states, it was felt by the attending physician that the most likely cause of his problem was a drug. Which would be the most likely one to consider?
  A. Atropine
  B. Narcotic withdrawal
  C. Ethanol withdrawal
  D. Amphetamine
  E. Methaqualone

22.16. Why is it important to make the diagnosis as quickly as possible?
  A. The mortality of amphetamine in overdose is 20%
  B. Sudden death from atropine overdose due to ventricular fibrillation is common
  C. Death from delirium tremors due to alcohol withdrawal is more common than death from acute overdose of amphetamine
  D. In overdoses of methaqualone, absorption is nearly complete at 3 hr postinjection
  E. Narcotic withdrawal can result in sudden death

22.17. The most important consideration in treatment that could result in a fatal reaction in this type of poisoning is
  A. convulsion secondary to cerebral edema
  B. disseminated intravascular coagulation
  C. dehydration
  D. cerebral hemorrhage
  E. hyperthermia

Questions 22.18–22.20: A 7-year-old girl began to complain of nausea and vomiting associated with abdominal pain the day prior to admission. There was progressive loss of control of her legs and she was not able to walk. A recent yearly preschool exam had declared her to be in excellent health. In the emergency room, gastroenteritis was diagnosed although she was afebrile. Clear liquid diet was prescribed. Vomiting continued. Diarrhea began and she became progressively restless. She was returned to ER and admitted to hospital. P 100, R 55, T 39°C, BP 85/50. Respirations were difficult and intubation was required with oxygen. She developed "twitching." A hemogram and lumbar puncture were negative.

22.18. Because of weakness, miosis, and profuse drooling despite her vomiting, the physician ordered an immediate
   A. serum phosphorus
   B. urine arsenic
   C. plasma cholinesterase
   D. urine coproprophyrine
   E. ferric chloride test of urine

22.19. Because of his strong suspicions regarding diagnosis, the antidote which he gives can also be used diagnostically. It is
   A. diphenhydramine
   B. pralidoxime
   C. atropine
   D. dimercaprol
   E. physostigmine

22.20. The laboratory level and response confirmed diagnosis. The dose should be
   A. 50 mg IV
   B. 1 g IV
   C. up to 5 mg IV
   D. 0.3 mg/kg IV
   E. 0.4 mg IV

Answers and Comments

22.1. (D) The bite of the brown recluse spider results in skin ulcerations, intravascular hemolysis, and even death. The venom of the *Loxosceles reclusa* is primarily cytotoxic. Initially there is endothelial damage to arterioles and venules, resulting in occlusion by thrombi, followed by tissue infarction. A circumferential zone of hemorrhage, stasis, and thrombi occurs with focal abscesses in the superficial fascia. The initial bite is painless, thus the victim is not aware of the envenomization. Several hours later, pain begins and is associated with a transient erythematous area at the site. The center becomes ischemic and blisters may form. Extravasated blood develops peripherally with edema. The central portion darkens and mummifies before sloughing, forming an open ulcer. The venom may continue to spread, undermining large areas of skin. Systemic symptoms may occur directly proportional to amount of venom, but not to the severity of skin lesion. These may occur 24 hr after bite and consist of fever, chills, malaise, nausea, vomiting, arthralgias, petechiae, hemolytic anemia, decreased platelets, hemoglobinuria, and shock (Ref. 1, pp. 523–525).

22.2. (A) The treatment of acetaminophen overdose is quite simple. A nomagram has been developed with plasma levels of toxic levels plotted with time. When this information is known, the antidote acetylcysteine can be given as recommended. If laboratory values will take a longer than anticipated time, an initial dose should be given and the decision regarding continuation of therapy made when laboratory values are known and can be evaluated.

Acetylcysteine may act by inhibiting the formation of the reactive intermediary of hepatic metabolism, by combining with it to prevent it from reacting with hepatic cellular protein, or by acting as a precursor of glutathion or sulfate and thus preventing the depletion of these detoxifying chemicals. It does seem to protect the liver from the toxic effects of acetaminophen. Oral administration is preferred to intravenous therapy. The drug goes directly to the liver after absorption (Ref. 5, pp. 118–141).

Antidotal Therapy—Acetylcysteine Administration

1. Initial (loading) dose should be: 140 mg/kg p.o.

2. Maintenance doses should be: 70 mg/kg p.o. every 4 hours for 17 total doses

Loading Dose:

Body Weight (kg)	20% Mucomyst (ml)	Diluent (ml)	2% solution (total ml)
100–110	75	225	300
90–99	70	210	280
80–89	65	195	260
70–79	55	165	220
60–69	50	150	160
50–59	40	120	160
40–49	35	105	140
30–39	30	90	120

Maintenance Dose: ½ amount used for loading dose

From: Management of Acetaminophen Overdose, 1985, McNeil Consumer Products Company, Fort Washington, PA, 19034.

22.3. **(E)** Activated charcoal is generally recognized to be an effective adsorbent of many drugs and other potentially toxic substances. If administered early and in sufficiently large amounts, it appreciably reduces the gastrointestinal absorption of such drugs as acetaminophen, aspirin, digoxin, phenobarbital, phenylpropanolamine, and phenytoin. There is now increasing evidence that activated charcoal not only inhibits drug absorption from the gastrointestinal tract, but can also increase the clearance of drugs that have been already absorbed and are in the systemic circulation. Because of the intrahepatic circulation of diazepam, tricyclics, and tetracyclics, patients with overdoses may benefit from repetitive doses (every 4–6 hr).

Recent studies have shown that oral activated charcoal increased theophylline clearance in normal volunteers (serum 10 mg/nl) and that even higher serum levels are rapidly reduced by oral charcoal. These have been reported in self-administered overdose and chronic use toxicity (Refs. 2, pp. 347–349, 418–427; 5, pp. 676–678; 6, 3130–3131).

22.4. **(E)** Deferoxamine is isolated as an iron chelate from a fungus and treated chemically to form the metal-free ligand which has high affinity for ferric ion, coupled with a low affinity for calcium ion. When given P.O., it combines with iron in the lumen of the gastrointestinal tract. The preferred route of administration in acute poisoning is IM. The iron complex is excreted in the urine (Ref. 2, pp. 1633–1634).

22.5. **(C)** Ethylene glycol is metabolized to toxic substances, including oxalic acid, by alcohol dehydrogenase. Ethyl alcohol competitively inhibits the enzymatic oxidation of the ethylene glycol, preventing formation of the more toxic compounds (Ref. 1, pp. 218–219).

22.6. **(D)** Jimson weed is a common weed used as a street drug. It contains 0.25–0.5% atropine and related alkaloids. The anticholinergic effects can be relieved by physostigmine, which readily crosses into the central nervous system compared to other related drugs (Ref. 3, pp. 343–345).

22.7. **(C)** The group of drugs identified as the tricyclic antidepressants (amitriptyline, imipramine, desipramine, and nortriptyline) block parasympathetic responses. The principal manifestations of poisoning are CNS stimulation and cardiac arrhythmias, which are major causes of fatalities (Ref. 3, pp. 254–258, 415–417).

22.8. (A) Methyl alcohol is metabolized by alcohol dehydrogenase to formic acid or formaldehyde. The former produces severe acidosis, with the urine pH reaching 5.0 (Ref. 3, pp. 161–163).

22.9. (D) Butyl nitrite, a popular drug used by inhalation to enhance sensation or sexual stimulation ("to get high") acts as all nitrites as a producer of methemoglobinemia when ingested. This can result in fatalities in young children (Ref. 3, pp. 75–76, 381–382).

22.10. (B) Clonidine is a potent antihypertensive with many diverse actions on the CNS. It initially is a direct stimulator of peripheral alpha adrenergic receptors and also a partial agonist producing significant peripheral alpha adrenergic blockage. Centrally sedation and decreased spontaneous motor activity occur. In overdose the most common findings are decreased or loss of deep tendon reflexes, drowsiness, bradycardia, hypothermia, hypotension, paralytic ileus, and pinpoint pupils (Ref. 2, pp. 797–799).

22.11. (E) Caustic alkali poisoning may result from the ingestion of a variety of household products (e.g., drain cleaners, ammonia, oven cleaners, certain detergents, and Clinitest). Sodium and potassium hydroxide in liquid or solid form results in transmural esophageal necrosis, which spreads insidiously to contiguous organs and requires vigorous early attention. Histologically these products combine with protein to form proteinates and with fats to form soap, thus producing (related to alkali concentration) deep penetrating burns on contact ("liquefactive necrosis"). On initial PE when this toxin is unknown, the lesions can be diagnostic. Acids result in charring or "coagulation necrosis" (Ref. 1, pp. 229–234).

22.12. (A) The most prominent toxic effects of phenytoin are referable to the central nervous system. Acute overdosage affects primarily the cerebellum and vestibular system. Tremors of the hands are common and mydriasis and hyperactive reflexes occur. In children, ataxia or lethargy may occur first. Nystagmus is initially on far lateral gaze. With high blood levels it may be present on forward gaze. Blood levels frequently are used to follow therapeutic levels. Sometimes correlations are variable; however, nystagmus occurs at 20 μg/ml, ataxia at 30 μg/ml, and mental changes at 40 μg/ml. Beyond that there is no correlation (Ref. 4, pp. 144–150).

22.13. (A) Naloxone is an excellent antidote. It does not have the depressant effects other narcotic antagonists do. It will correct the opiate effect in patients who have ingested alcohol or barbiturates and other sedatives. Because of this selectivity, it is an excellent and safe diagnostic tool. In addition to narcotics, it is an antagonist for pentazocine, proproxyphene, and possibly dextromethorphan (Ref. 4, pp. 257–262).

22.14. (B)	Pupillary Changes in Poisoning
Dilation of pupil (mydriasis)	Belladonna group, meperidine, alcohols, ether, chloroform, papaverine, sympathomimetics, parasympatholytics, antihistamines, gelsemium, cocaine, camphor, aconitine, benzene, barium, thallium, botulinal toxin, cyanide, carbon monoxide, carbon dioxide, phenytoin
Constriction of pupil (miosis)	Opium, morphine group, sympatholytics (ergot), parasympathomimetics, Dibenamine, barbiturates, chloral hydrate, picrotoxin, nicotine, caffeine, phenothiazines, ethanol, cholinesterase inhibitors, insecticide (organic phosphates and carbamates), clonidine

(Ref. 1, p. 6).

22.15. (D) Atropine changes heart rate without affecting cardiac output or blood pressure. It also causes bladder retention. Despite vasodilation, one of the major effects of atropine is inhibition of the activity of the sweat glands, so the skin is flushed, hot, and dry. Atropine raises systolic and lowers diastolic pressure. Withdrawal of barbiturates and related nonbarbiturate drugs results in anxiety, weakness, tremors, and orthostatic hypotension. Characteristically, patients faint frequently. Amphetamines may be injected, but most usually are used orally, as they are easily absorbed from the GI tract. The increased blood pressure, fever, and moist skin are important diagnostic signs and symptoms of amphetamines. Methaqualone is a depressant, without change in temperature or increase in blood pressure (Ref. 4, pp. 44−50).

22.16. (C) Death rarely occurs in clinical toxicity from amphetamine. It is estimated that delirium tremors occur in only 8% of all alcoholics, but the mortality rate may be as high as 20%. Atropine does cause cardiac arrhythmias (Ref. 4, pp. 44−50).

22.17. (E) The greatest morbidity and mortality are associated with heat stroke, resulting in cardiovascular collapse. Hypothermia measures are needed immediately. Sweating can also result in dehydration. Fluid therapy is essential (Ref. 4, pp. 44−50).

22.18. (C) Miosis associated with gastrointestinal symptoms of nausea, vomiting, diarrhea, and excessive salivation and weakness are associated with poisoning by the cholinesterase inhibitor group of insecticides. The clinical signs and symptoms are due to the enzyme acetylcholinesterase becoming bound to the insecticide, resulting in lowering of cholinesterase levels and in the accumulation of acetylcholine at the synapse, resulting in the clinical picture. The most helpful signs and symptoms are miosis and muscular fasciculation. Clinical signs occur when the cholinesterase level is less than 50% normal. This is the specific laboratory test for this type of poisoning (Ref. 4, pp. 276−291).

22.19. (C) Atropine blocks transmission at the synapse now being constantly stimulated by the acetylcholine. It is lifesaving and should be given as soon as possible. It may also reduce acetylcholine production in the nerve terminal. The victim of anticholinesterase poisoning is refractory to atropine; if used as a diagnostic aid, the indication of atropinization is pulse over 140 and dilated pupils (Ref. 4, pp. 276−291).

22.20. (C) For adults 2−5 mg IM or IV every 5−20 min during early therapy is recommended. For children under 12 the dose is 20−50 mg/kg, yet adult doses may be necessary. Inadequate early doses can be the difference between life and death (Ref. 4, pp. 276−291).

References

1. Arena, J.: *Poisoning, Toxicology—Symptoms—Treatment*, 4th Ed., Charles C Thomas, Springfield, IL, 1979.

2. Goodman, L.S. and Gilman, A.: *The Pharmacological Basis of Therapeutics*, 6th Ed., Macmillan, New York, 1980.

3. Driesbach, R.H.: *Handbook of Poisoning: Diagnosis and Treatment*, 10th Ed., Lange Medical Publications, Los Altos, CA, 1980

4. Osterhout, S.K.: *Case Studies in Poisoning*, Medical Examination Publishing, New York, 1981.

5. Hanson, William, Jr.: *Toxic Emergencies*, Churchill Livingstone, 1984

6. Levy, G.: Gastrointestinal clearance of drugs with activated charcoal, N. Engl. J. Med. 307, 1982.

7. True, R.J., Berman, J.M., and Mahutte, C.K.: Treatment of theophylline toxicity with oral activated charcoal. Crit. Care Med. 12 (2), 1984.

23

Pediatric Endocrinology
Wellington Hung, M.D., Ph.D.

DIRECTIONS: Each of the questions or incomplete statements below is followed by five suggested answers or completions. Select the **one** that is best in each case.

23.1. In a newborn with ambiguous external genitalia, the problem of greatest immediate importance is
A. hypoglycemia
B. sex assignment
C. adrenal insufficiency
D. urinary tract abnormalities
E. gonadal tumor

23.2. Gynecomastia
A. rarely occurs in the newborn male
B. tenderness is common
C. is unusual during adolescence
D. is usually associated with galactorrhea
E. treatment in the adolescent usually is surgical

23.3. Children with exogenous obesity
  A. are usually tall for their age
  B. have delayed sexual development
  C. are usually short for their age
  D. rarely are obese adults
  E. rarely have psychologic disturbances

DIRECTIONS: Each group of questions below consists of five lettered headings followed by a list of numbered words or statements. For each numbered word or statement, select the **one** lettered heading that is most closely associated with it. Each lettered heading may be selected once, more than once, or not at all.

  A. Chronic lymphocytic thyroiditis (Hashimoto's thyroiditis)
  B. Graves' disease
  C. Thyroid cancer
  D. Hyperthyroidism
  E. Colloid goiter

23.4. The most common cause of hypothyroidism in pediatric patients

23.5. Elevated serum TSH levels

23.6. The most common thyroid disease in pediatric patients

  A. Hypothyroidism
  B. Turner's syndrome
  C. Hypopituitarism
  D. Sexual precocity
  E. Congenital adrenal hyperplasia

23.7. 45, XO karyotype

23.8. Webbed neck and lymphedema of extremities

23.9. Coarctation of the aorta and idiopathic hypertension

    A. Turner's syndrome
    B. Isolated growth hormone deficiency
    C. Genetic short stature
    D. Constitutional delay in growth
    E. Cushing's syndrome

23.10. Plasma somatomedin-C is a good screening test

23.11. Symptomatic fasting hypoglycemia may occur

23.12. Diagnosis made by tests utilizing insulin, arginine, or L-dopa

---

DIRECTIONS: For each of the questions or incomplete statements below, **one or more** of the answers or completions given is correct. Select
    (A) if only 1, 2, and 3 are correct
    (B) if only 1 and 3 are correct
    (C) if only 2 and 4 are correct
    (D) if only 4 is correct
    (E) if all are correct

23.13. A 2½-year-old girl is brought to you for evaluation of bilateral breast development of 4-months duration (Figure 54). There are no other signs of sexual development. Which of the following should be included in the differential diagnosis?
    1. Ovarian tumor
    2. Premature thelarche
    3. Hypothalamic tumor
    4. Congenital adrenal hyperplasia

23.14. Signs and symptoms of hypothyroidism in the neonatal period are which of the following?
    1. Large tongue
    2. Prolonged jaundice
    3. Lethargy
    4. Birth weight less than 4000 g

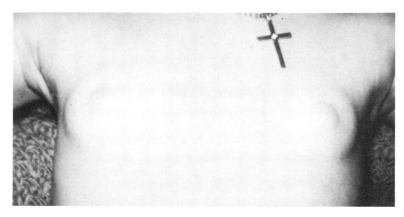

Figure 54

Answers and Comments

23.1. (C) A newborn with ambiguous external genitalia represents a medical emergency and requires immediate attention and investigation. The newborn may be at risk for the development of an adrenal crisis until the diagnosis of one of the forms of adrenal hyperplasia, associated with deficiency of glucocorticoid and mineralocorticoid synthesis and ambiguous genitalia, is ruled out (Ref. 1, pp. 1482–1487).

23.2. (B) Gynecomastia may occur in the newborn male and in up to two-thirds of adolescent males. During adolescence gynecomastia rarely persists for longer than 2 years and therapy usually consists of reassurance (Ref. 1, p. 1501).

23.3. (C) The child with exogenous obesity is usually taller than his/her peers and the bone age is slightly advanced. Puberty may begin early (Ref. 1, pp. 169–170).

23.4. (A)
23.5. (A)
23.6. (A) Chronic lymphocytic thyroiditis is the most common cause of thyroid disease in pediatrics and the most common cause of

acquired hypothyroidism. It is an autoimmune disease. Some patients who appear clinically euthyroid have elevated serum TSH levels, whereas some patients have clinical signs of frank hypothyroidism (Ref. 1, pp. 1461–1462).

23.7. (B)
23.8. (B)
23.9. (B) Turner's syndrome is a form of gonadal dysgenesis. The most common chromosomal anomaly in Turner's syndrome is a 45, XO karyotype. Girls with Turner's syndrome may have the following physical findings: short stature, congenital lymphedema, webbed neck, high arched palate, prominent ears, micrognathia, coarctation of the aorta, idiopathic hypertension, cubitus valgus, and multiple nevi (Ref. 1, pp. 1501–1502).

23.10. (B)
23.11. (B)
23.12. (B) Isolated growth hormone deficiency may result from congenital or acquired lesions of the hypothalamus and/or anterior pituitary gland. Retardation of growth may begin at birth. Symptomatic fasting hypoglycemia occurs in 10–15% of patients. Determination of plasma somatomedin-C levels is a good screening test for growth hormone deficiency but must be followed by growth hormone stimulation studies if the somatomedin levels are low. Provocative tests that cause the anterior pituitary to release growth hormone into the circulation utilize insulin, arginine, L-dopa, or glucagon (Ref. 1, pp. 1434–1437).

23.13. (A) The most common cause for breast development in a 2½-year-old girl is premature thelarche. Premature thelarche is the appearance of breast development before 8 years of age without any other evidence of precocious isosexual development. The breast development often regresses after several months to years, and no other signs of sexual maturation appear. There is no accelerated linear growth or bone maturation. No therapy is necessary. Since breast development may be the first stage of true sexual precocity or pseudosexual precocity, the patient must be followed for development of other signs of sexual precocity (Ref. 1, p. 1448).

23.14. (A) In most infants with congenital hypothyroidism, clinical manifestations during the early neonatal period are absent or mild and nonspecific. Signs and symptoms of hypothyroidism in the neonatal period include: large posterior fontanel, prolonged jaundice, macroglossia, constipation, circulatory mottling, lethargy, feeding problems, respiratory difficulties, umbilical hernia, hypothermia, and bradycardia (Ref. 1, pp. 1453–1457).

Reference

1. Behrman R.E. and Vaughan, V.C. (eds.): *Nelson Textbook of Pediatrics*, 12th Ed., W.B. Saunders, Philadelphia, 1983.

24

Pediatric Gastroenterology
William M. Liebman, M.D.

DIRECTIONS: Each of the questions or incomplete statements below is followed by five suggested answers or completions. Select the **one** that is best in each case.

24.1. Which of the following is the most common cause of acute diarrhea in infants and children?
A. Chemical
B. Bacteria
C. Parasite
D. Virus
E. None of the above

24.2. Which of the following is the most common cause of constipation in infants and children?
A. Anorectal anomaly
B. Hypothyroidism
C. Hirschsprung's disease
D. Lead poisoning
E. Functional

24.3. The most common cause of blood in the bowel movements of infants and children, 1 month−5 years of age, is
  A. Meckel's diverticulum
  B. colon polyp
  C. inflammatory bowel disease
  D. anal fissure/proctitis
  E. colon cancer

DIRECTIONS: The group of questions below consists of five lettered headings followed by a list of numbered words or statements. For each numbered word or statement, select the **one** lettered heading that is most closely associated with it. Each lettered heading may be selected once, more than once, or not at all.

For questions 24.4−24.6, refer to Table 1.

TABLE 1. Malabsorption—Clinical Evaluation

Step 1: Complete blood count
  Sedimentation rate
  Serum total protein and albumin
  Serum carotene
  Serum folate
  Urinalysis
  Stool WBC, occult blood, reducing substances, Sudan III stain, culture, and ova and parasites

Step 2: Quantitative stool fat (72 hr)
  Sweat test
  Quantitative immunoglobulins
  d-Xylose (5-hr urine; 0-, ½-, 1-, and 2-hour blood level)

Step 3: Upper gastrointestinal x-ray studies

Step 4: Breath tests (CO_2-C^{14}, C^{13}; hydrogen): fat, protein, carbohydrate

Step 5: Cr^{51}-albumin or ^{131}I-PVP excretion study (stool): protein loss

Step 6: Small intestinal biopsy and aspiration (histology, enzyme assays; culture, ova and parasites, enzymes, bile acids)

Step 7: Secretin−pancreozymin stimulation test (pancreas)
  Segmental perfusion studies (carbohydrate, protein)
  Gastric acid analysis

A. Malabsorption, gluten
B. Vomiting
C. Constipation
D. Jaundice (newborn)
E. Abdominal pain (recurrent)

24.4. Celiac disease

24.5. Gastroesophageal reflux

24.6. Neonatal hepatitis

DIRECTIONS: For each of the questions or incomplete statements below, **one or more** of the answers or completions given is correct. Select
    (A) if only 1, 2, and 3 are correct
    (B) if only 1 and 3 are correct
    (C) if only 2 and 4 are correct
    (D) if only 4 is correct
    (E) if all are correct
For questions 24.7–24.8, refer to Table 2.

24.7. Recurrent abdominal pain in children is characterized by
    1. low incidence of organic disease, 10–40%
    2. high incidence of peptic ulcer disease
    3. lack of relationship to time of day, meals, food types, and position
    4. good response to treatment with antacids or histamine-2 receptor antagonist, cimetidine

24.8. Infestation of the intestine with *Giardia lamblia* is associated with
    1. no symptomatology usually
    2. high percentage of cases with negative stool examinations
    3. nonspecific radiologic findings of the small intestine
    4. successful treatment with medication in practically all cases

TABLE 2. Evaluation of Recurrent Abdominal Pain

Step 1: Complete history (symptom, developmental, family, social, school)
Complete physical examination

Step 2: Initial laboratory studies
Complete blood count
Sedimentation rate
Urinalysis
Stool WBC, occult blood, and ova and parasites

Step 3: Urine culture
Urine and serum amylase
Upper gastrointestinal x-ray studies
Barium enema examination
Intravenous pyelogram

Step 4: Urine porphyrin screen
Heavy metal screen
Electroencephalogram
Pertechnetate isotope scan (Meckels' diverticulum)

Step 5: Gynecologic examination

Step 6: Upper endoscopy
Lower endoscopy

Step 7: Surgery (laparotomy)

Answers and Comments

24.1. **(C)** Viruses, particularly rotavirus (orbivirus, duovirus, reovirus), are the most common cause of acute diarrhea in infants and children. Acute gastroenteritis is produced, causing the typical patient to become suddenly ill with vomiting, fever, diarrhea, and generalized malaise. The illness usually lasts 1−8 days. Acute gastroenteritis is particularly prevalent during the winter months (Ref. 1, pp. 747−752).

24.2. **(E)** The most common cause of constipation with or without fecal retention is functional (idiopathic), accounting for at least 80−90% of cases. Organic lesions, such as Hirschsprung's disease, endocrinopathies, intestinal pseudoobstruction, hypothyroidism, and lead poisoning (chronic) only account for 10−20% of cases. Functional factors include the quality of the parent−child relationship, marital discord, the parental-cultural background (Ref. 2, pp. 105−110).

24.3. (D) The most common cause of gross blood in the bowel movements (hematochezia) of infants and children, 1 month−5 years of age, is anal fissure. The blood is usually small in amount, bright red, and is usually on the outside of the bowel movements (e.g., specks, streaks). Blood may also be seen on the diaper, toilet bowl, or toilet paper. Frequently, there is pain with defecation and possible withholding of fecal material. Direct examination of the anal canal is the most important study to perform; the knee−chest or left lateral position should be used. More than one tear may be present (Ref. 3, pp. 265−280).

24.4. (A) Celiac disease, along with cystic fibrosis, constitute the most common, specific causes of malabsorption in infants and children. Celiac disease is a small intestinal disorder resulting in clinical and chemical evidence of malabsorption and characterized by structural (histologic) abnormality of the small intestinal mucosa. The underlying etiology is a reactivity to gluten (wheat protein). The incidence is higher in Europe than the United States. Clinical manifestations include diarrhea, abdominal discomfort, irritability, slowed growth (weight more than height). Demonstration of steatorrhea (excessive fecal fat excretion), as well as other nutrient malabsorption, is usually present (over 80−85%). Treatment is highly effective and consists of a *gluten-free diet* (Ref. 4, pp. 639−642).

24.5. (B) Vomiting/spitting up is the most common manifestation of gastroesophageal reflux (GER) in infants and children. The vomitus usually contains undigested formula or food. The vomiting is more commonly nonprojectile, almost effortless, usually within 15−60 min after meals, and more likely in a reclining position. In older children, heartburn (pyrosis) is quite common. Nocturnal cough/wheezing (1−4%), hematemesis (10−25%), and slowed growth (30−50%) are other manifestations of GER in childhood. The underlying etiology is dysfunction of the lower esophageal sphincter (LES), the high pressure zone in the most distal portion of the esophagus, primary (LES only) or second (LES affected by another anatomic lesion, e.g., pyloric stenosis, peptic ulcer disease) (Ref. 5, pp. 135−141).

24.6. (D) Neonatal hepatitis accounts for 40−70% of cases of prolonged jaundice in the newborn. Associated infectious agents include cytomegalovirus (CMV), herpesvirus, rubella, echovirus 11, 14, and 19, hepatitis B virus (HBV), as well as toxoplasmosis sporozoon. The jaundice usually appears by 2 weeks of age, the stools becoming lighter and the urine darker. Appetite loss, decreased suck, decreased activity and alertness, as well as vomiting are frequent clinical observations. Hepatomegaly and variable splenomegaly occur. Laboratory results include mixed hyperbilirubinemia, significantly elevated transaminases (SGOT, SGPT), mildly elevated alkaline phosphatase and 5′ nucleotidase levels, and abnormal coagulation studies (PT, PTT). Isotope excretion studies, e.g., 99m-Tc-Pipida, ^{131}I-Rose Bengal, will demonstrate definite excretion into the intestines and stools. Liver biopsy (closed or percutaneous, open or surgical) will demonstrate findings consistent with inflammation and variable cholestasis, intrahepatic. Treatment is usually symptomatic, e.g., correction of fluid and electrolyte abnormalities, coagulation abnormalities. Prognosis can vary, from recovery to liver failure, death (Ref. 3, pp. 504−512; 6, 416−423).

24.7. (B) Recurrent abdominal pain (RAP) in children is a common, troublesome problem. Its incidence has been estimated at 9−15% of the general pediatric population. The etiology of RAP remains ill-defined, with confirmed organic factors, including primary acquired lactose intolerance, peptic ulcer disease, accounting for only 6−40% of cases. Psychologic factors have been most frequently implicated in the pathogenesis of RAP. No consistent relationship of RAP with meals, food types, bowel movements, position, activity, or time of day has been demonstrated. Associated symptomatology (e.g., nausea, vomiting, constipation) generally has not aided diagnosis or treatment. Laboratory, radiologic, and endoscopic studies have provided significant information only in the minority of cases. Selective use of such studies is mandatory. Treatment has focused mainly on support and counseling, because no specific medication (e.g., antacids, tranquilizers) has been significantly beneficial. Long-term follow-up has demonstrated a good outlook, although 15−35% of patients continue to have difficulty 10 or more years later (Ref. 7, pp. 31−53).

24.8. (E) Giardiasis is a frequent intestinal parasitic infestation, generally 5−10% of the population worldwide. Children *are* commonly affected. The clinical pattern can vary from no symptomatology (most common; 80−90%) to an "acute gastroenteritis" or chronic diarrheal, malabsorptionlike syndrome. *Giardia lamblia* is a flagellated protozoa; trophozoites are present in the upper small intestine. The cyst form is the means of transmission. Host susceptibility is variable, although altered immune responsiveness and achlorhydria increase such susceptibility. Stool examinations (zinc sulfate concentration smear; formal-ether smear) are negative in 30−50% of the cases (cysts). In the latter cases, duodenal intubation and aspiration, biopsy, or the string test (Enterotest-Pediatric) should be performed to demonstrate the presence of *Giardia lamblia*. Laboratory studies and radiologic findings are nonspecific. Treatment with medication is highly successful, approximating 70− 90% regardless of drug, e.g., quinacrine (Atabrine), drug of choice; metronidazole (Flagyl); and furazolidone (Furoxone) (Ref. 8, pp. 409−412; 9, pp. 279−280).

References

1. Hamilton, J.R., Gall, D.G., Kerzner, B., et al.: Recent developments in viral gastroenteritis. Pediatr. Cl. N. Am. 22, 1975.

2. Liebman, W.M.: Disorders of defecation in children: Evaluation and management. Postgrad. Med. 66, 1979.

3. Silverman, A. and Roy, C.C.: *Pediatric Clinical Gastroenterology*, 3rd Ed., C.V. Mosby, St. Louis, 1983.

4. Heiner, D.C. and Liebman, W.M.: Celiac syndrome. In *Pediatric Therapy*, 5th Ed., Shirkey, H.C. (Ed.), C.V. Mosby, St. Louis, 1975.

5. Berquist, W.E.: Gastroesophageal reflux in children: A clinical review. Pediatr. Ann. 11, 1982.

6. Liebman, W.M.: *Pediatric Gastroenterology Case Studies*, 2nd Ed., Medical Examination Publishing, New York, 1985.

7. Galler, J.R., Neustein, S., and Walker, W.A.: Clinical aspects of recurrent abdominal pain in children. Adv. Pediatr. 27, 1980.

8. Rosenthal, P. and Liebman, W.M.: Comparative study of stool examinations: Duodenal aspiration and entero-test-pediatric for giardiasis in children. J. Pediatr. 96, 1980.

9. Lerman, S.J. and Walker, R.A.: Treatment of giardiasis. Literature review and recommendations. Clin. Pediatr. 21, 1982.

25

Genetics

Raymond M. Russo, M.D., F.A.A.P.

DIRECTIONS: Each of the questions or incomplete statements below is followed by five suggested answers or completions. Select the **one** that is best in each case.

25.1. Congenital hypothyroidism may be the most prevalent cause of preventable mental retardation. What factor greatly decreases (by 30−50%) the risk of retardation caused by hypothryoidism?

- **A.** Efficient screening for phenylketonuria
- **B.** Application of thyroxine (T_4) radioimmunoassay
- **C.** The comparison of cord blood and filter paper spot screening methods
- **D.** Detection and treatment before 3 months of age
- **E.** None of the above

25.2. Which method provides the most comprehensive screening and identification of infants with primary hypothyroidism and those at risk for secondary hypothyroidism and TBG deficiency?

A. Primary TSH screening
B. Filter paper spot TSH testing of sample with low T_4 results
C. Cord blood T_4 followed by TSH measurement
D. Cord blood testing alone
E. None of the above

25.3. The likelihood that a pregnancy in which the serum α-fetoprotein is 2.5 times the median level will be affected with a neural tube defect is

A. 1 in 80 where the prevalence is 2 per 1000 births
B. 1 in 10 where the prevalence is 2 per 1000 births
C. 1 in 80 where the prevalence is 4.5 per 1000 births
D. 1 in 10 where the prevalence is 4.5 per 1000 births
E. 1 in 4 where the prevalence is 2 per 1000 births

DIRECTIONS: The group of questions below consists of five lettered headings followed by a list of numbered words or statements. For each numbered word or statement, select the **one** lettered heading that is most closely associated with it. Each lettered heading may be selected once, more than once, or not at all.

For questions 25.4−25.6, refer to Figure 55.

A. Turner's syndrome
B. Chromosomal anomalies
C. Neonatal hepatitis
D. Hydrocephalus
E. Congenital hypothyroidism

25.4. Primary TSH screening is effective for detection

25.5. Detected by measuring α-fetoprotein levels in amniotic fluid during the second trimester

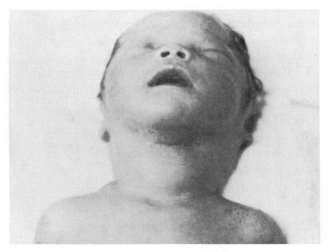

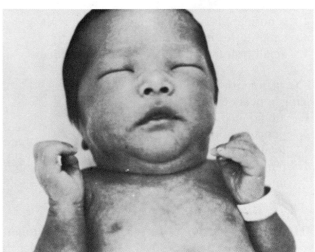

Figure 55

25.6. Detected 12 times more often in couples with a history of three or more spontaneous abortions

---

DIRECTIONS: For each of the questions or incomplete statements below, **one or more** of the answers or completions given is correct. Select

  (A) if only 1, 2, and 3 are correct
  (B) if only 1 and 3 are correct
  (C) if only 2 and 4 are correct
  (D) if only 4 is correct
  (E) if all are correct

25.7. Klinefelter's syndrome is characterized by
  1. normal testes, azoospermia, gynecomastia, and an XXY genotype
  2. a normal phenotypical male with an XXY genotype
  3. small testes in a fertile male
  4. small testes, sterility and sparse pubic hair

25.8. The major risk of placental aspiration for fetal blood sampling appears to be
  1. amnionitis
  2. puncturing the umbilical cord
  3. fetal blood loss into the amniotic cavity
  4. puncturing a major vessel near the insertion of the cord into the placenta

---

DIRECTIONS: This section of the test consists of a situation followed by a series of questions. Study the situation and select the **one** best answer to each question following it.

Questions 25.9–25.10: A 3-year-old girl being considered for adoption is referred to you for evaluation. She has a number of anomalies which give her an unusual facial appearance. She has an antimongolian slant to her palpebral fissures and hypoplasia of the malar bones. There are bilateral colobomas with eyelash deficiency medial to the colobomas. Ear tags, preauricular pits, large floppy ears, and a receding chin (hypoplastic mandible) complete the picture (Figure 56).

25.9. Which of the following conditions is NOT likely?
A. Nager acrofacial dysostosis
B. Osteogenesis imperfecta
C. Hypophosphatasia
D. Achondroplasia
E. Treacher Collins' syndrome

25.10. Before advising the prospective parents to adopt the child, which of the following functions would be LEAST crucial to test?
A. Hearing
B. Vision
C. Cardiovascular
D. Mental development
E. Muscular skeletal

Figure 56

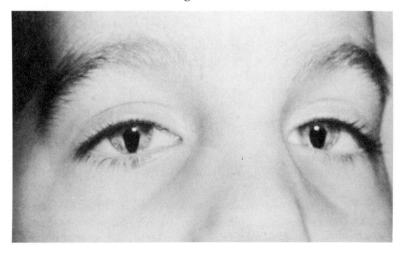

Answers and Comments

25.1. (D) It is clear that detection as early as possible, before 3 months of life, and subsequent treatment is the only choice that can significantly affect the incidence of mental retardation due to congenital hypothyroidism. It has been reported that 80% of infants with congenital hypothyroidism who are detected and treated before 3 months achieve an IQ of 90 or greater, whereas 50% or less reach that IQ level if treatment is delayed beyond 3 months. Screening of phenylketonuria will not assist the hypothyroid infant, nor will the results of thyroid screening tests unless therapy is also implemented (Ref. 1, pp. 423–430).

25.2. (B) Filter paper spot TSH testing when T_4 levels are low is the most comprehensive screening to identify congenital hypothyroidism. Primary TSH testing is applicable for primary hypothyroidism and has the lowest recall rate but is not as comprehensive. Cord blood testing for T_4 or cord blood T_4 followed by a TSH level is applicable to high density population screening where whole blood transport is feasible (Ref. 1, pp. 423–430).

25.3. (D) Where the prevalence of neural tube defect is 4.5 per 1000 births, the likelihood that a 2.5 greater than median serum α-fetoprotein level indicates an affected pregnancy is 1 in 10 (Ref. 2, pp. 619–629).

25.4. (E) TSH screening is useful in detecting primary hypothyroidism. The filter paper technique also helps identify neonates with secondary congenital hypothyroidism. Neither will detect Turner's syndrome, hepatitis, chromosomal anomalies, or hydrocephalus (Ref. 1, pp. 423–430).

25.5. (C) Although elevated levels of α-fetoprotein are associated with neural tube defects, neonatal hepatitis will also lead to an elevated level (Ref. 2, pp. 619–629).

25.6. (B) When three or more abortions have occurred for a mating couple, the incidence of chromosomal abnormalities in the conceptus is 12 times that of the general population. If this situation is encountered, it calls for expert genetic counseling. Examination of embryonic or fetal remains and the use of fetal tissue culture could be diagnostic. The opportunity to conduct these studies at the time of spontaneous abortion should not be overlooked (Ref. 3, pp. 593–618).

25.7. (C) Klinefelter's syndrome is characterized by small or undescended testes, sparse pubic hair, azoospermia, sterility, and gynecomastia. Mild mental deficiency may also be present. Normal-sized testes or fertility would not be characteristic of the syndrome. Treatment with testosterone can stimulate the development of pubic and facial hair, deepen the voice, and determine a more typically male fat distribution (Ref. 6, p. 118).

25.8. (C) The risk of fetal loss during placental aspiration to sample fetal blood is approximately 5–10%. The major cause of fetal death is puncturing the umbilical cord or a major blood vessel near the cord's placental insertion. A lesser risk has been amnionitis. Leakage of blood into the amniotic cavity increases the risk of amnionitis by providing a rich culture medium for bacterial organisms. Still, the major risk is cord or vessel puncturing (Ref. 4, pp. 631–642).

25.9. (E) The findings described are typical of Treacher Collins' syndrome. This is an autosomal dominant condition with variable expressivity. Some patients are missing one or both external auditory meati and may be deaf due to ear ossicle malformations. To rule this out, tomograms of the temporal bones should be done to evaluate the hearing mechanism. Mental retardation, commonly reported with the syndrome, may actually be due to conductive hearing loss. Nager acrofacial dyostosis is also characterized by mandibulofacial dyostosis but unlike Treacher Collins' syndrome is inherited as an autosomal recessive and causes preaxial upper limb deficiency and other anomalies. The findings are not characteristic of osteogenesis imperfecta, hypophosphatasia, or achondroplasia (Ref. 5, pp. 485–515).

25.10 (E) Because the hearing can be severely affected and may lead to mental development lag, both these functions are critical to test before advising adoption. The vision, because of coloboma, may be affected and there is the possibility of associated congenital heart lesions, particularly ventricular septal defect. The musculo-skeletal system is usually intact and is the least crucial to test (Ref. 5, pp. 485–515).

References

1. Fisher, D.A.: Neonatal thyroid screening. Pediatr. Cl. N. Am. 25, 1978.

2. Crandall, B.F., Lebherz, T.B., and Freihube, R.: Neural tube defects. Pediatr. Cl. N. Am. 25, 1978.

3. Miles, J.H. and Kaback, M.M.: Prenatal diagnosis of hereditary disorders. Pediatr. Cl. N. Am 25, 1978.

4. Leonard, C.O. and Kazazian, H.H.: Prenatal diagnosis of hemoglobinopathies. Pediatr. Cl. N. Am. 25, 1978.

5. Stewart, R.E.: Craniofacial malformations. Pediatr. Cl. N. Am. 25, 1978.

6. Burnhill, M.S.: The major disorders of sex chromatin formation. In *Sexual Development and Disorders in Childhood and Adolescence*, Russo, R.M. (Ed.), Medical Examination Publishing, New York, 1983.

26

Pediatric Hematology/ Oncology
Thomas D. Miale, M.D.

DIRECTIONS: Each of the questions or incomplete statements below is followed by five suggested answers or completions. Select the **one** that is best in each case.

26.1. Which of the following provides the best evidence of the cause of the anemia illustrated in Figure 57?
A. Low serum iron
B. Low transferrin saturation
C. High free erythrocyte protoporphyrin/hemoglobin ratio
D. Reticulocyte count and hemoglobin rise following iron therapy
E. Plasma ferritin

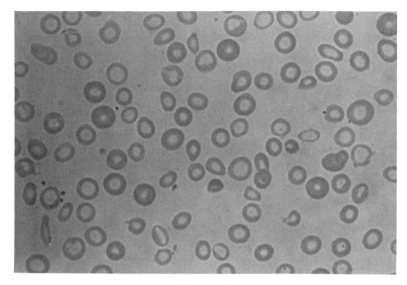

Figure 57

26.2. Which of the following is not characteristic of Burkitt's lymphoma in the non-African presentation?
  A. Translocation of a balanced reciprocal type of genetic material from the long arm of chromosome 8 to the long arm of chromosome 14
  B. Some implication that Epstein-Barr virus may be the etiologic agent
  C. Clinical findings of a growing jaw or orbital mass
  D. Common clinical presentation is an abdominal mass which is frequently associated with pain and intestinal obstruction and may lead to intussusception
  E. A neoplastic T-cell proliferation

26.3. Which infant formula is most often associated with megaloblastic anemia in the United States?
  A. Cow milk
  B. Human milk from a iron-deficient mother
  C. Human milk from a vitamin B_{12}-deficient mother
  D. Goat milk
  E. Soy-based formula

DIRECTIONS: The group of questions below consists of lettered headings followed by a list of numbered words or statements. For each numbered word or statement, select the **one** lettered heading that is most closely associated with it. Each lettered heading may be selected once, more than once, or not at all.

    A. Hypochromic microcytic anemia
    B. Normocytic normochromic anemia
    C. Macrocytic anemia

26.4. Sickle cell anemia

26.5. Sickle cell thalassemia

26.6. Special diets for phenylketonuria and maple syrup urine disease

---

DIRECTIONS: This section of the test consists of a situation followed by a series of questions. Study the situation and select the **one** best answer to each question following it.

Questions 26.7–26.8: A 3-year-old girl was found to have a palpable abdominal mass by her mother while bathing. A malignant tumor was found on surgical exploration. In retrospect, it was noted that one side of her body was somewhat larger than the other.

26.7. Statistically, the most likely pathologic diagnosis will be
    A. neuroblastoma
    B. teratocarcinoma
    C. Wilms' tumor
    D. sarcoma botryoides
    E. Burkitt's lymphoma

26.8. Another associated abnormality is
    A. aniridia
    B. café-au-lait spot
    C. pilonidal cyst
    D. fetal lobulations of the kidney
    E. accessory spleen

Answers and Comments

26.1. (D) While the alternative choices are compatible with iron deficiency, the most reliable index is the response of the anemia to iron, as documented by increases in reticulocyte and hemoglobin (Ref. 1, p. 81).

26.2. (E) The balanced translocation (t 8;14) is characteristic of Burkitt's lymphoma. However, it is seen in other human lymphomas, but not with the same frequency or specificity. The Epstein-Barr virus has been strongly implicated with the African type, while the relationship is less clear for the non-African type. The most common clinical presentations are growing jaw or orbital mass for the African type, and abdominal mass frequently associated with pain and obstruction and sometimes with intussusception at the ileocecal area, for the non-African type, respectively. Burkitt's lymphoma is usually a neoplastic B-cell proliferation. (Ref. 5, pp. 268–270).

26.3. (D) Goat milk anemia occurs in infants fed goat milk, which has a much lower folate content than cow milk. Despite many regulations requiring folate supplementation of processed goat milk sold in grocery stores, many families may still obtain goat milk directly from the source and, thereby, dietary goat milk anemia may result (Ref. 1, p. 113).

26.4. (B) In sickle cell anemia, the anemia is normocytic normochromic (Ref. 1, p. 184).

26.5. (A) In sickle cell thalassemia, the anemia is hypochromic microcytic (Ref. 3, p. 715).

26.6. (C) In phenylketonuria and maple syrup urine disease diets, the anemia is macrocytic secondary to folic deficiency (Ref. 3, p. 114).

26.7. (C) Classically, the child with Wilms' tumor or neuroblastoma is noticed by the mother while bathing the child. Wilms' tumor is the most common intraabdominal neoplasm in the children of this age and is associated with hemihypertrophy (Ref. 2, p. 636).

26.8. (A) Anomalies associated with Wilms' tumor include aniridia, hemihypertrophy. Of children with congenital aniridia, 7 of 28 have developed Wilms' tumor. Because of the abundance of nonocular defects also found in these children, the term "Wilms' tumoraniridia syndrome" has been applied (Ref. 4, p. 591).

References

1. Lanzkowsky, P.: *Pediatric Hematology-Oncology: A Treatise for the Clinician*, McGraw Hill, New York, 1980.

2. Levine, A.: *Cancer in the Young*, Masson, New York, 1982.

3. Nathan, D. and Oski, F. (eds.): *Hematology of Infancy and Childhood*, 2d Ed., W.B. Saunders, Philadelphia, 1981.

4. Sutow, W., Fernbach, D., and Vietti, T. (eds.): *Clinical Pediatric Oncology*, 3rd Ed., C.V. Mosby, St. Louis, 1984.

5. Quinn, J.J.: The lymphoproliferative disorders. In Altman, A.J. and Schwartz, A.D. (Eds.), *Malignant Diseases of Infancy, Childhood and Adolescence*, 2nd Ed., W.B. Saunders, Philadelphia, 1983.

27

Pediatric Infectious Diseases

Cheng T. Cho, M.D., Ph.D.

DIRECTIONS: Each of the questions or incomplete statements below is followed by five suggested answers or completions. Select the **one** that is best in each case.

27.1 Which of the following agents is the most common cause of acute otitis media in children?
  A. *Streptococcus pneumoniae*
  B. *Hemophilus influenzae* type b
  C. *Streptococcus pyogenes*
  D. *Staphylococcus aureus*
  E. *Candida albicans*

27.2. Invasive disease (e.g., meningitis) caused by *Hemophilus influenzae* type b is most common in children of ages
  A. under 1 month
  B. 3 months−3 years
  C. 4−7 years
  D. 8−10 years
  E. 11−15 years

27.3. Which of the following antimicrobial agents can enhance the production of kernicterus in a jaundiced newborn baby?
- **A.** Chloramphenicol
- **B.** Tetracycline
- **C.** Sulfonamide
- **D.** Novobiocin
- **E.** Nitrofurantoin

DIRECTIONS: Each group of questions below consists of five lettered headings followed by a list of numbered words or statements. For each numbered word or statement, select the **one** lettered heading that is most closely associated with it. Each lettered heading may be selected once, more than once, or not at all.

- **A.** *Pseudomonas aeruginosa*
- **B.** *Pneumocystis carinii*
- **C.** *Streptococcus pneumoniae*
- **D.** Group B streptococcus
- **E.** *Candida albicans*

27.4. Infection in a newborn baby

27.5. Infection in a child with cystic fibrosis

27.6. Infection in a child with sickle-cell anemia

- **A.** *Hemophilus influenzae* type b
- **B.** Group A streptococcus
- **C.** *Chlamydiae trachomatis*
- **D.** *Diplococcus pneumoniae*
- **E.** *Staphylococcus aureus*

27.7. The most common cause of acute epiglottitis

27.8. The major cause of conjunctivitis in newborn infant

27.9. The responsible agent for acute rheumatic fever

A. Molluscum contagiosum
B. *Pneumocystis carinii*
C. Toxoplasmosis
D. Hepatitis A
E. Meningococcal meningitis

27.10. Trimethoprim-sulfamethoxazole is the drug of choice for treatment

27.11. Human immune globulin (IG) has prophylactic value

27.12. Rifampin is the drug of choice for prophylaxis

DIRECTIONS: Each set of lettered headings below is followed by a list of numbered words or phrases. For each numbered word or phrase select
    (A) if the item is associated with A only
    (B) if the item is associated with B only
    (C) if the item is associated with both A and B
    (D) if the item is associated with neither A nor B

A. Transmitted from person to person
B. Transmitted from animal to human
C. Both
D. Neither

27.13. Herpes simplex virus (HSV)

27.14. Cytomegalovirus (CMV)

27.15. Varicella-zoster virus (V-Z)

27.16. Rotavirus

A. Common cause of pneumonia in children under 5 years old
B. Common cause of pneumonia in children over 5 years old
C. Both
D. Neither

27.17. *Mycoplasma pneumoniae*

27.18. *Streptococcus pneumoniae*

27.19. Respiratory syncytial virus

27.20. *Legionella pneumophila*

A. Often associated with eosinophilia in peripheral blood
B. Often associated with an elevated serum IgE
C. Both
D. Neither

27.21. Trichuriasis (whipworm infection)

27.22. Pertussis (whooping cough)

27.23. *Toxocara canis* and *T. cati* (visceral larva migrans)

DIRECTIONS: For each of the questions or incomplete statements below, **one or more** of the answers or completions given is correct. Select
- **(A)** if only 1, 2, and 3 are correct
- **(B)** if only 1 and 3 are correct
- **(C)** if only 2 and 4 are correct
- **(D)** if only 4 is correct
- **(E)** if all are correct

27.24. Inactivated vaccines are used in immunization against
1. polio
2. diphtheria
3. influenza
4. pneumococcal vaccine

27.25. Which of the following antituberculous drugs are often used in children?
1. Isoniazid
2. Rifampin
3. Paraaminosalicylic acid
4. Ethambutol

27.26. Live virus vaccines are used in immunization against
1. hepatitis B virus
2. measles
3. rabies
4. mumps

DIRECTIONS: This section of the test consists of situations, each followed by a series of questions. Study each situation and select the **one** best answer to each question following it.

Questions 27.27–27.29: A 13-year-old child enters the hospital because of cough and fever (39.8°C) for 1 week and skin rash for 4 days. There is pruritic maculopapular, hemorrhagic vesicular rash involving the palms, upper and lower extremities, with less involvement of the trunk and back and no facial lesions (Figure 58). Chest x-rays show pulmonary infiltrates (Figure 59).

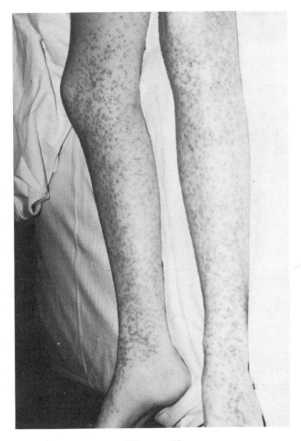

Figure 58

27.27. Based on the information, you would want to inquire about
    A. exposure to similar illness
    B. animal contacts
    C. history of measles vaccination
    D. headache
    E. change in vision

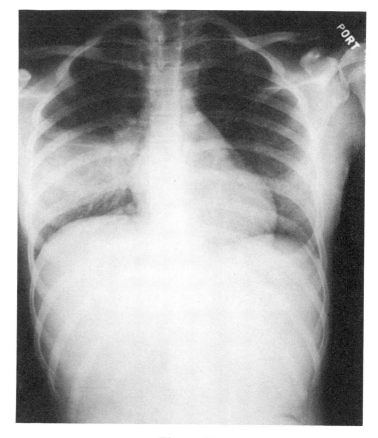

Figure 59

27.28. Your initial impression of this patient's problem should include
A. pneumococcal infection
B. Legionnaires' disease
C. atypical measles
D. measles
E. staphylococcal infection

27.29. You then proceed to obtain which of the following tests to confirm your impression?
  A. Throat culture for bacteria
  B. *Legionella* antibody levels
  C. Measles antibody levels
  D. Blood and skin cultures for bacteria
  E. Skin culture for viruses

Questions 27.30−27.32: This 14-month-old child is brought to the clinic because he has been very lethargic since morning. Mother thought he was more irritable and felt warm this morning. The child fell from his high chair yesterday and has vomited four times. On examination you find the child has a temperature of 39.8°C. His anterior fontanel is tense and bulging. His neck is not stiff. His pupils are reactive to light but not equal in size.

27.30. You would then proceed with which of the following?
  A. Perform a spinal tap
  B. Order a CAT scan of the head
  C. Order an EEG
  D. Order a skull x-ray
  E. Prescribe antipyretic and observe the child in the hospital

27.31. Based on the previous studies, you have ruled out subdural hematoma. You would then proceed with which of the following?
  A. Start antibiotics
  B. Perform a spinal tap
  C. Consult neurosurgeon
  D. Send the child home and observe the child at home
  E. Absolute bed rest

27.32. The most likely cause of this child's problem is
  A. head trauma
  B. meningitis
  C. brain tumor
  D. skull fracture
  E. drug ingestion

Questions 27.33—27.35: This 2-day-old male infant is found to have numerous discrete red-to-purplish macular rash over the face, trunk, and extremities. His liver is palpable 5 cm below the right costal margin and the spleen is palpable 4 cm below the left costal margin. You have included congenital infections in your differential diagnosis and you have reviewed the mother's record. She had a negative VDRL test before delivery and she had a rubella antibody (HI) titer of 1:20 during her previous pregnancy. You have ordered several laboratory tests to confirm your diagnosis. Four days later, the laboratory informed you that cytomegalovirus was isolated from the infant's urine.

27.33. Based on this information, the child has congenital
   A. syphilis
   B. rubella
   C. herpes simplex virus infection
   D. cytomegalovirus
   E. toxoplasmosis

27.34. Based on the previous information, what is the prognosis?
   A. Normal growth and development
   B. No risk to susceptible pregnant women
   C. Mental retardation
   D. Death during the first year
   E. Minor problems

27.35. The long-range problems in this infant should include
   A. need for antiviral therapy
   B. risk to susceptible pregnant women
   C. no risk to susceptible pregnant women
   D. no problem
   E. need for prophylactic antibiotics

Answers and Comments

27.1. (A) *S. pneumoniae (D. pneumoniae)* is the most frequently encountered in children with acute otitis media. The second most common organism is *H. influenzae* (Ref. 5, p. 60).

27.2. (B) Invasive disease caused by *H. influenzae* type b is most common in children 3 months—3 years old, it may occur in older children, and it is seen on occasion in adolescents and adults. Young children (those less than 4 years old) in contact with children who have had invasive disease caused by *H. influenzae* type b are at significant risk for serious infection from this organism (Ref. 1, p. 105).

27.3. **(C)** Kernicterus in premature infants has resulted from therapy with sulfisoxazole and from administration of excessive doses of vitamin K analogues to the infants or their mothers. Sulfonamide competes with bilirubin for binding to albumin (Ref. 5, p. 214).

27.4. **(D)** Neonatal sepsis is a relatively common and serious illness. Bacteria are the major causes of neonatal sepsis. Group B streptococci and *E. coli* are the two frequent causes of neonatal sepsis in recent years (Ref. 5, p. 206).

27.5. **(A)** Although *H. influenzae, E. coli, Proteus,* and other organisms are occasionally found in the respiratory tract of patients with cystic fibrosis, *S. aureus* and *P. aeruginosa* are the main organisms present and have a striking association with the disease (Ref. 2, p. 1992).

27.6. **(C)** Persons with sickle-cell anemia have a markedly increased susceptibility to pneumococcal meningitis and septicemia, like patients after splenectomy, and this is common in the first year of life. The increased risk stems from a deficiency of serum opsonins against pneumococci and the state of functional hyposplenia (Ref. 2, p. 1387).

27.7. **(A)** Acute epiglottitis is a dramatic, potentially lethal condition which occurs usually in children between the ages of 2 and 7 years and is usually caused by *H. influenzae* type b (Ref. 2, p. 765).

27.8. **(C)** Inclusion conjunctivitis may appear as congestion and edema, with minimal discharge developing 7−14 days after birth and lasting for 1−2 weeks. Recurrences may occur, even with adequate treatment (Ref. 1, p. 58).

27.9. **(B)** Rheumatic fever may properly be considered a complication of streptococcal infection of the upper respiratory tract. Although not all patients with acute rheumatic fever give a history of sore throat, evidence consistent with recent streptococcal infection can usually be obtained by careful laboratory examinations (Ref. 2, p. 683).

27.10. (B) *P. carinii* is ubiquitous in animals, particularly rodents. In developing countries, the disease frequently occurs in epidemic form and primarily affects malnourished infants and children. In developed countries, pneumocystosis is a significant complication of immunosuppression, particularly in patients with deficient cell-mediated immunity (Ref. 1, p. 177).

27.11. (D) All household contacts should receive 0.02 ml/kg IG as soon as possible after exposure. The use of IG more than 2 weeks after exposure or after onset of illness is not indicated (Ref. 1, p. 110).

27.12. (E) The source of meningococcal infections is the upper respiratory tract of humans only. Meningococcal infections may occur in closed communities, including day-care centers, nursery schools, and military recruit camps. Household and nursery school contacts may receive antibiotic prophylaxis as soon as possible, preferably within 24 hr of diagnosis of the primary case (Ref. 1, p. 140).

27.13. (A) Herpes simplex virus (HSV) is transmitted from person to person. HSV type 1 is believed to result from respiratory spread, whereas HSV type 2 usually occurs by venereal transmission (Ref. 1, p. 116).

27.14. (A) Many mammalian species are found to be infected with cytomegaloviruses, but there is little evidence for infection of one species with virus from another species in nature. Human CMV may be transmitted by blood transfusion, venereal spread, and breast feeding. Transmission from the infected maternal cervix to the newborn infant and household spread have been well documented (Ref. 1, p. 69).

27.15. (A) Humans are the only source of varicella-zoster virus infection. Person-to-person spread occurs presumably by direct contact or direct droplet infection. Airborne transmission has also been documented (Ref. 1, p. 286).

27.16. **(A)** Rotavirus infections are found in many animal species. However, human infection is believed to result only from human rotaviruses. Transmission is believed to occur by the fecal−oral route (Ref. 1, p. 228).

27.17. **(B)** *M. pneumoniae* is the single most frequent cause of pneumonia in school-aged children: it is an uncommon cause of pneumonia in infancy (Ref. 1, p. 145).

27.18. **(C)** *S. pneumoniae* is the most common cause of bacterial pneumonia, both in children and adults (Ref. 1, p. 327).

27.19. **(A)** Respiratory syncytial virus (RSV) infection is common in infants and young children, particularly during winter and early spring months. Bronchiolitis and pneumonia are common manifestations in older infants (Ref. 1, p. 219).

27.20. **(D)** In adults, severe pneumonia is a characteristic manifestation of Legionnaires' disease. However, clinical signs of *Legionella* infection have not been defined for children (Ref. 1, p. 125).

27.21. **(D)** Whipworm infection is frequently asymptomatic and without associated abnormalities in peripheral blood. The disease can be diagnosed by microscopic identification of the eggs in the feces (Ref. 1, p. 191).

27.22. **(D)** Whooping cough is associated with absolute lymphocytosis. Diagnosis is confirmed by culture of nasopharyngeal mucus obtained by swab and inoculated on special media (Bordet-Gengou with added penicillin) (Ref. 1, p. 199).

27.23. **(C)** *Toxocara* species are common roundworms of dogs and cats. Humans are infected by the ingestion of eggs containing infective larvae in soil or fomites. A history of pica, particularly the eating of soil, is common. Hypereosinophilia and hypergammaglobulinemia (IgE) with elevated titers of isohemagglutinins are presumptively diagnostic (Ref. 1, p. 186).

27.24. **(E)** Most bacterial vaccines and some viral vaccines are inactivated (or killed). The inactivated vaccines are incapable of replicating in the host; therefore, repeated doses and periodic booster doses are needed to maintain an adequate level of immunity. Both live (attenuated) and killed (inactivated) vaccines are available for polio virus vaccines (types 1, 2, and 3) (Ref. 1, p. 7).

27.25. (A) Ethambutol is an extremely effective antituberculous drug which has replaced paraaminosalicylic acid in most adults. However, ethambutol is not used in young children because of its side effect of optic neuritis. When ethambutol is used, careful, monthly visual examinations for acuity, visual fields, and color perception should be performed. Because cooperation on the part of the child is essential for adequate testing, it cannot be used safely in small children (Ref. 1, p. 270).

27.26. (C) Measles and mumps virus vaccines are live (attenuated) vaccines and do not require multiple doses or frequent booster. Hepatitis B virus and rabies vaccines are inactivated vaccines; therefore, multiple doses are needed to achieve protective levels of immunity (Ref. 1, p. 6).

27.27. (C) Atypical measles may occur after exposure to natural measles in some individuals who received killed measles vaccine in the United States between 1963 and 1967. It was used in Canada until 1970. Patients with atypical measles are acutely ill with fever and a rash that is most pronounced peripherally. The rash is usually maculopapular, but it may be hemorrhagic, urticarial, or vesicular. The patient may have pulmonary involvement, occasionally in the absence of skin lesions (Ref. 1, p. 133).

27.28. (C) At the present time, atypical measles is seen mainly in adolescents and young adults because killed vaccine has not been available for more than 10 years (Ref. 1, p. 134).

27.29. (C) Patients with atypical measles do not appear to be contagious. Extremely high titers of antibody appear rapidly in the patient's serum (Ref. 1, p. 134).

27.30. (B) The child has signs of increased intracranial pressure (tense and bulging anterior fontanel) and possibly a focal CNS lesion (pupils are not equal in size). Because of the history of trauma, it is important to rule out a subdural hematoma or other intracranial lesions by a CAT scan (Ref. based on the author's clinical experience).

27.31. (B) A spinal tap to rule out bacterial meningitis is essential in a febrile child with lethargy and bulging anterior fontanel (Ref. based on the author's clinical experience).

27.32. (B) An acutely ill child with fever, irritability, lethargy, vomiting, and a tense, bulging anterior fontanel are indications of CNS infection, either bacterial or viral (Ref. based on the author's clinical experience).

27.33. (D) Isolation of cytomegalovirus (CMV) from infant's urine during the first week of life indicates congenital CMV infection. Recovery of the virus after 1 month of life indicates either congenital infection or infection acquired perinatally. Intrauterine CMV infection is the most common congenital infection, occurring in approximately 1% of all live births, as evidenced by the presence of viruria during the first days of life. CMV causes a wide range of clinical syndromes, ranging from asymptomatic infection to severe, even fatal, disease (Ref. 5, p. 181).

27.34. (C) Most infants with symptomatic CMV infection have some degree of encephalitis, as evidenced by the frequent development of microcephaly. Mental retardation, spastic diplegia, seizures, optic atrophy, blindness, and deafness are common (Ref. 5, p. 185).

27.35. (B) At the present time, there is no antiviral agent that can be used to treat the infections. This patient may excrete CMV for many months or years. Therefore, it is prudent to attempt to reduce risks to susceptible pregnant women or severely immunocompromised patients by at least preventing direct contact with this infant (Ref. 1, p. 70).

References

1. Report of the Committee on Infectious Diseases, American Academy of Pediatrics, Evanston, IL, 1982.

2. Vaughan, V.C., III, McKay, R.J., Jr., and Behrman, R.I.: *Nelson Textbook of Pediatrics*, W.B. Saunders, Philadelphia, 1979.

3. Rudolph, A.M.: *Pediatrics*, 16th Ed., Appleton-Century-Crofts, New York, 1977.

4. Feigin, R.D. and Cherry, J.D.: *Textbook of Pediatric Infectious Diseases*, W.B. Saunders, Philadelphia, 1981.

5. Cho, C.T. and Dudding, B.A.: *Pediatric Infectious Diseases*, Medical Outline Series, Medical Examination Publishing, New York, 1978.

6. Krugman, S. and Katz, S.L.: *Infectious Diseases in Children*, 7th Ed., C.V. Mosby, St. Louis, 1981.

28

Neonatology
Raymond M. Russo, M.D., F.A.A.P.

DIRECTIONS: Each of the questions or incomplete statements below is followed by five suggested answers or completions. Select the **one** that is best in each case.

28.1. What is the mechanism of fetal growth potential reduction?
- **A.** Hypoxia
- **B.** Interference with hyperplastic and hypertrophic growth
- **C.** Interference with the hyperplastic growth phase characterized by no growth cessation, but rather a persistently slow growth rate and reduced absolute size from the first trimester
- **D.** Impairment of transplacental nutrient supplies associated with hypertensive disorders where, pathophysiologically, arteriography has revealed small size and slow filling of uterine arteries
- **E.** Neonatal asphyxia

28.2. What group of symptoms are characteristic of massive meconium aspiration syndrome?
   A. Mesenteric vasoconstriction, intestinal ischemia, and transient hyperperistalsis
   B. Increased gastrointestinal motility and anal sphincter dilation
   C. Rapid, irregular respiratory efforts with REM sleep, accompanied by small alterations of pulmonary volume
   D. Tachypnea and mild cyanosis
   E. Irregular and gasping respiration, profound cyanosis, hyperinflated chest, and a roentgenogram showing nonuniform, coarse, patchy infiltrates radiating from the hila into the peripheral lung fields

28.3. Severe forms of respiratory distress syndrome are associated with the acute onset of group B streptococcal disease in which of the following ways?
   A. Respiratory distress syndrome is prerequisite to the onset of group B streptococcal disease
   B. Group B streptococcal disease is a primary cause of respiratory distress syndrome
   C. Respiratory distress syndrome is the tertiary stage of acute onset of group B streptococcal disease
   D. Acute onset of group B streptococcal disease is clinically indistinguishable from severe forms of respiratory distress syndrome
   E. None of the above

DIRECTIONS: The group of questions below consists of five lettered headings followed by a list of numbered words or statements. For each numbered word or statement, select the **one** lettered heading that is most closely associated with it. Each lettered heading may be selected once, more than once, or not at all.

   A. Hyperaminoacidemia
   B. Hyperammonemia
   C. Hyperbilirubinemia
   D. Hyperglycemia
   E. Hypertriglyceridemia

28.4. During parenteral alimentation there is a common problem in a low birth-weight infant receiving large amounts of glucose via central venous catheter

28.5. Reported in infants receiving protein hydrolysate

28.6. Reported to be associated with mental retardation. Parenteral dose should be less than 2.5 g/kg/day

---

DIRECTIONS: For each of the questions or incomplete statements below, **one or more** of the answers or completions given is correct. Select
- **(A)** if only 1, 2, and 3 are correct
- **(B)** if only 1 and 3 are correct
- **(C)** if only 2 and 4 are correct
- **(D)** if only 4 is correct
- **(E)** if all are correct

28.7. Which of the following provide clinical clues to a diagnosis of congenital hypothyroidism in the newborn?
1. Large fontanels
2. Poor feeding and cry
3. Prolonged physiologic jaundice
4. A surge in the level of thyrotropin 48 hr postpartum

28.8. Bronchopulmonary dysplasia (BPD) is characterized by
1. progressive symptoms over weeks to months occurring in infants recovering from respiratory distress syndrome, pneumonia, or meconium aspiration
2. edema, massive atelectasis, pulmonary fibrosis, and emphysema
3. symptoms and signs of hypoxia with small changes in ambient oxygen
4. cor pulmonale in the fibrotic stage

DIRECTIONS: This section of the test consists of a situation followed by a series of questions. Study the situation and select the **one** best answer to each question following it.

Questions 28.9–28.10: A newborn with Apgar scores of 6 and 9 is noted to have petechiae over the trunk (Figure 60). The infant is restless and jittery. Temperature is 98.6°F (38°C).

Figure 60

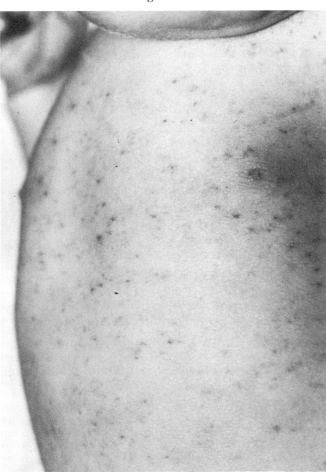

28.9. Which of the following clinical entities is most likely to cause petechiae in the neonate and must be considered in the differential diagnosis?
  A. Neonatal hypoglycemia
  B. Torch syndrome
  C. Severe maternal anemia
  D. Fetal alcohol syndrome
  E. Meningococcal sepsis

28.10. Of the following procedures, which one would most likely help establish the diagnosis?
  A. Hemoglobin
  B. Blood culture
  C. Skull x-ray
  D. Blood glucose
  E. Maternal hemoglobin

Answers and Comments

28.1. **(C)** It is important to distinguish between two essentially different mechanisms of intrauterine growth retardation: reduction in fetal growth potential and reduction in fetal growth support. In the former, growth is compromised by constitutional limitations, chromosomal anomalies, or congenital infections like rubella. The basic problem is interference with the hyperplastic phase of growth. Growth does not stop; it slows. In the latter, the constitutional potential for normal growth exists, but nonfetal factors cause growth to slow or stop altogether. Hypoxia, asphyxia, or impairment of transplacental nutrients are all examples of problems with fetal growth support. Reduction in fetal growth potential is characterized by interference withh hyperplastic growth; problems of fetal growth support include interference with hypertrophic growth as well (Ref. 1, pp. 431–454).

28.2. **(E)** Massive meconium aspiration is a life-threatening condition. The respiratory effort is seriously affected, with gasping and profound cyanosis the observable outcome. Roentgenogram findings showing patchy infiltrate radiating from the hilum serve to distinguish this condition from respiratory distress syndrome. Tachypnea and mild cyanosis may occur with minimal meconium aspiration but not with the massive variety. Gastrointestinal tract effects are not characteristic of meconium aspiration (Ref. 2, pp. 463–479).

28.3. (D) Although it is becoming increasingly obvious that respiratory distress syndrome cannot be distinguished clinically from acute onset group B streptococcal disease, many misconceptions remain to be dispelled. Respiratory distress is not a prerequisite to the onset of group B streptococcal disease, nor is it caused by group B streptococcal organisms (Ref. 3, pp. 501–508).

28.4. (D) Of the many complications arising from parenteral alimentation, hyperglycemia is one of the most common in low birthweight neonates. It leads to osmotic diuresis and subsequent dehydration and can be avoided with additional insulin (Ref. 4, pp. 547–556).

28.5. (B) Protein hydrolysate can cause hyperammonemia; so can L-amino acid mixtures. Adding 0.5–mM/kg/day arginine corrects the problem (Ref. 4, pp. 547–556).

28.6. (A) When adding amino acids, it is well to remember that too high a blood level is associated with mental retardation and is believed to be causative. Total protein infusion should be calculated to be no more than 2.5 gm/kg/day (Ref. 4, pp. 547–556).

28.7. (A) Large fontanels, poor feeding and cry, and prolonged physiologic jaundice are all common findings in congenital hypothyroidism. Others are: depressed nasal bridge, eyelid swelling, nasal congestion, large tongue, umbilical hernia, coarse dry skin, and bradycardia. There should not be a surge in the thyrotropin normally in the first few hours postpartum; normal levels should return by 48 hr. This is not a parameter to establish a diagnosis of congenital hypothyroidism (Ref. 5, pp. 529–535).

28.8. (E) All the signs and symptoms of progressive lung disease caused by the combined result of prolonged oxygen administration and the barotrauma of assisted ventilation can occur. The result may be a fibrotic end stage with cor pulmonale and respiratory failure. Prevention may be achieved by early weaning from oxygen therapy and assisted ventilation. Careful fluid management, nutritional support and treatment of a concomitant patent ductus arteriosus is helpful as well (Ref. 6)

28.9. (B) Neonatal hypoglycemia does not, per se, cause petechiae, although restlessness and jitteriness are features of low blood sugar in the newborn. The Torch syndrome, (which stands for *T*oxoplasmosis, *O*ther [diseases], *R*ubella, *C*ytomegalovirus, and *H*erpes simplex) can cause thrombocytopenia with resultant petechiae formation. All of these conditions can infect the fetus in utero with a chronic inflammatory process. Other common manifestations are a small size for gestational age, hepatosplenomegaly, icterus, and bony changes. Maternal anemia would not account for petechiae formation in the newborn unless maternally derived antiplatelet antibodies were responsible. Restlessness would not be expected to form part of the clinical picture in this case. None of the stigmata of fetal alcohol syndrome are described, although restlessness can be encountered. The syndrome does not produce petechiae. Meningococcal sepsis can produce all of the clinical findings described. However, the meningococcus is almost never encountered in the newborn period and would have to be considered highly unlikely (Ref. 7, pp. 194–195).

28.10. (C) A hemoglobin would not shed much light on the cause of petechiae. Thrombocytopenia would not be reflected in a lowered hemoglobin unless a pancytopenia or extensive hemorrhaging also occurred. Chronic uterine infection can lead to anemia as well, however. A blood culture would be useful to help identify bacterial causes of neonatal sepsis. Unless viral studies were done, the procedure would not establish the diagnosis of Torch syndrome diseases. A skull x-ray may be very helpful in establishing the diagnosis of congenital toxoplasmosis or cytomegalovirus infection, because intracranial calcifications can be seen in both cases. The blood glucose would not necessarily be markedly depressed in the Torch syndrome spectrum of diseases. Maternal hemoglobin would not be helpful in establishing a diagnosis of Torch syndrome in the fetus (Ref. 7, pp. 194–195).

References

1. Cook, L.N.: Intrauterine and extrauterine recognition and management of deviant fetal growth. Pediatr. Cl. N. Am. 24, 1977.

2. Bacsik, R.D.: Meconium aspiration syndrome. Pediatr. Cl. N. Am. 24, 1977.

3. Miller, T.C.: Emergency treatment of group b streptococcal disease. Pediatr. Cl. N. Am. 24, 1977.

4. Lorch, V. and Lay, S.A.: Parenteral alimentation in the neonate. Pediatr. Cl. N. Am. 24, 1977.

5. Katoyan, M.: Aspects of perinatal endocrinology. Pediatr. Cl. N. Am. 24, 1977.

6. Bateman, D.: In *Textbook of Pediatrics*, Russo, R.M. and Allen, J.E. (Eds.), Medical Examination Publishing, New York, 1985.

7. Alistair, P.: *Neonatology Case Studies*, 2d Ed., Medical Examination Publishing, New York, 1982.

29

Pediatric Nephrology
Charles E. Hollerman, M.D.

DIRECTIONS: Each of the questions or incomplete statements below is followed by five suggested answers or completions. Select the **one** that is best in each case.

29.1. A 5-year-old boy is admitted to the hospital with the diagnosis of idiopathic nephrotic syndrome of childhood. A renal biopsy is performed. Light microscopy of the biopsy specimen is illustrated in Figure 61. The pathologic diagnosis based on the biopsy is
 A. membranoproliferative glomerulonephritis
 B. membranous glomerulonephritis
 C. chronic glomerulonephritis
 D. focal segmental glomerulonephritis
 E. minimal glomerulonephritis

29.2. Ten days following an upper respiratory infection, a 2-year-old patient presents with oliguria, pallor, and hypertension. Laboratory studies reveal hemoglobin levels of 5 g/dl, burr cells, depressed serum complement levels, and azotemia. The most likely diagnosis is
 A. acute poststreptococcal glomerulonephritis
 B. anaphylactoid purpura (Henoch-Schönlein) nephritis
 C. acute pyelonephritis
 D. hemolytic−uremic syndrome
 E. IgG−IgA nephropathy (Berger's disease)

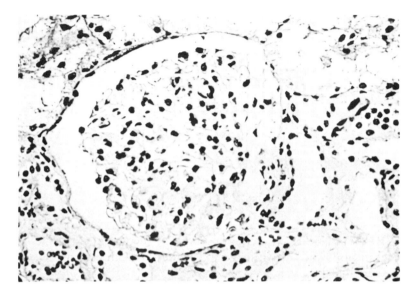

Figure 61

29.3. Cystic diseases of the kidney are commonly heritable conditions. A nonhereditary cystic disease is
  A. infantile–childhood polycystic disease
  B. adult polycystic disease
  C. infantile microcystic disease
  D. nephronophthisis
  E. medullary sponge kidney

DIRECTIONS: For each of the questions or incomplete statements below, **one or more** of the answers or completions given is correct. Select
  (A) if only 1, 2, and 3 are correct
  (B) if only 1 and 3 are correct
  (C) if only 2 and 4 are correct
  (D) if only 4 is correct
  (E) if all are correct

29.4. Appropriate conservative (nondialysis, nonparenteral alimentation) therapy for a pediatric patient with acute oliguric parenchymal renal failure would include
1. fluids at 300 cc/m^2/day plus replacement of urinary output
2. daily weights
3. 1 g/kg body weight high biologic protein/day
4. prophylactic antibiotic therapy

29.5. The term chronic pyelonephritis has given way to a new term: reflux nephropathy. Which of the following may be associated with reflux nephropathy?
1. Intrarenal reflux
2. Focal glomerulosclerosis
3. Hypertension
4. Proteinuria

Answers and Comments

29.1. (E) Idiopathic nephrotic syndrome of childhood (lipoid nephrosis) occurs predominantly in boys, with the majority of cases occurring between 1−5 years of age. In minimal glomerular diseases or lipoid nephrosis, light microscopy (as in Figure 61) reveals a normal-appearing glomerulus (*center*). There may be occasional clusters of interstitial foam cells also seen in the illustration (*upper right*) (Refs. 1, pp. 15−17: 2, p. 1495).

29.2. (D) A patient with hemolytic−uremic syndrome may have a preceding gastroenteritis, flu-like syndrome, or acute upper respiratory infection some days to 2 weeks prior to clinically presenting with oliguria, hemolytic anemia (with associated pallor), uremia (azotemia), and hypertension. Thrombocytopenia may or may not be present. Fragmented, helmet-shaped burr cells are characteristically seen. The serum complement level, which is depressed in acute poststreptococcal glomerulonephritis, may be transiently depressed in patients with hemolytic−uremic syndrome. The serum complement levels are characteristically normal in acute pyelonephritis, IgG−IgA nephropathy, or anaphylactoid purpura nephritis (Ref. 2, pp. 1512−1514).

29.3. (E) Infantile–childhood polycystic kidney is an autosomal recessive disease, whereas adult polycystic kidney is an autosomal dominant disease. Nephronophthisis may be inherited apparently as an autosomal dominant, recessive, or even sex-linked disease. Infantile microcystic disease (congenital nephrotic syndrome) is an autosomal recessive disease. Medullary sponge kidney is not inherited (Ref. 2, pp. 1500, 1526, 1530–1531).

29.4. (A) Insensible water loss in acute renal failure falls from the usual level of 600–900 cc/m^2/day to 300 cc/m^2/day. To this insensible water loss must be added fluids for replacement of urinary losses. Daily weighing of these patients is mandatory for monitoring of fluid balance. A weight loss of 0.5–1% of body weight daily is indicative of proper therapy. Protein intake is encouraged in children with acute renal failure. The recommended intake is 1 g high biologic value protein (milk, eggs, cheese, meats)/kg body weight/day. Prophylactic antibiotics are not indicated; antibiotics should be used for the treatment of identified infection (Refs. 2, pp. 1533–1534; 3, pp. 467–474; 4, pp. 416–421).

29.5. (E) Intrarenal reflux is possible if the papilla have circular, rather than slitlike, orifices. In human kidneys, about 1/7 of the papillae are of the circular type and predominate at the poles of the kidney. Hence "pyelonephritic" scarring occurs most commonly at these sites. Focal glomerulosclerosis may occur in reflux nephropathy, with proteinuria sufficient to occasionally produce a nephrotic syndrome. The mechanism(s) responsible for the lesion is/are unknown. Hypertension may be associated; indeed, some authors believe reflux nephropathy may be the most common cause of hypertension in childhood (Ref. 4, pp. 229–230, 235–237).

References

1. Jenis, E.H. and Lowenthal, D.T.: *Kidney Biopsy Interpretations*, F.A. Davis, Philadelphia, 1977.

2. Vaughn, V.C., III, McKay, R.J., Behrman, R.E., and Nelson,

W.E.: *Nelson Textbook of Pediatrics*, 11th Ed., W.B. Saunders, Philadelphia, 1979.

3. Edelmann, C.M., Jr.: *Pediatric Kidney Disease*, Little Brown, Boston, 1978.

4. Hollerman, C.E.: *Pediatric Nephrology*, Medical Outline Series, Medical Examination Publishing, New York, 1979.

30

Pediatric Neurology
Lawrence W. Brown, M.D.

DIRECTIONS: Each of the questions or incomplete statements below is followed by five suggested answers or completions. Select the **one** that is best in each case

---

30.1. All of the following statements about Reye's syndrome are true EXCEPT

    A. Reye's syndrome is a disorder of unknown etiology usually associated with preceding bacterial infection

    B. prior aspirin treatment has been implicated as a risk factor in the development of Reye's syndrome

    C. typical laboratory findings include elevated serum transaminases, prolonged prothrombin time, and high blood ammonia

    D. characteristic pathologic features of fatty degeneration of the liver are produced by disruption of mitochondrial function

    E. intracranial pressure monitoring is indicated in all comatose patients with Reye's syndrome

30.2. Migraine is the most common paroxysmal disorder of the brain in the pediatric age. Which of the following findings is seen in the majority of the affected children?
   A. Significant EEG abnormalities
   B. Positive family history for migraine
   C. Transient hemiplegia
   D. Onset of symptoms before 5 years of age
   E. Attacks triggered by minor head injury

30.3. Which of the following statements is NOT true about status epilepticus?
   A. Status epilepticus in the child should always be considered a medical emergency
   B. Status epilepticus can be precipitated by sudden discontinuance of anticonvulsant medication
   C. Intravenous diazepam is a common initial treatment in status epilepticus in the neonate
   D. Lead intoxication can be a cause of status epilepticus in childhood
   E. Respiratory arrest is a complication of intravenous diazepam administration

---

DIRECTIONS: The group of questions below consists of five lettered headings followed by a list of numbered words or statements. For each numbered word or statement, select the **one** lettered heading that is most closely associated with it. Each lettered heading may be selected once, more than once, or not at all.

Choose the most frequently associated anticonvulsant with its significant adverse effect.

   A. Ethosuximide (Zarontin)
   B. Phenobarbital
   C. Carbamazepine (Tegretol)
   D. Valproic acid (Depakene)
   E. Phenytoin (Dilantin)

30.4. Hyperactivity

30.5. Acute hepatic failure

30.6. Lymphadenopathy (pseudolymphoma)

DIRECTIONS: For each of the questions or incomplete statements below, **one or more** of the answers or completions given is correct. Select
(A) if only 1, 2, and 3 are correct
(B) if only 1 and 3 are correct
(C) if only 2 and 4 are correct
(D) if only 4 is correct
(E) if all are correct

30.7. Transient sleep disorders common in the preschool child include
1. obstructive sleep apnea
2. somnambulism (sleepwalking)
3. narcolepsy
4. pavor nocturnus (night terrors)

30.8. Common clinical signs of acutely increased intracranial pressure in infants include
1. lethargy
2. strabismus
3. full fontanel
4. papilledema

DIRECTIONS: This section of the test consists of situations, each followed by a series of questions. Study each situation and select the **one** best answer to each question following it.

Question 30.9: A 20-month-old black boy awoke with a temperature of 39.4°C and developed episodes of generalized clonic seizures followed by persistent flaccid weakness of his right arm and leg.

30.9. The differential diagnosis of this child includes all of the following conditions EXCEPT
   A. sickle cell disease
   B. acute bacterial meningitis
   C. arteriovenous malformation
   D. simple febrile seizure
   E. battered child syndrome

Question 30.10: A 9-week-old infant is hospitalized with a brief history of poor feeding, bilateral facial weakness, and progressive weakness (Figure 62). Routine studies including complete blood count, electrolytes, calcium, chest x-ray, and lumbar puncture are all normal. An edrophonium (Tensilon) test produces no improvement.

30.10. The most likely diagnosis is
   A. Guillain-Barré syndrome
   B. botulism
   C. viral encephalitis
   D. myasthenia gravis
   E. poliomyelitis

Figure 62

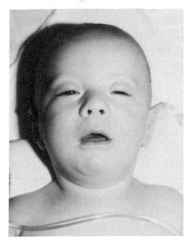

Answers and Comments

30.1. (A) Reye's syndrome is a generalized hepatoencephalopathy, which usually follows a nonspecific respiratory or gastrointestinal illness. The most frequently identified pathogens are influenza B and varicella, although many other viruses have been implicated. Although aspirin has not been directly linked to the development of Reye's syndrome, epidemiologic evidence is accumulating that it is a strong risk factor. Aspirin should be avoided in children with viral illnesses according to the U.S. Surgeon General, the Academy of Pediatrics, the Food and Drug Administration, and the Centers for Disease Control (Ref. 2, pp. 402–406).

30.2. (B) The family history is positive in 70–80% of pediatric migraine sufferers, suggesting a genetic vasomotor instability. Nonspecific EEG abnormalities are occasionally found, but paroxysmal tracings are definitely uncommon. Complicated migraine with pronounced neurologic findings are fortunately rare. Only 1 out of 5 patients has the first attack before the age of 5 years. There are many factors which can trigger migraine in the susceptible patient, and trivial head injury is an unusual example (Ref. 2, pp. 658–662).

30.3. (C) In neonatal status epilepticus, diagnosis of the underlying abnormality and its specific therapy is more important than treatment of the seizures with anticonvulsants. Intravenous phenobarbital is the most generally accepted medication for treatment of prolonged seizures in this age group. Diazepam is infrequently used because of the short duration of action necessitating addition of phenobarbital or phenytoin for prolonged seizure protection (Ref. 1, pp. 1064–1070).

30.4. (B)
30.5. (D)
30.6. (E) A paradoxical hyperactivity syndrome can be seen in up to 40% of young children on phenobarbital. Idiosyncratic fulminant liver failure is a rare but potentially fatal complication seen with valproic acid. The most common side effects with phenytoin include nystagmus, gingival hyperplasia, hirsutism, and acne; occasionally, lymphadenopathy with histologic features indistinguishable from lymphoma can be associated (Ref. 1, pp. 1045–1047).

30.7. (C) Although brief asymptomatic episodes of central apnea are universal in infancy, obstructive apnea is rarely benign or transient. Narcolepsy most often begins in the late teenage years or early adulthood. Both night terrors and sleepwalking are common transient disorders of arousal from stage 4 sleep seen most frequently in toddlers (Ref. 1, pp. 206–213).

30.8. (A) The clinical signs of acutely increased intracranial pressure are similar in the infant and older child, except that papilledema is infrequent in infants with open sutures; other common signs of raised intracranial pressure in the infant include vomiting, separated sutures, and altered vital signs. Enlarged head circumference and signs of herniation are occasional findings (Ref. 1, pp. 190–195).

30.9. (D) Acute infantile hemiplegia is caused by any condition which can lead to cerebrovascular occlusion. Trauma, CNS infection, cyanotic congenital heart disease, and arteriovenous malformations account for most of the identifiable causes. By definition, a simple febrile seizure is a brief, generalized convulsion without focal component (Ref. 3, pp. 1592–1594).

30.10. (B) Infant botulism is a recently described disorder in which intestinal germination of spores leads to elaboration of botulinal toxin. Characteristic clinical features include constipation, followed by progressive neuromuscular weakness with cranial nerve involvement. Congenital myasthenia gravis is an extremely rare condition, which is excluded by the negative Tensilon test. The normal lumbar puncture eliminates the other listed diagnoses (Ref. 4, pp. 273–275).

References

1. Swaiman, K.F. and Wright, F.S.: *The Practice of Pediatric Neurology*, 2d Ed., C.V. Mosby, St. Louis, 1982.

2. Menkes, J.H.: *Textbook of Child Neurology*, 3rd Ed., Lea & Febiger, Philadelphia, 1985.

3. Behrman, R.E. and Vaughan, V.C.: *Nelson Textbook of Pediatrics*, 12th Ed., W.B. Saunders, Philadelphia, 1983.

4. Bell, W.E. and McCormick, W.F.: *Neurologic Infections in Children*, 2d Ed., W.B. Saunders, Philadelphia, 1981.

31

Pediatric Nutrition
Raymond M. Russo, M.D., F.A.A.P.

DIRECTIONS: Each of the questions or incomplete statements below is followed by five suggested answers or completions. Select the **one** that is best in each case.

31.1. Mature human milk contains 0.1 mg of iron per 100 ml of which?
- **A.** 20–30% is absorbed by normal infants
- **B.** 30–40% is absorbed by normal infants
- **C.** 50–70% is absorbed by normal infants
- **D.** 80–100% is absorbed by normal infants
- **E.** An unpredictable percentage is absorbed by normal infants

31.2. Which of the following statements best characterizes the group of children most subject to "nursing bottle" caries?
- **A.** Neonates sensitive to cow's milk
- **B.** One- to 2-year-old children sensitive to cow's milk
- **C.** One- to 4-year-old children who live in areas where the fluoride level of the drinking water is below 1 ppm optimal level
- **D.** Three- to 4-year-old children who continue to use the nursing bottle as a pacifier at bedtime
- **E.** One- or 2-year-old children who drink sugar-sweetened beverages from a nursing bottle

447

31.3. What are the dangers posed to infants by mothers feeding them according to Zen macrobiotic diets?
  A. Shorter stature and lighter weight than matched controls
  B. Rickets and beriberi
  C. Rickets, beriberi, scurvy, and energy deficiency
  D. Energy inadequacy, vitamin B_{12} deficiency, and anemia
  E. Energy and protein deficiency, vitamin and mineral inadequacies, dehydration, and starvation ketosis

---

DIRECTIONS: The group of questions below consists of five lettered headings followed by a list of numbered words or statements. For each numbered word or statement, select the **one** lettered heading that is most closely associated with it. Each lettered heading may be selected once, more than once, or not at all.

  A. Carbohydrate malnutrition
  B. Vitamin and mineral deficiencies
  C. General malnutrition
  D. Protein malnutrition
  E. Protein and iron deficiency

31.4. Results in atrophy of liver, spleen, bone marrow, and lymphoid tissues from which phagocytes and lymphocytes originate

31.5. Thymus atrophy, findings that peripheral lymph nodes, tonsils, spleen, and circulating lymphocytes are reduced, and an increased susceptibility to tuberculosis, moniliasis, herpes simplex, chickenpox, and measles

31.6. Particularly likely to depress cellular immunity

DIRECTIONS: The set of lettered headings below is followed by a list of numbered words or phrases. For each numbered word or phrase select

(A) if the item is associated with A only
(B) if the item is associated with B only
(C) if the item is associated with A and B
(D) if the item is associated with neither A nor B

For questions 31.7–31.9, refer to Figure 63.

A. Congenital heart disease
B. Myelomeningocele
C. Both
D. Neither

31.7. Obesity can impair the child's ambulation potential to such a degree that he must spend his lifetime in a wheelchair

Figure 63

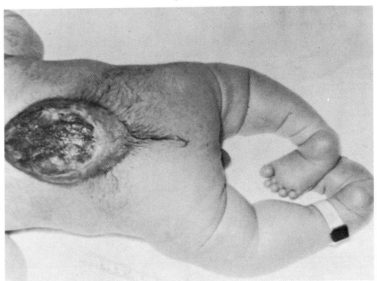

31.8. Severely impaired linear growth

31.9. Body fat comprises a greater proportion of body mass than otherwise normal

---

DIRECTIONS: For each of the questions or incomplete statements below, **one or more** of the answers or completions given is correct. Select

   (A)   if only 1, 2, and 3 are correct
   (B)   if only 1 and 3 are correct
   (C)   if only 2 and 4 are correct
   (D)   if only 4 is correct
   (E)   if all are correct

31.10. What factors define and confirm the diagnosis of iron deficiency anemia in full-term infants between the ages of 6 months and 3 to perhaps 5 years (Figure 64).

   1. Hemoglobin concentration below 11 g/dl
   2. The presence of microcytosis, a mean corpuscular volume of less than 70 μm^3 as determined on the Coulter model S
   3. Hypochromia, a mean corpuscular hemoglobin concentration less than 30%
   4. A serum iron level below 200 $\mu g/dl$

31.11. A simple office procedure for assessing body fat stores consists of

   1. subtracting body weight in total water immersion from standard body weight
   2. measuring the upper arm muscle circumference
   3. calculating the height and dividing it by the expected height-for-age (50th percentile) × 100
   4. measuring the triceps skinfold thickness

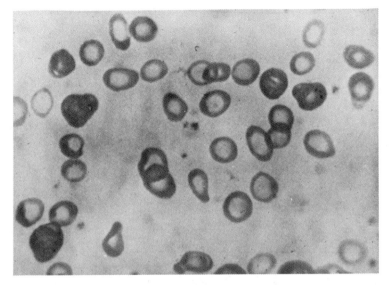

Figure 64

31.12. Secondary to counseling the mother to bring her child to the dentist for preventative dental services when he or she is no older than 3, the pediatrician might also offer which of the following as dietary guidance for the prevention of caries?

1. Reduce the use of spinach because the high iron content contributes to the decalcification of teeth

2. Absolutely forbid the between-meal eating of any baked goods, confections, and beverages that are sweetened with sugar

3. Discourage starchy foods such as pretzels, crackers, pizza, popcorn, corn chips

4. Encourage fibrous carboyhdrates such as raw fruits and vegetables which require vigorous chewing

---

DIRECTIONS: This section of the test consists of a situation followed by a series of questions. Study the situation and select the **one** best answer to each question following it.

Questions 31.13–31.15: You are called to the emergency room to see an unmarried teenager's 2-month-old son who has his first generalized seizure. You learn that the mother received little prenatal care and has yet to take her child to a physician for routine pediatric care because her "son has always been a normal, healthy child." The baby has been fed undiluted evaporated milk for the past 2 weeks in the belief that "a stronger formula would make him grow faster." Your examination reveals a poorly reactive, somnolent baby.

31.13. A serum electrolyte determination is likely to show
  A. hypocalcemia
  B. hypokalemia
  C. hyperkalemia
  D. hyponatremia
  E. hypernatremia

31.14. Which of the following would also be likely to be elevated in the blood?
  A. Glucose
  B. Urea
  C. Total bilirubin
  D. Alkaline phosphatase
  E. Iron

31.15. Associated clinical findings would most likely include which of the following?
  A. Plethora
  B. Pallor
  C. Depressed reflexes
  D. Maculopapular eruption
  E. Diarrhea

Answers and Comments

31.1. (C) Normal infants will absorb a predictable percentage of iron from mature mother's milk. This percentage varies from 50–70%. It should be realized that iron absorption in the infant's gut can be adversely affected by the introduction of foods containing different iron salts, such as cow's milk or cow's milk formulas. Thus, if supplemental feedings of cow's milk formulas are offered to a breast-fed baby, iron supplementation is warranted (Ref. 1, p. 139).

31.2. (D) The 3- or 4-year-old child still being given the nursing bottle as a pacifier is the most likely candidate for nursing bottle caries. Milk sensitivity does not cause this problem at any age. Fluoride in the drinking water may prevent caries and certainly will not cause them. Overadministration of fluoride (fluorosis) leads to dental mottling instead. A 1- or 2-year-old who drinks sugar-sweetened beverages from a nursing bottle, but whose teeth are not subjected to a continuous exposure to the sweetened liquid, has a much lower risk for developing caries (Ref. 2, pp. 141–155).

31.3. (E) While infants fed Zen macrobiotic diets may be of shorter stature and lighter weight than normal, they are more specifically prone to energy/protein/vitamin/mineral deficiencies, dehydration, and starvation ketosis. Vitamin deficiency states or anemia are not as prominent a part of the picture (Ref. 3, pp. 189–201).

31.4. (D) Although general malnutrition may adversely affect cellular immune response, protein malnutriton most specifically results in atrophy of spleen, liver, and lymphoid tissues. Carbohydrate malnutrition and vitamin, mineral, or iron deficiency states certainly have adverse effects but do not cause the same degree of spleen, liver, and lymphatic compromise (Ref. 4, pp. 241–252).

31.5. (C) General malnutrition has been reported to lead directly to thymus and lymphatic tissue atrophy, as well as an increase in specific infectious diseases. In addition, the diseases tend to be more severe and to give rise to an increased number of complications and an elevated mortality rate (Ref. 4, pp. 241–252).

31.6. (E) The combination of protein and iron deficiencies is particularly likely to depress cellular immunity. Carbohydrate, vitamin, and mineral deficiencies do not affect cellular immunity to the same degree (Ref. 4, pp. 241–252).

31.7. (B) Children with congenital heart disease are at no particular risk for obesity. Often, weight gain and somatic growth are compromised by a serious heart lesion. However, children with myelomeningocele are often confined to wheelchairs and are relatively inactive. Because obesity is a product of calorie intake less expenditure, the inactive individual has a tendency to gain excessive amounts of weight. Add to this the potential of an overindulgent parent who overfeeds the child, and obesity can be a disadvantageous outcome, to the point that it may interfere with the ambulation potential and lead to permanent dependence on the wheelchair (Ref. 5, pp. 157–174).

31.8. (C) Myelomeningocele, as well as congenital heart disease, will impede linear growth. Almost any serious organic heart disease in infancy will reflect itself in suboptimal linear growth. The reason for this is related to persistently less than normal tissue perfusion. Myelomeningocele, on the other hand, involves spinal nerves in the lower section of the cord. The paresis and/or paralysis this gives rise to prevents normal musculoskeletal growth and the attainment of normal stature (Ref. 5, pp. 157–174).

31.9. (B) It has been demonstrated that body fat comprises a greater proportion of body mass in children with meningocele than the general pediatric population. This may cause an underestimate of the extent of obesity if standard weight-for-height criteria are used (Ref. 5, pp. 157–174).

31.10. (A) A hemoglobin concentration below 11 g/dl, the presence of microcytosis, and hypochromia are hallmarks of iron deficiency anemia. The serum iron level can also be useful but is not usually above 40 μg/dl (Ref. 6, pp. 85–94).

31.11. (D) Measuring triceps skinfold thickness is a simple, practical office method of assessing body fat stores. Calibrated calipers are available for this purpose. Weighing in total water immersion would hardly be a simple office procedure. Measuring the upper arm muscle circumference is a way of assessing lean body mass. Calculating the height and dividing by expected height × 100 gives the weight-for-height deficit not body fat store (Ref. 7, pp. 195–196).

31.12. (C) The essential advice a practitioner should impart to parents of young children is contained in responses 2 and 4. Starchy foods such as pretzels and pizza will not cause caries and may be encouraged as alternatives to sugar-containing foods, keeping in mind the issue of weight control where appropriate. A vegetable like spinach should not have any serious dental side effects. Fluoride supplements, when the drinking water is not fluoride treated, may also be recommended (Ref. 2, pp. 141–155).

31.13. (E) Hypocalcemia is encountered in the early neonatal period when infants are given high calcium loads with their formula. However, neonatal tetany causes twitching, jitteriness, and muscle spasms, and at 2 months of age the infant is a bit too old for transient hypothyroidism. Hypokalemia usually occurs in the course of protracted, severe diarrhea, or renal disease. It would be unlikely to encounter potassium disturbances with no other indication of illness. Hyperkalemia is associated with renal diseases and iatrogenic causes. There is little reason to believe that this infant has an excessive serum potassium load. Diarrhea, excessive vomiting, suctioning, or lack of NaCl intake all may lead to hyponatremia. This condition is unlikely with this history. Infants fed excessively concentrated or unmodified formulas are exposed to a dangerously high solute load. The kidney can concentrate urine to a lesser degree in neonates than older infants. For this reason, sodium retention may occur and, over the course of several days, lead to hypernatremia. The symptoms of hypernatremia include seizures, lethargy, a doughy feel to the abdomen. The disorder is life threatening and may cause permanent central nervous system sequelae (Ref. 8, pp. 49–61).

31.14. (B) Glucose is usually not affected markedly by feeding concentrated formula. Davis and Saunders have demonstrated increased urea levels in infants fed concentrated or unmodified formula. What adverse effects this might have is not clear. Total bilirubin should be normal by 2 months of age in the absence of hemolysis and liver disease. It would be unlikely for the infant to present with a seizure and no other indications of hyperbilirubinemia. Alkaline phosphatase is not likely to have contributed to a seizure in this infant. Increased solute load will not lead to markedly deranged values. Serum iron, if maternally derived amounts were normal, is not likely to be abnormally low at 2 months. Feeding concentrated formula should not affect the serum value to any great degree (Ref. 8, pp. 49–61).

31.15. (C) Plethora is associated with neonates born of diabetic mothers. This 2-month-old with hypernatremia is more likely to be pale. Pallor could be a part of the clinical picture, but it is not the most likely choice. Because excessive sodium retention leads to acute brain swelling, not only is seizure activity to be expected, but also depressed or hyperactive reflexes may be. There is no association between hypernatremia and cutaneous eruptions. Diarrhea may lead to hypernatremic dehydration, but, in this case, the cause is excessive intake of solute, not loss of dilute fluid. Hypernatremia, on this basis, does not cause diarrhea (Ref. 8, pp. 49−61).

References

1. Lawrence, R.A.: Infant nutrition. Pediatrics in Review 5:133−140, 1983.

2. Nizel, A.E.: Preventing dental caries: The nutritional factors. Pediatr. Cl. N. Am. 24, 1977.

3. Robson, J.R.K.: Food faddism. Pediatr. Cl. N. Am. 24, 1977.

4. Brown, R.E.: Interaction of nutrition and infection in clinical practice. Pediatr. Cl. N. Am. 24, 1977.

5. Rickard, K., Brady, M.S., and Gresham, E.L.: Nutritional management of the chronically ill child. Pediatr. Cl. N. Am. 24, 1977.

6. Woodruff, C.W.: Iron deficiency in infancy and childhood. Pediatr. Cl. N. Am. 24, 1977.

7. Suskind, R.M. and Varma, R.N.: Assessment of nutritional status of children. Pediatrics in Review 5:195−202, 1984.

8. Jelliffe, E.F.P.: Infant feeding practices: Associated iatrogenic and commerciogenic diseases. Pediatr. Cl. N. Am. 24, 1977.

32

Pediatric Ophthalmology
Henry S. Metz, M.D.

DIRECTIONS: Each of the questions or incomplete statements below is followed by five suggested answers or completions. Select the **one** that is best in each case.

32.1. Exotropia (outward drifting eyes or "wall-eyed") (Figure 65)
   A.   is a normal finding in many children
   B.   never requires therapy
   C.   may be seen as an intermittent deviation
   D.   is not associated with amblyopia
   E.   is not associated with any potential for fusion

32.2. Amblyopia (lazy eye) may be caused by all of the following EXCEPT
   A.   strabismus
   B.   anisometropia (unequal refractive error in the two eyes)
   C.   anisocoria (unequal pupillary size)
   D.   congenital cataract
   E.   significant, unilateral upper lid ptosis

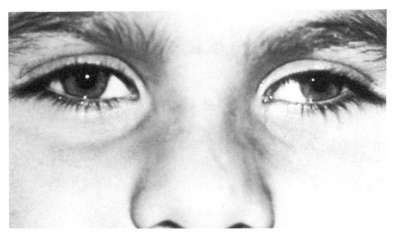

Figure 65

32.3. Cataract in childhood may be caused by all of the following
EXCEPT
   A. galactosemia
   B. ocular trauma
   C. long-term systemic steroid therapy
   D. strabismus
   E. maternal rubella during pregnancy

DIRECTIONS: For each of the questions or incomplete statements below, **one or more** of the answers or completions given is correct. Select
   (A) if only 1, 2, and 3 are correct
   (B) if only 1 and 3 are correct
   (C) if only 2 and 4 are correct
   (D) if only 4 is correct
   (E) if all are correct

32.4. Leukocoria (white pupillary reflex in a child) may be caused by
1. retinoblastoma
2. cataract
3. retrolental fibroplasia (RLF)
4. glaucoma

32.5. The findings of congenital glaucoma include
1. enlarged cornea
2. hazy cornea
3. increased intraocular pressure
4. photophobia (sensitivity to light)

Answers and Comments

32.1. (C) Exotropia frequently begins in childhood with an intermittent pattern, the child having straight eyes part of the time and drifting outward part time (especially with fatigue). A parallel position of the eyes is normal, not an outward deviation. Although amblyopia is less common than is exotropia, monocular (nonalternating) exotropes can be amblyopic. Treatment is needed both to obtain a parallel eye position and prevent amblyopia. Because many exotropes begin with an intermittent pattern, fusion is often a goal that can be achieved with therapy (Ref. 1, pp. 314–326).

32.2. (C) Amblyopia can be caused when an eye is deviated (and suppressed), when unequal refractive error results in a blurred image in one eye, and by deprivation of clear image formation (cataract, ptosis, corneal scarring, anterior chamber or vitreous hemorrhage). Unequal pupillary size does not result in diminished vision in one eye (Ref. 4, pp. 59–68).

32.3. (D) Cataracts can be caused by ocular injury, steroid therapy, certain maternal infections during pregnancy (rubella, CMV), and metabolic disease (galactosemia, diabetes). Although strabismus may be caused by unilateral cataract in childhood, it is not the cause of cataract (Ref. 5, pp. 549–566).

460 / Pediatrics

32.4. (A) Retinoblastoma, opacity of the lens, and RLF (white, updrawn membrane associated with oxygen therapy in the premature infant) can all be responsible for a white reflex of the pupil. Congenital glaucoma patients generally have a dark pupil (Ref. 2, pp. 90–116).

32.5. (E) In addition to raised intraocular pressure, infants with congenital glaucoma often have corneal enlargement (diameter greater than 11 mm), corneal haze (secondary to edema), and light sensitivity (secondary to corneal edema). Examination of the anterior chamber frequently reveals abnormal mesodermal tissue in the angle (Ref. 3, pp. 233–263).

References

1. Burian, H. and von Noorden, G.: *Binocular Vision and Ocular Motility*, 2nd Ed., C.V. Mosby, St. Louis, 1980.

2. Reese, A.B.: *Tumors of the Eye*, 3rd Ed., Harper & Row, New York, 1976.

3. Kwitko, M.L.: *Glaucoma in Infants and Children*, Appleton-Century-Crofts, New York, 1973.

4. Helveston, E.M. and Ellis, F.D.: *Pediatric Ophthalmology Practice*, C.V. Mosby, St. Louis, 1980.

5. Harley, R.D.: *Pediatric Ophthalmology*, 2nd Ed., W.B. Saunders, Philadelphia, 1983.

33

Pediatric Otolaryngology
W. Frederick McGuirt, M.D.

DIRECTIONS: Each of the questions or incomplete statements below is followed by five suggested answers or completions. Select the **one** that is best in each case.

33.1. The most common congenital anomaly of the branchial arch system is which of the following?
A. First branchial cleft cyst
B. Thyroglossal duct cyst
C. Second branchial cleft cyst
D. Cystic hygroma
E. Third branchial cleft cyst

33.2. The most reliable diagnostic sign for identifying a neck mass as a thyroglossal duct cyst is
A. purulent drainage
B. transillumination of the mass
C. elevation of the mass with tongue protrusion
D. a midline location of the mass
E. compressibility of the mass

33.3. A 13-year-old boy is diagnosed as having a second branchial cleft cyst and is advised to have it surgically removed. At the operation, the surgeon would expect to find which of the following relationships?

A. The cyst tract would pass inferior and medial to cranial nerve XII

B. The cyst tract would pass inferior and medial to the internal and external carotid arteries

C. The cyst tract would pass between the internal and external carotid arteries

D. The cyst tract would enter the pyriform sinus of the pharynx

E. The cyst tract would enter the ventricle of the larynx

DIRECTIONS: Each group of questions below consists of lettered headings followed by a list of numbered words or statements. For each numbered word or statement, select the lettered heading or headings that are most closely associated with it. Each lettered heading may be selected once, more than once, or not at all.

For questions 33.4–33.7, refer to Figure 66.

Questions 33.4–33.10:

A. Type A tympanogram
B. Type B tympanogram
C. Type C tympanogram

33.4. Perforated tympanic membrane

33.5. Normal middle ear

33.6. Secretory otitis media

TYMPANOGRAM

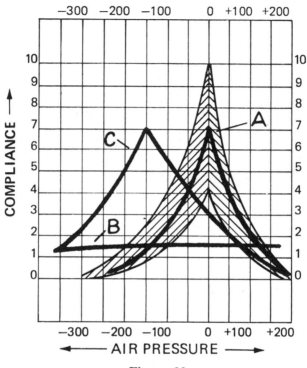

Figure 66

33.7. Intermittent eustachian tube dysfunction

   A. Air conduction and bone conduction curves on audiometry superimposed at less than 5 dB threshold
   B. Air conduction curve indicates higher threshold than bone conduction by audiometry
   C. Air conduction and bone conduction threshold curves superimposed at 40 dB
   D. Air conduction threshold curve higher than bone conduction threshold curve, which is at 40 dB
   E. Air conduction threshold curve at lower threshold than bone conduction threshold curve

33.8. Conductive hearing loss

33.9. Sensorineural hearing loss

33.10. Mixed hearing loss

   A. Relative frequency is greater in children than in adults
   B. Sex incidence is equal in children
   C. Worse prognosis in children than in adults
   D. Therapy is by surgical excision
   E. None of the above

33.11. Parotid gland malignant tumors

33.12. Thyroid gland malignant tumors

33.13. Nasopharyngeal carcinoma

DIRECTIONS: For each of the questions or incomplete statements below, **one or more** of the answers or completions given is correct. Select

   (A) if only 1, 2, and 3 are correct
   (B) if only 1 and 3 are correct
   (C) if only 2 and 4 are correct
   (D) if only 4 is correct
   (E) if all are correct

33.14. Vocal nodules causing hoarseness in the prepubertal child
   1. most commonly result from vocal abuse
   2. are treated by surgical removal
   3. occur at the junction of the anterior and middle thirds of the vocal cords
   4. are treated by prolonged voice rest

33.15. Which of the following are indications for tonsillectomy?
   1. Cor pulmonale secondary to tonsillar hypertrophy
   2. Peritonsillar abscess
   3. Recurrent tonsillitis
   4. Chronic tonsillitis

DIRECTIONS: This section of the test consists of situations, each followed by a series of questions. Study each situation and select the **one** best answer to each question following it.

Questions 33.16–33.18: An 8-week-old infant presents at the emergency room with a 4- to 5-day history of constant, slowly progressive respiratory distress associated with inspiratory stridor and sternal retractions. He had been born of an uncomplicated pregnancy and delivery, had an Apgar score of 10 at birth, and went home on the second postdelivery day.

33.16. The differential diagnosis would NOT include
    A. laryngomalacia
    B. congenital subglottic stenosis
    C. congenital subglottic hemangioma
    D. acquired subglottic stenosis
    E. laryngeal cyst

33.17. What findings would be most helpful in arriving at your differential diagnosis?
    A. Presence of a cleft uvula
    B. Umbilical hernia
    C. Webbed digits of hands
    D. Birthmark (strawberry hemangioma) of buttocks
    E. Red hair

33.18. The diagnostic test of preference in infant airway obstructive disorders is
    A. CT scan of neck
    B. fluoroscopy of the neck
    C. soft tissue x-rays of neck
    D. indirect laryngoscopy
    E. direct laryngoscopy

Questions 33.19–33.21: A 5-year-old boy falls from his bicycle and strikes his chin on a parked car. He had no loss of consciousness. He is brought to the emergency room bleeding from the chin and mouth and has an open-bite deformity, but he is too uncooperative to be examined adequately.

33.19. The evaluation should begin with which of the following?
  A. Mandible x-ray
  B. Cervical spine x-ray
  C. Dental consultation
  D. An examination under anesthesia with closing of the wounds
  E. CBC

33.20. The most common mandible fracture sustained under this circumstance will be
  A. angle fracture
  B. midbody fracture
  C. coronoid process fracture
  D. subcondylar neck fracture
  E. symphyseal fracture

33.21. The subcondylar neck fracture is treated with a Barton's bandage and a soft diet for 3 weeks. The long-term potential problem to look for is
  A. asymmetrical mandibular growth and development
  B. no future problem
  C. premature loss of second and third molar teeth
  D. permanent numbness in V_{III} distribution
  E. temporomandibular joint syndrome

Answers and Comments

33.1. (C) Thyroglossal duct cysts and cystic hygromas are not derived from the branchial arch systems. The second branchial cleft and groove account for 95% of branchial cleft defects (Ref. 1, p. 48).

33.2. (C) One of the most important findings that will help distinguish a thyroglossal duct cyst from other neck masses is upward movement of the mass when the patient protrudes his tongue. This movement is caused by the retained fibrous tract from the foramen cecum to the thyroglossal duct cyst (Ref. 1, p. 20).

33.3. (C) The relationship to nerves and blood vessels is the determining factor in identifying the origin of a branchial cleft cyst or fistula. All vestiges of branchial clefts are found ventral to cranial nerve XII. Thus, any mass or structure that lies dorsal to cranial nerve XII is not of branchial origin. The tract of the second branchial cleft cyst classically passes between the internal and external carotid arteries to enter the pharynx at the tonsillar fossa (Figure 67) (Ref. 1, pp. 47–49).

Figure 67

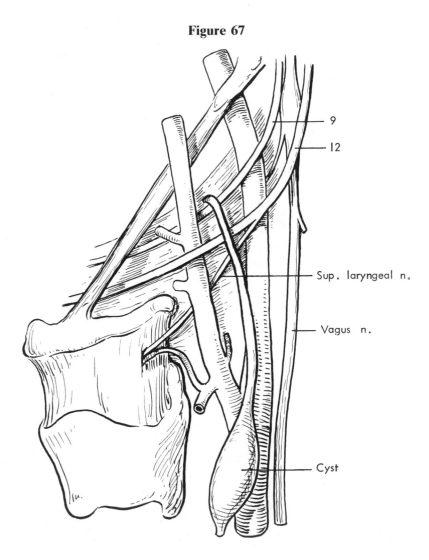

33.4. (B)

33.5. (A)

33.6. (B)

33.7. (C) The tympanogram plots a function of middle ear compliance versus changing air pressure in the external auditory meatus. A tympanogram with a well-defined compliance peak at or near atmospheric identifies a normal middle ear condition. That is the so-called type A pattern. A type B or flat tympanogram has no discernible compliance peak and is usually consistent with secretory otitis media or a perforated eardrum. A normal-shaped pattern with the compliance peak shifted to the left is a type C tympanogram, and it indicates a negative middle ear pressure due to an abnormally functioning eustachian tube (Ref. 1, pp. 180−181).

33.8. (B)

33.9. (C)

33.10. (D) The normal bone conduction threshold curve, which is representative of the sensorineural hearing capability, should be less than 5 dB for the normal population. When the air conduction threshold curve is higher than the bone conduction threshold curve, one is said to have a conduction component to the hearing loss. If this occurs in addition to an elevated bone conduction threshold curve, there is said to be a mixed hearing loss. When the air and bone conduction threshold curves are superimposed, but at an elevated threshold level above approximately 5 dB, a sensorineural hearing loss is present. Clinically, an air conduction curve at a lower threshold than the bone conduction curve is not possible (Ref. 2, pp. 95−99).

33.11. (A,D) From 15−25% of parotid tumors in adults are malignant, whereas 60% of solid salivary masses in children are malignant. The prognosis of specific parotid neoplasms in children is not unlike that of the same neoplasms in adults (Ref. 1, pp. 427−431).

33.12. (A,B,D) The distribution of the various histologic types of thyroid malignant cancers is different between children and adults. Papillary carcinoma accounts for one-half to two-thirds of all adult thyroid neoplasms but is even more prevalent in the pediatric population and represents up to 70% of cases. In children, however, the sex distribution is nearly equal, whereas women are two to three times more likely than men to develop papillary carcinoma. It is not uncommon for both adults and children to have prolonged periods in seemingly symbiotic relationships with their tumors. Prolonged survival in the young patient is attributed to increased host resistance and a less aggressive tumor (Ref. 1, pp. 435–439).

33.13. **(E)** Nasopharyngeal carcinoma occurs more frequently in male patients, especially those who are black and in their teens. Its therapy is by radiation to the primary site alone and the prognosis is essentially the same as in adults for a similar stage of the disease (Ref. 1, pp. 475–478).

33.14. **(B)** Classically, vocal nodules are located at the junction of the middle and anterior thirds of the vocal cords because that is the point of maximal resonance and cord excursion. They develop from local trauma, especially from excessive shouting and yelling. Childhood vocal nodules are reversible lesions and respond to vocal training that does not include prolonged voice rest. Surgical removal should be avoided at least until into the postpubertal period (Ref. 1, pp. 210–213).

33.15. **(E)** Cor pulmonale due to tonsillar hypertrophy is rare, but it is a true entity and one of the absolute indications for tonsillectomy. Peritonsillar abscess may indicate an immediate tonsillectomy for drainage or a delayed tonsillectomy after drainage in the child with a history of recurrent tonsillitis. Recurrent and chronic tonsillitis are again relative indications; their significance lies in the definitions of recurrent and/or chronic (Ref. 1, p. 289).

33.16. **(D)** All of these lesions must be considered in the differential diagnosis of airway problems in the newborn, but with no history of intubation at birth, acquired subglottic stenosis can be ruled out in this particular patient. Laryngomalacia is the most common cause of airway problems in children, with vocal cord paralysis the second most common cause. The delayed appearance of partial airway obstruction in this child is most often seen with a congenital subglottic problem (Ref. 1, pp. 384–385).

33.17. **(D)** The presence of a vascular birthmark or hemangioma should alert one to the possibility of a congenital subglottic hemangioma in the child with delayed onset of airway obstruction. Fifty percent of children with subglottic hemangioma will have hemangiomas elsewhere (Ref. 1, pp. 387–388).

33.18. **(E)** While fluoroscopy and soft tissue x-rays of the neck can be quite helpful in diagnosing these airway disorders, the only way to confirm the diagnosis is by direct laryngoscopy (Ref. 1, p. 386).

33.19. **(B)** Although all the responses are appropriate, the first consideration must be the integrity of the cervical spine, especially in the patient such as this who will need a general anesthetic for adequate evaluation and treatment. The greater elasticity of the skeleton usually necessitates a greater force to induce a fracture and, likewise, the larger cranium-to-body ratio predisposes the cervical spine to greater instability. Cervical spine x-rays should be taken before any manipulative examination of the child's face and jaw is done (Ref. 1, p. 485).

33.20. **(D)** A direct blow to the chin with posterior displacement most commonly results in a subcondylar neck fracture with an open-bite deformity (Ref. 1, p. 487).

33.21. **(A)** The most serious complication in terms of long-term morbidity in this child is asymmetrical mandibular development arising from interference with the mandibular–condylar growth center. That interference may cause deviation of the chin toward the side of the fracture and cause problems with bite and occlusion (Ref. 1, p. 487).

References

1. McGuirt, W.F.: *Pediatric Otolaryngology—Case Studies, 2nd Ed.*, Medical Examination Publishing, New Hyde Park, 1984.

2. Newby, H.A.: *Audiology*, Appleton-Century-Crofts, New York, 1958.

34

Pediatric Pulmonary Medicine

Albin B. Leong, M.D.

DIRECTIONS: Each of the questions or incomplete statements below is followed by five suggested answers or completions. Select the **one** best in each case.

34.1. The lateral view of a barium swallow in a 2-month-old infant (Figure 68) represents which of the following causes of recurrent lung infiltrates?
   A. Gastroesophageal reflux
   B. Foreign body
   C. Alpha-1-antitrypsin deficiency
   D. Tracheoesophageal fistula
   E. Cystic fibrosis

34.2. The most common type of bacterial pneumonia in childhood is
   A. group A streptococcus
   B. *Staphylococcus aureus*
   C. pneumococcus *(Streptococcus pneumoniae)*
   D. *Hemophilus influenzae* type b
   E. group B streptococcus

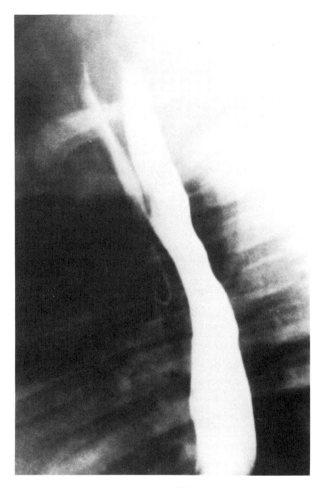

Figure 68

34.3. All of the following are descriptive of the childhood respiratory tract EXCEPT

    A. the greatest incidence of upper respiratory infections occurs from 1 through 7 years of age

    B. kyphoscoliosis and neuromuscular conditions are the most common causes of restrictive lung disease

    C. the major portion of alveoli develop after birth

    D. respiratory frequency (rate) decreases from infancy to adulthood

    E. bronchospasm does not occur in infants less than 6 months of age

DIRECTIONS: The group of questions below consists of five lettered headings followed by a list of numbered words or statements. For each numbered word or statement, select the **one** lettered heading that is most closely associated with it. Each lettered heading may be selected once, more than once, or not at all.

    A. Influenza virus
    B. Parainfluenza virus
    C. Respiratory syncytial virus
    D. *Corynebacterium diphtheriae*
    E. *Hemophilus influenzae* type b

34.4. Laryngotracheobronchitis (croup)

34.5. Epiglottitis

34.6. Bronchiolitis

DIRECTIONS: For each of the questions or incomplete statements below, **one or more** of the answers or completions given is correct. Select
    (A) if only 1, 2, and 3 are correct
    (B) if only 1 and 3 are correct
    (C) if only 2 and 4 are correct
    (D) if only 4 is correct
    (E) if all are correct

34.7. An almost 2-year-old toddler presents with a 3-day onset of cough and fever, markedly decreased breath sounds over the right hemithorax with some wheezes and decreased expansion, and the chest radiograph shown in Figure 69. Common aspects of the diagnosis and immediate treatment of bronchial foreign bodies include
    1. prevalence in the right lung
    2. hemoptysis
    3. endoscopy
    4. pulmonary physiotherapy

DIRECTIONS SUMMARIZED

A	B	C	D	E
1,2,3 only	1,3 only	2,4 only	4 only	All are correct

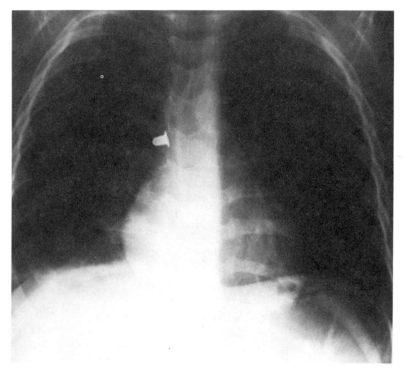

Figure 69

34.8. Risk factors for sudden infant death syndrome (SIDS) include
1. low socioeconomic status
2. male sex
3. low birth weight
4. formula ("bottle") feeding

DIRECTIONS: This section of the test consists of a situation followed by a series of questions. Study the situation and select the **one** best answer to each queston following it.

Questions 34.9 – 34.10: A 9-month-old white boy presents with a history of recurrent "bronchitis" manifested by fever with a congested cough since about 2 months of age. In addition, there is a history of chronic diarrhea, which was felt to be "greasy" in appearance and foul-odored. Your examination reveals a thin, malnourished-appearing infant with weight of 15 lb, a temperature of 39.8°C rectally, a respiratory rate of 50, with physical signs including coughing, bilateral rales, and a protuberant abdomen. Further questioning of the parents reveals two maternal siblings and a paternal uncle with cystic fibrosis.

34.9. Supportive evidence for the diagnosis of cystic fibrosis includes all of the following EXCEPT
  A. elevation of the sweat electrolyte concentrations of sodium and chloride
  B. defective pancreatic endocrine function
  C. positive family history, usually autosomal recessive pattern
  D. chronic pulmonary disease
  E. meconium ileus

34.10. Other features of cystic fibrosis include all of the following EXCEPT
  A. airway reactivity
  B. intestinal obstruction
  C. vitamin B deficiency
  D. nasal polyposis
  E. pulmonary infections with *Pseudomonas aeruginosa*

Answers and Comments

34.1. (D) The radiograph depicts movement of barium across a fistula into the trachea. There is no atresia, so this patient has an "H-type" tracheoesophageal fistula. This type usually presents with recurrent aspiration pneumonia and represents a type of congenital anomaly that can cause chronic lung infiltrates (Ref. 1, pp. 893–894, 1074–1078; 2, pp. 945–947).

34.2. (C) Pneumococcal pneumonia accounts for over 90% of childhood bacterial pneumonias. It usually occurs in late winter and early spring due to frequency at these times of viral respiratory infections, which are the most common predisposing causes of childhood bacterial pneumonias (Ref. 1, pp. 1048–1050).

34.3. (E) Smooth muscle, though thin, does exist in the smaller airways of the newborn. Growth occurs slowly until about 4 years of age, when it begins to increase in proportion to lung growth. Infants are thus capable of having bronchospasm (Ref. 1, pp. 991–992; 2, pp. 1377–1378).

34.4. (B) Laryngotracheobronchitis is caused primarily by viruses, with over two-thirds of all cases due to parainfluenza virus. There is usually a prodrome of an upper respiratory infection for several days prior to onset of the characteristic "brassy" or "seal-like" cough and inspiratory stridor (Ref. 1, pp. 1034–1037).

34.5. (E) In contrast to croup, epiglottitis is usually a rapidly progressive and more severe, life-threatening infection, with only a minority of cases having a prodrome greater than a few hours. The etiology is almost always *H. influenzae* type b. Therefore, therapy includes appropriate antibiotics, as well as establishing an airway (Ref. 1, pp. 1034–1037).

34.6. (C) Bronchiolitis is a common viral illness afflicting the lower respiratory tract of infants. The causative agent is respiratory syncytial virus in the majority of cases, with a peak incidence in the winter through early spring months (Ref. 1, pp. 1044–1045).

34.7. (B) Because the right main stem bronchus is shorter and wider with a less acute angle of origin from the trachea, bronchial foreign bodies are more apt to be located in the right middle and lower lobes. Hemoptysis is rare. Treatment includes endoscopy, with removal of the object as soon as feasible. Pulmonary physiotherapy, on the other hand, may dislodge the foreign object with impaction in the subglottic area and consequent acute asphyxia. Thus, this form of treatment is contraindicated (Ref. 1, pp. 1038–1040).

34.8. (A) Demographic studies of infants dying of SIDS indicate increased risk with prematurity, low birth weight, male sex, low socioeconomic status, twins, and race (with greater incidence, for example, occurring in blacks versus whites by about 3–4 times). There is no evidence supporting a difference between formula-fed versus breast-fed infants (Ref. 1, pp. 1770–1773; 2, pp. 768–772, 1390–1394).

34.9. (B) Diagnostic criteria for cystic fibrosis usually require an abnormal sweat test with either chronic pulmonary disease or pancreatic exocrine dysfunction. Although pancreatic endocrine manifestations such as diabetes mellitus may occur, these are usually late signs. Meconium obstruction in the newborn is relatively rare but is almost always associated with cystic fibrosis. It is estimated that 5–10% of CF patients present in this manner (Ref. 1, pp. 1086–1099; 2, pp. 1433–1440).

34.10. (C) There are a number of protean features of cystic fibrosis including respiratory problems (e.g., staphylococcal and pseudomonas pneumonias, especially, reactive airways, chronic cough, bronchiectasis, atelectasis, nasal polyposis, sinusitis, clubbing, pneumothoraces), gastrointestinal (e.g., meconium ileus, intestinal obstruction, intussusception, pancreatitis, cholelithiasis, pancreatic insufficiency with malabsorption [but not of water soluble vitamins], resultant diabetes mellitus, liver cirrhosis), as well as other signs including metabolic alkalosis, heat prostration, and infertility. Later complications include hemoptysis and cor pulmonale (Ref. 1, pp. 1086–1099; 2, pp. 1433–1440).

References

1. Behrman, R.E., Vaughan, V.C., III, and Nelson, W.E.: *Nelson Textbook of Pediatrics*, 12th Ed., W.B. Saunders, Philadelphia, 1983.

2. Rudolph, A.M., Hoffman, J.I.E., and Axelrod, S.: *Pediatrics*, 17th Ed., Appleton-Century-Crofts, New York, 1982.

35

Pediatric Radiology
Alan E. Oestreich, M.D.

DIRECTIONS: Each of the questions or incomplete statements below is followed by five suggested answers or completions. Select the **one** that is best in each case.

35.1. A round density in the lung of a child, as in Figure 70 (*arrowheads*), is most likely due to
   A. metastatic neuroblastoma
   B. acute bacterial pneumonia
   C. ectopic thyroid
   D. cavitating tuberculosis
   E. bronchogenic carcinoma

35.2. This child in the second decade of life has unilateral hip pain. Which of the following statements is INCORRECT (Fig. 71)?
   A. The abnormality is likely to have occurred within the last 48 hours
   B. The condition requires orthopedic treatment
   C. A line along the outer left femur neck does not intersect the head
   D. The child is nearing the stage of growth plate closure
   E. This is an example of slipped femoral capital epiphysis.

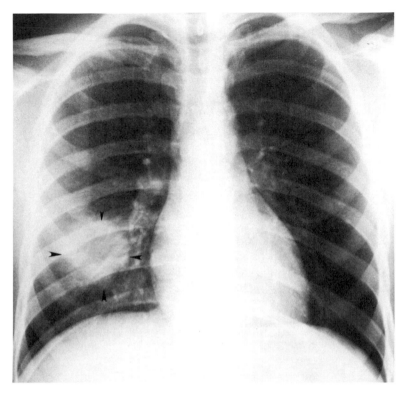

Figure 70

Answers and Comments

35.1. (B) The most common round, soft tissue density in the lung of a *child* is acute pneumonia, usually bacterial. However, a round shadow is one of the less common manifestations of pneumonia. In sheep-raising areas, *Echinococcus* is another common cause (Ref. 1, pp. 98–102).

35.2. (A) is the proper answer. This slipping of the left femoral capital epiphysis (SCFE) is accompanied by a small dense *(white)* zone of the medial proximal neck, a reaction that takes many weeks to develop. The line along the outer neck (Klein's line) normally *(as*

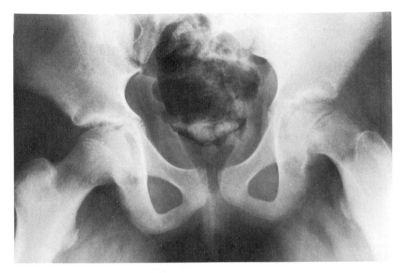

Figure 71

on the right) intersects the head; here it does not, indicating a slip. The normal right growth plate is narrow, indicating its closure will occur relatively soon, which is the typical maturation stage for SCFE. Pinning across the left growth plate or ablation of the plate by bone pegs is needed to avoid progression of the slip (Ref. 1, pp. 182–183).

References

1. Oestreich, A.E.: *Pediatric Radiology*, Medical Outline Series, 3rd Ed., Medical Examination Publishing, New York, 1984.

36

Pediatric Rheumatology

Aram S. Hanissian, M.D.

DIRECTIONS: Each of the questions or incomplete statements below is followed by five suggested answers or completions. Select the **one** that is best in each case.

36.1. Which of the following clinical features does NOT occur in systemic lupus erythematosus (Figure 72).
   A. Glomerulonephritis
   B. "Butterfly" skin rash
   C. Mononeuritis multiplex
   D. Deforming arthritis
   E. Thrombocytopenic purpura

36.2. Raynaud's phenomenon (vasospasm on cold exposure resulting in blue and white discoloration of hands and feet) is present in all of the following EXCEPT
   A. scleroderma, generalized
   B. acute rheumatic fever
   C. systemic lupus erythematosus
   D. mixed connective tissue disease
   E. dermatomyositis

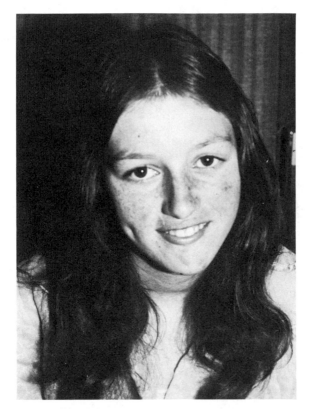

Figure 72

Answers and Comments

36.1. (D) Nondeforming arthritis is one of the 14 provisional criteria for the diagnosis of systemic lupus developed by the American Rheumatism Association. It occurs in up to 78% of all children with SLE. The arthritis may be mono- or oligoarticular or it may be manifested as generalized joint stiffness with periarticular inflammation and very little effusion. The arthritis usually does not cause joint deformity or ankylosis (Refs. 1, pp. 315–321; 2, pp. 287–294).

36.2. (B) This condition does not cause vasospasm of peripheral vessels. Presence of Raynaud's phenomenon usually indicates a diffuse connective tissue disease (Ref. 3).

References

1. Cassidy, J.T., Sullivan, D.B., Petty, R.E., and Ragsdale, C.: Lupus nephritis and encephalopathy: Prognosis in 58 children. Arthritis Rheum. (Suppl), 20, 1977.

2. King, K.K., Kornreich, H.K., Bernstein, B.H., Simpson, B.H., and Hanson, V.: The clinical spectrum of systemic lupus erythematosus in childhood. Arthritis Rheum. (Suppl), 20, 1977.

3. Bulletin on the Rheumatic Diseases, Vol. 33, No. 5, 1–8, 1983.

37

Pediatric Urology
Stephen A. Koff, M.D.

DIRECTIONS: For each of the questions or incomplete statements below, **one or more** of the answers or completions given is correct. Select

    (A)   if only 1, 2, and 3 are correct
    (B)   if only 1 and 3 are correct
    (C)   if only 2 and 4 are correct
    (D)   if only 4 is correct
    (E)   if all are correct

37.1. Fusion of the labia minora (labial fusion) may occur in young girls and require which of the following therapies
    1.   no treatment
    2.   surgical incision
    3.   manual separation
    4.   application of estrogen-containing cream

37.2. Based on current knowledge, the optimum age for performing orchidopexy is before the age of
    1.   puberty
    2.   8
    3.   5
    4.   2

486 / Pediatrics

A	B	C	D	E
1,2,3 only	1,3 only	2,4 only	4 only	All are correct

DIRECTIONS SUMMARIZED

37.3. The infant shown in Figure 73 is likely to have which of the following genitourinary tract abnormalities?
1. Hydroureteronephrosis
2. Hypospadias
3. Cryptorchidism
4. Horseshoe kidney

Answers and Comments

37.1. (E) All are correct. Trauma, irritation, or inflammation may cause the delicate labial epithelium to agglutinate and adhere. Fusion results and appears as a thin translucent line that proceeds upward from the posterior fouchette to just below the clitoris where it may cover the urethral meatus.

Labial adhesions are not seen after puberty because estrogen excretion causes cornification of the labial epithelium, which results in spontaneous separation of adhesions. Therefore, treatment is not necessary for most cases of incomplete fusion. Application of estrogen-containing cream, used for 2 weeks or less, will hasten the separation process and may be required to reassure the family that the genitalia are normal. Manual separation or surgical incision are painful procedures that may be required in severe cases, which fail to respond to estrogens, but should be carried out under anesthesia (Ref. 1, p. 901).

37.2. (D) Beginning at about age 2 and developing progressively thereafter, the undescended testis is subjected to loss of spermatogonia and thickening of seminiferous tubular basement membrane. These adverse effects may be eliminated be early orchidopexy (Ref. 2, p. 188).

37.3. (B) The prune belly syndrome consists of a triad which includes: deficiency of abdominal wall musculature, urinary tract

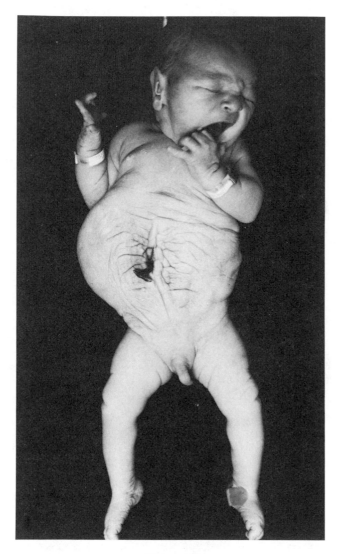

Figure 73

dilation with hydroureteronephrosis, and cryptorchidism. Although the abdominal wall defect is often the most obvious anomaly, its severity bears no direct correlation to the degree of urinary tract distortion (Ref. 1, pp. 805-824).

References

1. Kelalis, P.P. and King, L.R.: *Clinical Pediatric Urology*, 2nd Ed., W.B. Saunders, Philadelphia, 1985.

2. Belman, A.B. and Kaplan, G.W.: *Genitourinary problems in pediatrics, vol 23*. In *Major Problems in Clinical Pediatrics*, W.B. Saunders, Philadelphia, 1981.

OBSTETRICS
AND
GYNECOLOGY

38

Perinatology
Leslie Iffy, M.D.

DIRECTIONS: Each of the questions or incomplete statements below is followed by five suggested answers or completions. Select the best choice(s) in each case.

38.1. The genetic code is based on which of the following systems?
   - **A.** A sequence of four amino acids determining the development of a new protein molecule
   - **B.** A triplet system of three successive nucleotides serving as a code for a single amino acid
   - **C.** The bars connecting the spirals of the double-stranded helix of RNA coding for new nucleotides
   - **D.** Both A and B
   - **E.** None of the above

38.2. Figure 74 depicts normal and abnormal cell divisions. The abnormal type of cell division is conducive to which of the following anomalies?
   - **A.** Down's syndrome
   - **B.** Turner's syndrome
   - **C.** Asherman's syndrome
   - **D.** A and B
   - **E.** B and C

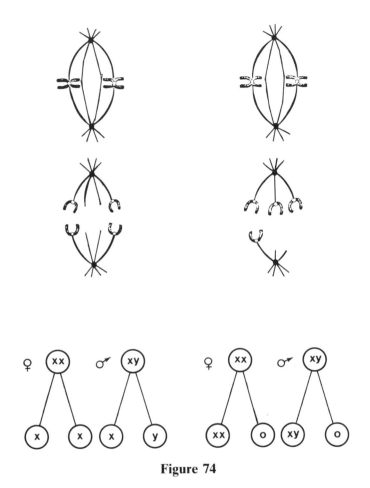

Figure 74

38.3. Multiple gestations are associated with increased frequency with the following complications
  A. growth retardation secondary to twin transfusion in identical twins
  B. growth retardation of heterozygous twin, or twins, in the third trimester
  C. fetal development defect
  D. all of the above
  E. A and C only

38.4. Maternal exposure to 100 rads of ionizing irradiation directed at the pelvis 5 days following conception most likely entails the following consequence
   A. no harm to the migrating ovum
   B. developmental defect involving the central nervous system
   C. limb reduction defect
   D. embryonic death or survival without teratogenic effect
   E. hydatidiform mole

38.5. Which of the following organs or systems is the main site of hemopoiesis during the second trimester of prenatal life?
   A. Bone marrow
   B. Spleen
   C. Lymph nodes
   D. Placenta
   E. None of the above

38.6. Velamentous insertion of the umbilical cord is relatively frequently associated with which of the following anomalies or complications?
   A. Fetal developmental defects
   B. Hemorrhage from vasa previa
   C. Preeclamptic toxemia
   D. A and B
   E. B and C

38.7. The risk–benefit ratio of genetic amniocentesis is determined with awareness of the following risk factor(s)
   A. development of amnionitis
   B. fetomaternal transfusion
   C. injury to the umbilical cord
   D. abortion
   E. all of the above

38.8. Figure 75 shows the rate of frequency in relation to maternal age of which of the following gestational, or reproductive, abnormalities (prorated to 1000 pregnancies)?
   A. Preeclamptic toxemia
   B. Gestational diabetes
   C. Congenital fetal malformations
   D. Fetal manifestations of phenylketonuria (PKU)
   E. Fetal rubella syndrome

Figure 75

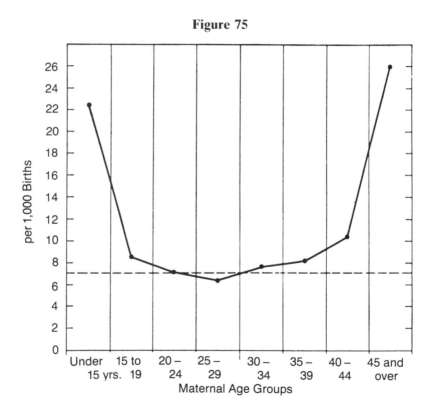

38.9. Neural tube defects can be detected in early gestation by which of the following tests or procedures?
  A. Assessment of hCG levels by β subunit immunoassay
  B. Measurement of α-fetoprotein concentration in the amniotic fluid
  C. Performing maternal chromosome studies for evidence of Robertsonian translocation
  D. By serial evaluation of estriol (E_3) levels in the maternal blood
  E. None of the above

38.10. All of the following drugs (or vitamins) are known to possess teratogenic effects when administered in usual therapeutic doses to the mother during the time of embryonic organogenesis EXCEPT
  A. tetracycline
  B. streptomycin
  C. diethylstilbestrol
  D. pyridoxine
  E. diphenylhydantoin

38.11. The characteristic clinical manifestations of congenital toxoplasmosis include which of the following?
  A. Chorioretinitis
  B. Cerebral calcifications
  C. Fetal macrosomia
  D. B and C
  E. A and B

38.12. "Fetal alcohol syndrome" (FAS) causes a variety of clinical manifestations, including which of the following?
  A. Intrauterine growth retardation
  B. Cranial and facial abnormalities
  C. High fetal weight for gestational age due to excessive caloric intake
  D. A and B
  E. B and C

38.13. Spontaneous first trimester abortion is frequently associated with which of the following abnormalities?

  A. Fetal chromosomal defects, such as trisomy, monosomy, or triploidy
  B. Fetal anatomic developmental abnormalities, such as those of the central nervous system
  C. Increased incidence of severe maternal morning sickness before termination of pregnancy
  D. Increasing pregnanediol levels in the maternal plasma
  E. A and B

DIRECTIONS: Each group of questions below consists of five lettered headings followed by a list of numbered words or statements. For each numbered word or statement, select the **one** lettered heading that is most closely associated with it. Each lettered heading may be selected once, more than once, or not at all.

Figure 76 shows the possible sites of ectopic implantation. These various types of ectopic gestation may be divided into five major groups (A−E). For questions 38.14−38.15, select the appropriate group assignments of the described cases of ectopic pregnancy based upon the information provided.

  A. Tubal pregnancy
  B. Ovarian pregnancy
  C. Abdominal pregnancy
  D. Cervical pregnancy
  E. Uterine (angular and diverticular) gestation

38.14. Presents with uterine bleeding, simulating early abortion. May be mistaken for malignant growth. Treatment may require hysterectomy

38.15. May not be diagnosed until gestation is advanced and fetus is viable. Surgical treatment may be difficult. Placenta may have to be left behind to avoid severe operative hemorrhage

Figure 77 depicts the 10th and 90th percentiles of fetal weight in relation to gestational age. These standards define "high weight for gestational age," "appropriate weight for gestational age," and

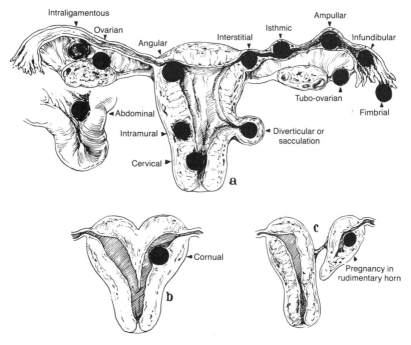

Figure 76

"low weight for gestational age" infants. For questions 38.16–38.18, choose from the five listed "high-risk" categories the ones that are most likely to be associated with high, appropriate, or low birth weights for gestational age.

A. Severe maternal essential hypertension; pregnancy at 36 weeks

B. Twin gestation at 33 weeks

C. Gestational diabetes diagnosed at 38 weeks; no previous dietary control during pregnancy

D. Mild preeclamptic toxemia (blood pressure 130/90 mm Hg) first diagnosed at 38 weeks gestation during a regular visit

E. Maternal mitral insufficiency at term; class I category according to the New York Heart Association (no evidence of circulatory insufficiency even when patient is fully active)

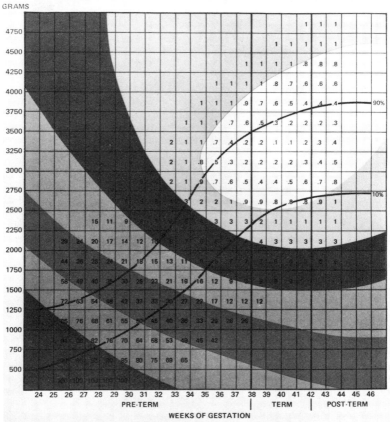

Figure 77

38.16. High weight for gestational age

38.17. Appropriate weight for gestational age

38.18. Low weight for gestational age

DIRECTIONS: The set of lettered headings below is followed by a list of numbered words or phrases. For each numbered word or phrase select
    (A) if the item is associated with A only
    (B) if the item is associated with B only
    (C) if the item is associated with both A and B
    (D) if the item is associated with neither A nor B

  A. An increased incidence of intraventricular hemorrhage leading to neonatal death or permanent mental or physical disability
  B. A high incidence of respiratory distress syndrome during the early neonatal period
  C. Both
  D. Neither

38.19. Breech delivery at 42 weeks' gestation of a primigravida. A male fetus weighing 3800 g is born following assisted breech delivery using the Mauriceau's maneuver. Apgar score at birth: 5

38.20. Spontaneous delivery at 31 weeks' gestation of a 1500 g female fetus. Episiotomy done before birth. Apgar score at birth: 7

38.21. Delivery at 38 weeks' gestation of a multigravida by lower segment transverse cesarean section on account of placenta previa diagnosed by ultrasound. Amniocentesis the day before the operation indicated L/S ratio: 3.0. Phosphatidylglycerol (PG) was demonstrated. No antepartum bleeding was recorded prior to surgery

DIRECTIONS: For each of the questions or incomplete statements below, **one or more** of the answers or completions given is correct. Select
(A) if only 1, 2, and 3 are correct
(B) if only 1 and 3 are correct
(C) if only 2 and 4 are correct
(D) if only 4 is correct
(E) if all are correct

38.22. Oxytocin can be used legitimately in clinical obstetric practice for which of the following indications?
 1. Elective induction of labor in nulliparous gravidas at or near term
 2. For induction of labor at 36 weeks in case of premature rupture of the membranes
 3. For stimulation of labor to achieve early delivery in case of evidence of fetal distress in the deceleration phase of labor
 4. For induction of labor at 37 weeks' gestation in case of progressive preeclampsia

38.23. The labor of a multiparous woman is considered abnormal under which of the following circumstances?
 1. When cervical dilation at the maximum slope of the first stage of labor progresses at a rate of 0.5−1 cm/hr
 2. When the second stage lasts longer than 60 min
 3. When the head descends at the rate of 0.5 cm/hr during the second stage of labor
 4. When the membranes fail to rupture spontaneously before full dilation of the cervix

38.24. Arrest of labor secondary to cephalopelvic disproportion (CPD) may entail which of the following consequences?
 1. Secondary inertia due to uterine exhaustion
 2. Type II fetal heart rate deceleration patterns due to hypoxia
 3. Uterine rupture
 4. Sacculation of the uterus due to extreme attenuation of the lower uterine segment during labor

38.25. In the presence of breech presentation, vaginal delivery can be attempted in a multiparous woman at 39 weeks' gestation unless which of the following complications is known to be present?
1. Deflexion of the fetal head with "star gazing" position
2. Intermediate degree of pelvic contraction
3. Estimated fetal weight of 4000 g or larger
4. Frank breech presentation

38.26. Prolapse of the cord has a demonstrated cause–effect relationship with which of the following?
1. Artificial rupture of the membranes in the presence of floating head
2. Labor in the presence of transverse lie
3. Occurrence of severe variable decelerations following the rupture of the membranes
4. A 50% or higher probability of fetal death if delivery is delayed for more than 1 hr

---

DIRECTIONS: This section of the test consists of situations, each followed by a series of questions. Study each situation and select the **one** best answer to each question following it.

Questions 38.27 – 38.28: A 22-year-old primigravida developed evidence of hypertension (140/92 mm Hg) at 34 weeks' gestation. This was an elevation of 30/20 mm Hg compared to the blood pressure at the time of the first visit. There was protein (+ +) in the urine. She gained 4 kg since the last visit 2 weeks earlier. Deep tendon reflexes were normal. There was moderate arterial spasm on fundoscopy. Her face was puffy. She could not remove her wedding ring. The estimated fetal weight was 2000 g. Presentation was vertex, station −1 cm. The pelvis was found adequate. The urine output during the first 24 hr was 1600 ml and it contained 0.5 g of protein.

38.27. The most probable diagnosis is
    A. essential hypertension
    B. preeclamptic toxemia
    C. pheochromocytoma
    D. acute pulmonary congestion due to circulatory failure
    E. chronic nephrosis

38.28. The most appropriate management in this case is which of the following?

    A. Immediate delivery by cesarean section

    B. Hospitalization with rest, close maternal and fetal monitoring, and delivery by the most expeditious means when lung maturity has been demonstrated or if signs and symptoms indicate progression of the disease

    C. Use of hypotensive agents, such as Apresoline, and delivery at term

    D. Intensive digitalization and delivery within 3 days

    E. Administration of a diuretic agent, such as mannitol, and induction of labor by cervical insertion of *Laminaria* the next day

Questions 38.29–38.30: At 33 weeks' gestation, a 31-year-old primigravida develops painless, brisk vaginal bleeding that she estimates consistent with 200 ml (a large cupful). On examination, the presenting vertex is floating. The estimated fetal weight (EFW) is 2000 g. The bleeding no longer is active. On monitoring, the fetal heart is about 150/min. The pattern is reactive. Maternal hemoglobin (Hb) is 13.5 g. The hematocrit (Hct) is 35%. On inspection, the cervix is closed and looks healthy. There is no leakage of amniotic fluid noted. The abdomen is soft and not tender. The blood pressure is 120/75 mm Hg. The pulse rate is 84/min. The patient's general condition is satisfactory. Bleeding and clotting factors are within the range of normal.

38.29. The most probable diagnosis is

    A. placenta previa

    B. abruption of the placenta

    C. invasive cervical cancer

    D. bleeding from aberrant vessel of the placenta

    E. contact bleeding from cervical erosion

38.30. The preferred management of this condition is
  A. immediate induction of labor with oxytocin
  B. artificial rupture of the membranes and induction with vaginal application of prostaglandin
  C. expectative management until further bleeding or evidence of lung maturity on amniocentesis performed at about 36 weeks' gestation, then delivery by cesarean section
  D. immediate vaginal examination in the examination room for a differential diagnosis and further management depending on the findings
  E. returning the patient home with appropriate instructions

Answers and Comments

38.1. (B) The genetic code is based on a triplet system where three nucleotides code any one of 20 amino acids (Ref. 1, pp. 7–8).

38.2. (D) The depicted anomaly is nondysjunction. Two of the quoted chromosome defects are caused by nondysjunction of autosomal (A) or sex (B) chromosomes (Ref. 1, pp. 31–33).

38.3. (D) The incidence of malformations and that of growth retardations with both etiologic factors are increased in twin pregnancies (Refs. 1, p. 1171; 2, p. 617).

38.4. (D) During the preimplantation stage of embryonic development teratogenic insults usually have an "all or none" effect. If the embryo survives, in all likelihood the development will be unimpaired (Ref. 1, p. 126).

38.5. (E) The yolk sac, liver, and bone marrow are the main sites of hemopoiesis in the first, second, and third trimesters respectively (Ref. 1, pp. 174–175).

38.6. (D) Abnormal insertion of the cord appears to reflect disturbed early development and is related to both anomalies and complications quoted in choices A and B (Ref. 1, p. 207).

38.7. **(E)** Although all of them are small, the listed complications do occur occasionally following amniocentesis (Ref. 2, p. 164).

38.8. **(C)** Very young and advanced maternal age both predispose to congenital chromosomal and anatomic defects, excluding those that are related to intrauterine infection or other iatrogenic noxae that may affect the fetus in utero (Refs. 1, pp. 358, 398; 3).

38.9. **(B)** Elevation of α-fetoprotein concentration in the maternal plasma or in the amniotic fluid is highly suggestive of neural tube defects. It may also be increased in relation to other congenital abnormalities, such as hydrocephaly, Rh isoimmunization, or in case of intrauterine death (Ref. 1, pp. 402–403).

38.10. **(D)** An increasing number of drugs have been shown to possess embryotoxic effects in recent years. It is considered advisable, therefore, to avoid the use of drugs in pregnancy unless strongly indicated. Repeated trials have failed to show such effect by vitamin B_6 (pyridoxine), thus its continued use for the treatment of hyperemesis gravidarum (Ref. 1, pp. 461–481, 1155).

38.11. **(E)** Toxoplasmosis is capable of causing extensive damage to the central nervous system (CNS), including involvement of organs and systems quoted under choices A and B (Refs. 1, p. 507; 4, p. 89).

38.12. **(D)** FAS may manifest with a variety of signs and symptoms. Growth retardation is an almost invariable feature of the clinical picture because excessive ethanol consumption is conducive to a form of malnutrition (Ref. 1, p. 543).

38.13. **(E)** Early abortion frequently is associated with chromosomal and anatomic defects. There is no positive relationship between hyperemesis and spontaneous abortion. Pregnanediol levels tend to decrease (Ref. 1, p. 557).

38.14. **(D)** Cervical pregnancy is a rare form of ectopic gestation. Surgical management may be difficult. Invasion of cervical stroma by chorionic villi may resemble invasive cervical cancer (Ref. 1, p. 628).

38.15. (C) Abdominal gestation is another rare form of ectopic pregnancy. Removal of placenta may entail extreme difficulty and may induce life-endangering hemorrhage. Diagnosis may be delayed due to relative paucity of symptoms in early gestation (Ref. 1, pp. 627–628).

38.16. (C) Gestational diabetes in the absence of dietary control is likely to cause fetal macrosomia (Ref. 5, pp. 135–139).

38.17. (E) Well-compensated maternal cardiac valve defect is not likely to affect fetal growth (Ref. 6, p. 593).

38.18. (A) Prolonged maternal hypertension is conducive to severe growth retardation secondary to inadequate uterine blood flow and reduced fetomaternal exchange of oxygen and nutrients. Mild hypertension of short duration, such as the early stage of preeclampsia, is less likely to have such an effect (Ref. 1, pp. 1241–1290).

38.19. (A) Breech delivery of a large fetus, particularly when pregnancy is prolonged, carries high risks in terms of fetal damage. A variety of circumstances, including primigravida state, add to the risks involved (Ref. 1, pp. 907–924).

38.20. (C) Prematurity is highly conducive to various manifestations of cerebral hemorrhage. Careful management of labor reduces, but does not eliminate, this risk. The same comment applies to respiratory distress syndrome (Refs. 1, pp. 1601–1607; 7, pp. 970–973).

38.21. (D) Cesarean section in general reduces the likelihood of cerebral damage in many clinical situations. Respiratory distress is most unlikely to follow once fetal lung maturity is demonstrated by L/S ratio and PG studies (Ref. 1, pp. 1488–1490).

38.22. (C) Regulations by the Federal Drug Administration advise against use of oxytocin for elective induction of labor. Fetal distress amounts to a contraindication to the use of oxytocin (Ref. 1, pp. 804–805, 927, 1035–1037, 1282).

38.23. **(A)** By definition, the labor curve is abnormal if the cervix of the multiparous parturient dilates less than 1.5 cm/hr at the maximum slope stage of labor or when the head fails to descend during the second stage. (Ref. 8, pp. 89−103).

38.24. **(A)** Uterine inertia, late decelerations, and, on rare occasions, uterine rupture are causatively related to CPD. Sacculation of the uterus is an independent anomaly that develops during pregnancy rather than in the course of labor (Ref. 1, pp. 841, 940, 1422−1423).

38.25. **(A)** Maternal pelvic contraction, large fetal head, or gross deflexion each warrant abdominal delivery. Frank breech presentation facilitates cervical dilatation and, therefore, is a relatively favorable factor for vaginal delivery (Refs. 1, pp. 917−922, 1521−1527; 6, pp. 657−659).

38.26. **(E)** Any condition that prevents obstruction of the pelvic inlet by a large fetal part (preferably the head) is conducive to prolapse of the cord. Cord compression causes variable fetal heart rate decelerations and, in the absence of help, fetal death (Refs. 1, pp. 951−957; 5, pp. 270−274).

38.27. **(B)** The clinical picture is the classic manifestation of preeclamptic toxemia (Ref. 5, pp. 290−293).

38.28. **(B)** The immediate treatment of preeclampsia calls for hospitalization and bed rest; most patients improve temporarily following admission to the hospital. Unless worsening of symptoms demands early delivery, conservative management should be attempted until lung maturity is demonstrated by amniocentesis (Ref. 6, pp. 542−544).

38.29. **(A)** The described clinical picture is most consistent with bleeding from placenta previa, a diagnosis that requires confirmation by ultrasound (Ref. 1, pp. 1085−1120).

38.30. **(C)** The optimum treatment for placenta previa is delivery by cesarean section at about 36 weeks' gestation, preferably after demonstrated lung maturity. Significant episodes of bleeding may necessitate earlier surgical intervention (Ref. 9, pp. 359−368).

demonstrated lung maturity. Significant episodes of bleeding may necessitate earlier surgical intervention (Ref. 9, pp. 359–368).

References

1. Iffy, L. and Kaminetzky, H.A.: *Principles and Practice of Obstetrics & Perinatology*, J. Wiley, New York, 1981.

2. Iffy, L. and Charles, D.: *Operative Perinatology and Invasive Perinatal Techniques*, Macmillan, New York, 1984.

3. Jongbloet, P.H. and Zwetz, J.H.J.: Preovulatory overripeness in the human subject. Internat. J. Gynaecol. Obstet. 14:111, 1976.

4. Charles, D.: *Infections in Obstetrics and Gynecology*, W.B. Saunders, Philadelphia, 1980.

5. Langer, A. and Iffy, L.: *Perinatology Case Studies*, 2nd Ed., Medical Examination Publishing, New Hyde Park, New York, 1985.

6. Pritchard, J.A., MacDonald, P.C., and Gant, N.F.: *Williams Obstetrics*, 17th Ed., Appleton-Century-Crofts, Norwalk, Connecticut, 1985.

7. Avery, G.B.: *Neonatology. Pathophysiology and Management of the Newborn*, 2nd Ed., Lippincott, Philadelphia, 1981.

8. Friedman, E.A.: *Labor: Clinical Evaluation and Management*, 2nd Ed., Appleton-Century-Crofts, New York, 1978.

9. Iffy, L. and Langer, A.: *Perinatology Case Studies*, Medical Examination Publishing, Garden City, New York, 1978.

39

Obstetrics
Ralph W. Hale, M.D.

DIRECTIONS: Each of the questions or incomplete statements below is followed by five suggested answers or completions. Select the **one** that is best in each case.

39.1. The neonatal mortality rate is expressed as the number of neonatal deaths per
- **A.** 1000 births
- **B.** 1000 live births
- **C.** 1000 population
- **D.** 1000 pregnancies
- **E.** 1000 women in the population

39.2. A patient whose karyotype is represented in Figure 78 would have which of the following diagnoses?
- **A.** Testicular feminization
- **B.** Ovarian dysgenesis
- **C.** Kleinfelter's syndrome
- **D.** Superfemale
- **E.** Down's syndrome

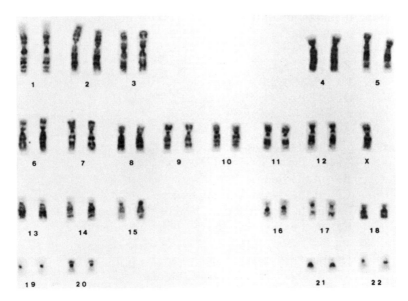

Figure 78

39.3. An autosomal dominant characteristic in only the male partner is found in what percentage of offspring?
- **A.** 10%
- **B.** 25%
- **C.** 50%
- **D.** 75%
- **E.** 100%

39.4. The most common karyotype of a patient with Down's syndrome is
- **A.** 5/21 translocation
- **B.** 18-trisomy
- **C.** 14/21 translocation
- **D.** 21-trisomy
- **E.** 13-trisomy

39.5. Implantation of the blastocyte occurs how many days after fertilization?
   A. 1–2
   B. 3–5
   C. 6–8
   D. 9–10
   E. 12–14

39.6. Fertilization of the ovum by the sperm usually occurs
   A. on the surface of the ovary
   B. in the fimbria
   C. at the uterotubal junction
   D. in the proximal one-third of the fallopian tube
   E. in the distal two-thirds of the fallopian tube

39.7. The major function of hCG appears to be
   A. to maintain the corpus luteum
   B. stimulation of decidua formation
   C. to initiate implantation
   D. to initiate breast development
   E. determination of fetal viability

39.8. Alpha-fetoprotein analysis of amniotic fluid is helpful in which of the following conditions?
   A. Trisomy-21
   B. Neural tube disease
   C. Cri-du-chat syndrome
   D. Gaucher's syndrome
   E. Glucose-6-phosphate dehydrogenase deficiency

39.9. Which of the following measurements of respiratory function does NOT change during pregnancy?
   A. Tidal volume
   B. Residual volume
   C. Expiratory reserve volume
   D. Inspiratory reserve volume
   E. Timed vital capacity

39.10. The most common cause of anemia in a pregnant woman is
   A. sickle-cell trait
   B. sickle-cell anemia
   C. iron deficiency
   D. β thalassemia
   E. folic acid deficiency

39.11. During pregnancy, the blood volume has its greatest increase
   A. during the middle of the first trimester
   B. at the beginning of the second trimester
   C. at the end of the second trimester
   D. during the middle of the third trimester
   E. during labor

39.12. Positive manifestations of pregnancy include
   A. quickening
   B. a cyanotic (blue) cervix
   C. persistent elevation of the basal body temperature
   D. uterine soufflé
   E. palpation of fetal movements

39.13. Which of the following pregnancy tests would be most reliable in a patient whose last menstrual period occurred 6 weeks ago?
   A. Immunoassay for hemagglutination inhibition
   B. Induction of rabbit ovulation (A-Z test)
   C. Radio receptor assay
   D. Assay for β-hCG
   E. Induction of toad ejaculation (toad test)

39.14. A patient has her last normal menstrual period on May 21. Her estimated date of delivery would be
   A. February 28
   B. March 21
   C. March 28
   D. February 21
   E. March 14

39.15. In evaluation of the bony pelvis the obstetric conjugate is the measurement of
  A. anterior–posterior diameter of the midpelvis
  B. interspinous distance
  C. transverse plane of the inlet
  D. distance between the ischial tuberosities
  E. anterior posterior diameter of inlet

39.16. Which of the following drugs has a risk-benefit ratio that makes its indicated use acceptable during pregnancy
  A. Tetracycline
  B. Podophyllin
  C. Alcohol
  D. Meclizine
  E. Heparin

39.17. The most frequently reported cause of spontaneous abortion is
  A. chromosomal abnormalities
  B. trauma
  C. Rh incompatibility
  D. inadequate progesterone
  E. maternal infection

39.18. The major cause of death in patients with tubal ectopic pregnancy is
  A. pulmonary embolism
  B. bowel obstruction
  C. hyponatremia
  D. hemorrhage
  E. infection

39.19. Follow-up of a patient with hydatidiform mole would include
  A. pelvic examination at 3-month intervals
  B. weekly hCG assays until remission
  C. an intravenous pyelogram or CAT scan
  D. a 5-day course of actinomycin D
  E. monthly hCG assays until remission

39.20. In a pregnant patient who has a known Rh° (D) sensitization, the proper method of managing a subsequent pregnancy is to
  A. give mini-doses of Rh antibody at 12, 20, 28, and 34 weeks
  B. obtain a maternal antibody evaluation at 12, 28, and 36 weeks
  C. give promethazine therapy at 2−4-week intervals
  D. measure amniotic fluid bilirubin at 22−24 weeks
  E. carefully follow changes in serum bilirubin levels

39.21. During the third trimester, placenta previa should always be suspected in the presence of
  A. sudden, sharp abdominal pain
  B. painless vaginal bleeding
  C. premature rupture of the membranes
  D. a loud soufflé over the anterior uterine wall
  E. unengaged head

39.22. Premature placental separation may be associated with
  A. trauma
  B. placenta previa
  C. prolonged labor
  D. breech presentation
  E. premature rupture of the membranes

39.23. In a patient with pregnancy-induced hypertension, which of the following symptoms is considered the most ominous?
  A. Visual disturbances
  B. Epigastric pain
  C. Proteinuria of 1 g/L
  D. Weight gain of 3 lb in 3 days
  E. Headache

39.24. Which of the following blood values would be abnormal for a pregnant woman?
  A. Hemoglobin of 12.4 g/dl
  B. WBC 12,500/cu mm
  C. Serum iron 100 μg/dl
  D. Platelets 135,000/cu mm
  E. Sedimentation rate 40 mm/hr

39.25. Your primigravida patient has been noted to have the fetal monitor pattern shown in Figure 79 while in active labor at 6 cm dilation and +1 station. Your working diagnosis should be
    A. uteroplacental insufficiency
    B. severe fetal distress
    C. congenital heart block
    D. head compression
    E. umbilical cord compression

39.26. A characteristic of true labor is
    A. progressive cervical effacement and dilatation
    B. progressively increasing uterine pain
    C. increasing frequency and duration of contraction
    D. increasing amount of show
    E. suprapubic and groin pain

39.27. The second stage of labor begins with
    A. internal rotation
    B. expulsion of the fetus
    C. complete cervical dilatation
    D. expulsion of the placenta
    E. descent of the presenting part

Figure 79

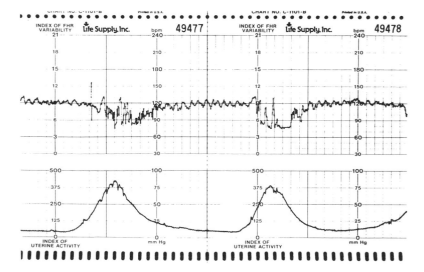

39.28. During a forceps delivery of a diabetic mother, it is noted that the head is delivered with ease but the remainder of the baby appears to be prevented from delivery. Your first diagnosis should be
- **A.** hydrocephalus
- **B.** shoulder dystocia
- **C.** omphaalocele
- **D.** siamese twins
- **E.** uterine atony

39.29. In the presence of thickly meconium-stained amniotic fluid, without fetal distress, the physician should
- **A.** initiate positive-pressure breathing as soon as delivery is complete
- **B.** perform an immediate cesarean section
- **C.** obtain a scalp pH
- **D.** suction the oropharynx as soon as the head delivers and before the shoulder drops
- **E.** heparinize the baby immediately upon delivery

39.30. Immediate delivery of the infant is indicated when
- **A.** meconium-stained fluid is observed
- **B.** the patient has been completely dilated for 2 hr
- **C.** a bradycardia lasting for 30 sec after each uterine contraction is present
- **D.** a pulsating umbilical cord is palpated next to the fetal head at 6 cm dilatation
- **E.** a scalp pH of 7.275 is obtained

39.31. In a primigravida patient who is at term and having a "painful labor" at 4-5 cm, the best form of analgesia would be
- **A.** continuous paracervical
- **B.** meperidine, 100 mg, plus promethazine 25 mg
- **C.** pudendal block
- **D.** intermittent nitrous oxide
- **E.** epidural block

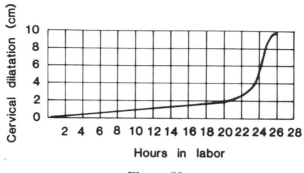

Figure 80

39.32. Given the labor curve shown in Figure 80, the most likely diagnosis would be
  A. uterine inertia
  B. secondary arrest of labor
  C. prolonged latent phase
  D. prolonged second stage
  E. primary dysfunctional labor

39.33. The placenta shown in Figure 81 would be diagnosed as
  A. circumvallate
  B. membranaceous
  C. accreta
  D. bilobed
  E. velamentous insertion

39.34. The lecithin/sphingomyelin ratio is considered to have reached maturity when the ratio has reached at
  A. 0.5
  B. 2.0
  C. 1.5
  D. 1.0
  E. 0.1

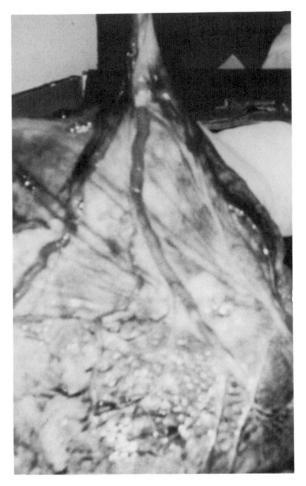

Figure 81

DIRECTIONS: Each group of questions below consists of five lettered headings followed by a list of numbered words or statements. For each numbered word or statement, select the **one** lettered heading that is most closely associated with it. Each lettered heading may be selected once, more than once, or not at all.

A. Two or more cell types from the same zygote
B. A chromosome number deviating from normal by an exact multiple
C. A chromosome number deviating from normal and from an exact multiple
D. A multiple of a basic number of chromosome
E. Two or more genetically different cell types, each from different zygotes

39.35. Mosaic

39.36. Aneuploid

39.37. Chimera

A. Growth hormone
B. Maternal cholesterol
C. Serum thyroxine
D. Insulin release
E. Serum estrogens

39.38. Maternal levels decreased during pregnancy

39.39. Results in production of progesterone

A. Nonpregnant
B. First trimester
C. Second trimester
D. Third trimester
E. Postpartum

39.40. Maximum blood volume obtained

39.41. Vena cava compression syndrome

39.42. Fibrinogen level 500 mg/100 ml

    A. Diagonal conjugate
    B. Biischial diameter
    C. Intertuberous diameter
    D. Symphysis−sacral distance
    E. Obstetric conjugate

39.43. Shortest anterior−posterior diameter of the pelvic inlet

39.44. Smallest diameter of the midplane

39.45. Outlet measurement

    A. Vaginal bleeding
    B. Ovarian enlargement
    C. Preeclampsia
    D. Hyperthyroidism
    E. Nausea and vomiting

39.46. Ultimately occurs in virtually all cases of hydatidiform mole

39.47. An uncommon but serious complication of hydatidiform mole

39.48. Occurs in 15% of patients with hydatidiform mole

    A. Placenta previa
    B. Premature placental separation, mild
    C. Premature placental separation, severe
    D. Uterine rupture
    E. Vasa previa

39.49. Presence of fetal hemoglobin

39.50. External bleeding, maternal hemoglobin

39.51. Coagulopathy

    A. Pregnancy-induced hypertension
    B. Essential hypertension
    C. Pheochromocytoma
    D. Lupus erythematosus
    E. Eclampsia

39.52. Renal cortical necrosis

39.53. Paroxysmal hypertension

39.54. Proteinuria of 20 g/L

    A. Hydramnios
    B. Oligohydramnios
    C. Intrauterine growth retardation
    D. Rh hemolytic disease
    E. Diabetes mellitus

39.55. Esophageal atresia

39.56. Fetal congestive heart failure

39.57. Fetal macrosomia

    A. Anterior parietal bone presentation
    B. Posterior parietal bone presentation
    C. Midline sagittal suture
    D. Deflexion of the vertex
    E. Marked flexion of the vertex

39.58. Posterior ansynclitism

39.59. Second stage

39.60. Anterior asynclitism

    A. Uterus becomes globular and firmer
    B. Prolonged steady blood loss
    C. Elevated temperature on the first postpartum day
    D. Persistent vulvar pain
    E. Ritgen maneuver

39.61. Hematoma

39.62. Delivery of fetal head

39.63. Placental separation

    A. Lacerations
    B. Uterine atony
    C. Hematomas
    D. Placenta accreta
    E. Retained placental fragment

39.64. Most common cause of postpartum hemorrhage

39.65. Postpartum hemorrhage occurring more than 24 hr after delivery

39.66. Usually requires a hysterectomy

DIRECTIONS: Each set of lettered headings below is followed by a list of numbered words or phrases. For each numbered word or phrase select

    (A)   if the item is associated with A only
    (B)   if the item is associated with B only
    (C)   if the item is associated with both A and B
    (D)   if the item is associated with neither A nor B

    A. Levels of 90,000 mIU/ml hCG at 3 lunar months
    B. Levels of 5 μg/ml human placental lactogen at 9 lunar months
    C. Both
    D. Neither

39.67. Normal pregnancy

39.68. Stimulates lipolysis, inhibits gluconeogenesis

39.69. Suppresses lactation

    A. Proteinuria of greater than 1+
    B. 750−2000 IU of hCG in the urine
    C. Both
    D. Neither

39.70. Positive immunologic pregnancy test

39.71. Negative immunologic pregnancy test

39.72. Hydatidiform mole

    A. Vaginal bleeding
    B. Hydropic degeneration
    C. Both
    D. Neither

39.73. Spontaneous abortion

39.74. Choriocarcinoma

39.75. Maternal rubella

    A. Previously sensitized Rh($-$) mother
    B. Initially sensitized Rh($-$) mother
    C. Both
    D. Neither

39.76. Weekly antibody titers

39.77. Amniocentesis and Δ O.D_{450} analysis

39.78. Postpartum should receive anti-D immune globulin

    A. 28$-$32 weeks
    B. Labor at 40 weeks
    C. Both
    D. Neither

39.79. Onset of decompensation in a pregnant cardiac patient

39.80. Greatest risk of death in a pregnant cardiac patient

39.81. Physiologically, period of least cardiac stress

    A. A reduction in the fetal heart rate of 40 beats/ min synchronous with uterine contraction
    B. Scalp pH of 7.188
    C. Both
    D. Neither

39.82. Normal finding

39.83. Indicative of fetal distress

39.84. Frequently associated with maternal cardiac decompensation

    A. An A-P diameter of the inlet of 11 cm or greater
    B. Prominent ischial spines
    C. Both
    D. Neither

39.85. Gynecoid pelvis

39.86. Platypelloid pelvis

39.87. Android pelvis

DIRECTIONS: For each of the questions or incomplete statements below, **one or more** of the answers or completions given is correct. Select
  (A) if only 1, 2, and 3 are correct
  (B) if only 1 and 3 are correct
  (C) if only 2 and 4 are correct
  (D) if only 4 is correct
  (E) if all are correct

39.88. Figure 82 represents the genitalia of a 2-day-old infant. The defect may be caused by
  1. 21-hydroxylase deficiency
  2. 17 β-hydroxydehydrogenase deficiency
  3. 11 β-hydroxylase deficiency
  4. 13-hydroxylase deficiency

39.89. During pregnancy
  1. urinary 17-ketosteroids are elevated
  2. serum estradiol levels are lowered
  3. serum dehydroepiandrosterone levels are lowered
  4. serum estriol levels are increased

39.90. As pregnancy progresses in a normal patient
  1. renal plasma flow increases by 30−40%
  2. calcium stores are decreased
  3. circulating leukocytes are increased
  4. heart rate is decreased

39.91. An infection that may affect the fetus during early pregnancy and cause an abnormality is
  1. tuberculosis
  2. hepatitis
  3. chickenpox
  4. rubella

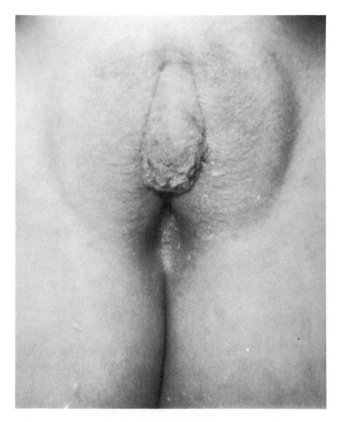

Figure 82

39.92. Diagnostic symptoms and findings of an ectopic (tubal) pregnancy include
1. abdominal pain
2. scanty, persistent vaginal bleeding
3. a pelvic or adnexal mass
4. negative pregnancy test

39.93. A hCG determination is indicated with a recent history of hydatidiform mole and
1. pelvic pain
2. enlarged uterus
3. late onset of menarche
4. intermenstrual spotting

		DIRECTIONS SUMMARIZED		
A	B	C	D	E
1,2,3	1,3	2,4	4	All are
only	only	only	only	correct

39.94. Treatment of abruptio placenta (premature separation) should include
1. immediate cesarean section
2. rupture of the membranes
3. double setup examination
4. evaluation of fibrinogen and fibrinolysin levels

39.95. Laboratory studies on the serum of patients with pregnancy-induced hypertension reveal the
1. hematocrit is stable
2. BUN is decreased
3. fibrinogen is decreased
4. uric acid is elevated

39.96. During labor, the pregnant woman should
1. be given only a liquid diet
2. be given antacids
3. have no more than two vaginal examinations
4. be allowed to sit in a chair or walk in the early stages

39.97. An episiotomy
1. will reduce tears of the pelvic floor
2. will reduce the time of the second stage
3. will usually heal without complications
4. should always be performed in the midline

39.98. Involution of the uterus
1. is not associated with pain in multiparous patients
2. is rarely present before the first week postpartum
3. is frequently associated with endometritis
4. reduces uterine size so that it weighs about 500 g at 1 week

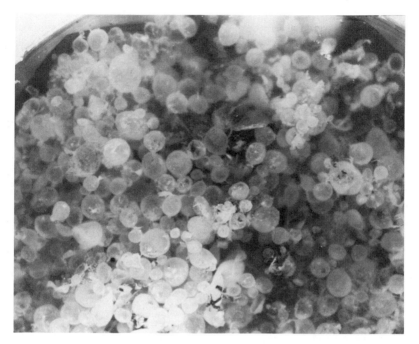

Figure 83

DIRECTIONS: This section of the test consists of situations, each followed by a series of questions. Study each situation and select the **one** best answer to each question following it.

Questions 39.99–39.100: Your patient is seen in the emergency room by you, stating that she has missed two menstrual periods and just passed a large amount of bloody tissue. The tissue appears in Figure 83.

39.99. Your immediate treatment should be
   A.   methotrexate chemotherapy
   B.   total abdominal hysterectomy
   C.   suction curettage
   D.   observation unless bleeding increases
   E.   intravenous estrogens

39.100. At the completion of therapy, you should also
  A. begin maintenance methotrexate therapy
  B. switch to actinomycin-D therapy
  C. order weekly hCG assays
  D. start oral estrogens
  E. encourage a repeat pregnancy as soon as possible

Questions 39.101 – 102: A 19-year-old patient is seen in your office for evaluation of a 20-week pregnancy. On examination, pelvic measurements reveal the following: diagonal conjugate of 11 cm, angulation increased to the forepelvis, and iliopectineal lines nearly straight; the widest transverse diameter is near the sacrum. Her sacrosciatic notch is narrow, and the subpubic arch is narrowed.

39.101. You would describe this pelvis as
  A. gynecoid
  B. anthropoid
  C. platypelloid
  D. android
  E. ethnoid

39.102. Based on your examinatioin, you would anticipate that
  A. she would have no problem with labor and delivery of an average-sized baby
  B. unless she has a small baby, she may have CPD
  C. her second stage would be very short
  D. engagement will take place early
  E. the vertex will automatically assume an OA position

Questions 39.103 – 39.104: A 22-year-old gravida 2 para 1 abO is seen in your office complaing of a sharp left lower quadrant pain. Her last normal menstrual period was 6 weeks ago. She is sexually active and uses an IUD (intrauterine device) for contraception. Her past history reveals an episode of pelvic infection 3 years ago and an allergy to penicillin. Further history reveals the pain is gradually increasing in severity and she noted the onset of vaginal bleeding this morning. Her examination reveals a temperature of 99.2°F, pulse of 86, and blood pressure of 110/68. The only positive findings include hypoactive bowel sounds, some guarding with left lower quadrant pain. The pelvic examination reveals dark blood in the vault and a uterus that is normal in size. There is pain but no mass in the left adnexal area. Laboratory studies reveal a hemoglobin of 11 g and a hematocrit of 33%. Her leukocyte count is 12,500/mm³. The urine is normal and a urine pregnancy test is negative.

39.103. The next test/procedure that you should perform would be
  A. diagnostic laparoscopy
  B. dilatation and curettage
  C. serum beta hCG radioimmunoassay
  D. culdocentesis
  E. ultrasonography

39.104. Based upon the most likely diagnosis, you should
  A. observe the patient at bed rest
  B. begin hormonal suppressive therapy
  C. perform an emergency laparotomy
  D. start high doses of an antibiotic
  E. repeat the laboratory studies in 4 hr

Question 39.105: A 29-year-old gravida 4 para 2 ab 1 Rh negative patient is seen in your office for consultation. Her past history reveals that her previous child was jaundiced and that she had "positive titers" during her pregnancy. She is not at 30 weeks' gestation and an amniocentesis at 28 weeks revealed amniotic fluid that was reported as .024 Δ O.D.$_{450}$. Based on your interpretation of the results (Figure 84), answer the following question.

39.105. Your initial treatment should be
  A. immediate delivery
  B. repeat amniocentesis immediately
  C. 2 cc of anti-D immune globulin immediately
  D. observation and repeat amniocentesis in 2−3 weeks
  E. observation and induction of labor at 36 weeks

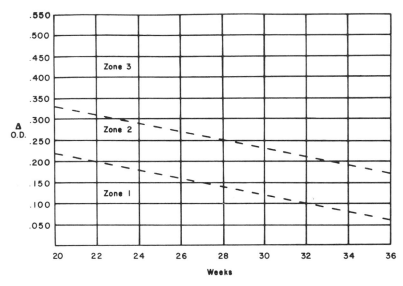

Figure 84

Question 39.106:. You have obtained the following laboratory results from your 34-year-old primigravida, who is at 30 weeks' gestation and has a persistent blood pressure of 150/100.

Hgb	15.0 g%
Hct	45%
BUN	18 mg/dl
Uric acid	15 mg/dl
Fibrinogen	550 mg/dl
Urine protein	4 g/24 hr

39.106. Based on the laboratory results, the patient has which of the following diseases?
A. Pregnancy-induced hypertension
B. Chronic renovascular hypertension
C. Acute glomerulonephritis
D. Pheochromocytoma
E. Lupus nephritis

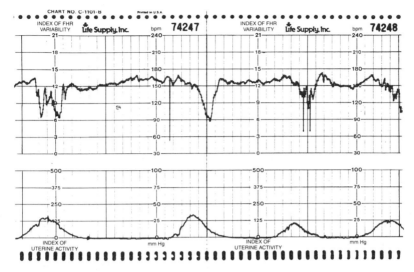

Figure 85

Question 39.107: The fetal monitor strip (Figure 85) was obtained from your patient who is in active labor and was last examined 10 min ago. She was 5 cm dilated, 0 station at that time. Her past history reveals that this is her second pregnancy. She has had an uneventful course and started labor 4 hr ago. Her membranes ruptured 1 hr ago and the fluid was clear.

39.107. Based on this pattern, which is repetitive, your management should be
  A. immediate cesarean section
  B. position to the left side and start O_2
  C. begin intravenous pitocin
  D. encourage the patient to begin pushing
  E. begin tocolytic therapy

Questions 39.108 – 39.109: Your patient is a 24-year-old gravida 2 para 1 who began labor at term. She had the onset of labor 4 hr ago and rapidly progressed to complete dilation. Delivery was spontaneous and uncomplicated over a midline episiotomy with local anesthesia. At the completion of repair of the episiotomy, you notice that the patient is continuing to have a slow, steady flow of bright red blood.

39.108. Your initial diagnosis is
    A. uterine rupture
    B. retained placenta
    C. inverted uterus
    D. a coagulation defect
    E. uterine atony

39.109. Immediate treatment would consist of
    A. a uterine currettage
    B. intravenous fibrinogen
    C. intrauterine packing
    D. uterine massage
    E. observation and accurate pad evaluation

Question 39.110. Mrs. Jones is a 28-year-old gravida 3 para 2 who has an estimated delivery date of June 5. She has had an uneventful pregnancy and her previous babies delivered within 1 week of her due date. She is seen on June 20 in your office. Examination reveals a normal blood pressure. The estimated fetal size is 8 lb. McDonald's measurement is 33 cm (it was 32 on the last two exams). Fetal heart tones are normal. The cervix is 1 cm, 50% effaced, and -1 station. A contraction stress test is ordered, which shows the following pattern (Figure 86).

39.110. Based on your interpretation, you should
    A. repeat the test in 24 hr
    B. perform a cesarean section
    C. begin induction of labor with oxytocin
    D. reassure the patient and reschedule another test in 1 week
    E. perform amniocentesis for L/S ratio

Questions 39.111 – 39.112: Approximately 4 hr ago, you delivered a normal newborn spontaneously with a pudendal block and a midline episiotomy. Careful inspection and evaluation of the cervix, vagina, and uterus revealed no apparent problems. The nurse has just called to inform you that your patient is now complaining of severe pain in the lower vaginal area. Her pulse is 84, temperature 98.8°F, and blood pressure 110/68. Her uterus is firm and lochia is normal.

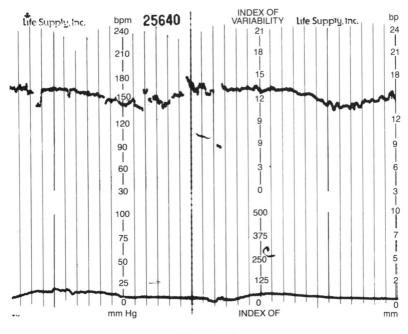

Figure 86

39.111. Based on this information your most likely diagnosis is
 A. uterine rupture
 B. vulvar hematoma
 C. retained placenta
 D. urinary retention
 E. uterine inversion

39.112. Your management should be
 A. prepare for immediate hysterectomy
 B. morphine 15 mg and reevaluate in 4 hr
 C. start intravenous oxytocin
 D. catheterization of the bladder
 E. explore the episiotomy site

Question 39.113: You have just delivered a normal newborn male at 40 weeks' gestation. On initial examination, the baby has a heart rate of 90; there is a weak cry and minimal chest expansion; the baby has some flexion in response to flicking of the sole; his color is blue; and he lies limply when held.

39.113. Your Apgar score would be
  A. 2
  B. 3
  C. 4
  D. 5
  E. 6

Question 39.114: At 5 min the baby has a vigorous cry; the heart rate is 140; there is some flexion of the extremities; the trunk is pink, but the extremities are blue; and the baby cries when he is stimulated on the sole of the foot.

39.114. The Apgar score would be
  A. 3
  B. 5
  C. 7
  D. 8
  E. 9

Answers and Comments

39.1. (B) Neonatal mortality rates are based upon the number of neonatal deaths per 1000 live births. A neonatal death refers to a live born infant that dies within the first 30 days of life (Ref. 3, p. 2).

39.2. (B) This karyotype has only one X chromosome in the sex chromosome section. The manifestation of this patient is phenotypic female (Ref. 2, p. 36).

39.3. (C) The effect of an autosomal dominant characteristic manifests itself whenever present and it is transmitted to 50% of all offspring based on mendelian genetics (Ref. 2, pp. 31–32).

39.4. (D) Down's syndrome (mongolism) is a result of an extra chromosome. A trisomy of chromosome 21 occurs in 95% of patients. A translocation of chromosome 21 and another chromosome, usually the D group, accounts for 5% (Ref. 2, p. 38).

39.5. (C) The fertilized ovum is moved by a peristaltic action of the fallopian tube. During this time, a series of division occurs which results in blastocyst formation. It takes 6−7 days for this transport to take place and then the zygote begins to implant (Ref. 1, p. 78).

39.6. (E) The ovum is met by sperm in the distal portion of the fallopian tube, where fertilization occurs. The fertilized ovum (zygote) then spends a 6−7 day period of transport (Ref. 2, p. 295).

39.7. (A) The developing placenta (syncytiotrophoblast) begins producing hCG as soon as implantation occurs. Its major function is luteotropic and serves to maintain the corpus luteum (Ref. 2, p. 344).

39.8. (B) A maternal serum α-fetoprotein of greater than 2.5 standard deviations at 16−18 weeks is suggestive of neural tube disease. An amniotic fluid analysis is therefore indicated. If the amniotic fluid level is 3 or more standard deviations above normal it is reasonable to assume that a neural tube defect exists (Ref. 1, p. 601).

39.9. (E) During pregnancy, several components of lung volume are changed. None of these changes affect the timed vital capacity and, therefore, this is a key measurement of respiratory function during pregnancy (Ref. 2, p. 327).

39.10. (C) About 95% of all pregnant women with anemia will have iron deficiency anemia. However, those of black ancestry or Mediterranean/Asiatic ancestry must be evaluated for sickle-cell disease or thalassemia. Folic acid deficiency occurs in only 1:200 to 400 women (Ref. 1, p. 892).

39.11. (C) The increases in fluid and red cell volume occur slowly in the first trimester. The rate increases rapidly during the second trimester and by the end of the second trimester has increased by about 50%. Only a slight rise occurs during the third trimester (Ref. 2, p. 331).

39.12. **(E)** Positive manifestations of pregnancy must be based upon an objective finding of a fetus. These include heart sounds, palpation of fetal parts, x-ray, ultrasound, electronic monitoring, and radioimmunoassay (Ref. 1, p. 607).

39.13. **(D)** The major problem with all pregnancy tests is the cross reaction of LH and hCG. The radioimmunoassay of the β-hCG is the most accurate test currently available (Ref. 3, pp. 214–215).

39.14. **(A)** The average length of pregnancy is 266 days. This is estimated by subtracting 3 months from the last normal menstrual period and then adding 7 days (Ref. 2, p. 362).

39.15. **(E)** The obstetric conjugate is the shortest distance between the sacral promontory and the pubic symphysis. It is one of the most important measurements of the obstetric pelvis (Ref. 3, p. 222).

39.16. **(E)** Use of any drugs in pregnancy is risky; therefore the potential benefit must be compared to the risk. Heparin has no known risk to the fetus (Ref. 1, p. 647).

39.17. **(A)** Studies of spontaneous abortion reveal that at least 50–60% are the result of chromosomal abnormalities (Ref. 2, p. 379).

39.18. **(D)** Tubal ectopic pregnancy is associated with rupture and profuse bleeding. This results in intraperitoneal bleeding and exsanguination if untreated (Ref. 1, p. 721).

39.19. **(B)** Retention of viable trophoblastic tissue in a patient with a hydatidiform mole is best determined by hCG determinations, preferably by a β-hCG radioimmunoassay, at weekly intervals until absent (Ref. 2, p. 400).

39.20. **(D)** Once a Rh(−) patient becomes sensitized, maternal antibody titers have little value. There is only one safe way to follow the patient and that is by amniotic fluid levels. Currently, there is no evidence that Rh D antibody (Rhogam) or promethazine (Phenergan) have any value in a sensitized patient (Ref. 3, pp. 773–777).

39.21. (B) Painless vaginal bleeding is the main characteristic of placenta previa (Ref. 2, pp. 444).

39.22. (A) Although the etiology is usually unknown, trauma is a precipitating factor in some cases (Ref. 2, p. 449).

39.23. (B) Epigastric pain occurring in a patient with pregnancy-induced hypertension is followed frequently by convulsions (Ref. 3, p. 527).

39.24. (D) Normal blood values during pregnancy include a hemoglobin of $12-13$ g/dl, a WBC of $10-30,000/mm^3$, a serum iron of $60-120$ μg/dl, a sedimentation rate of $10-60$ mm/hr, and a platelet count of $230-400,000/mm^3$ (Ref. 2, p. 482).

39.25. (D) A reduction of the fetal heart rate that is a mirror image of the contraction pattern is a result of vagal stimulation associated with fetal head compression (Ref. 2, p. 816).

39.26. (A) The only evaluation of true labor is by measurement of changes in the cervix, specifically dilatation and effacement (Ref. 3, pp. 313–314).

39.27. (C) The first stage of labor ends and the second stage begins when the cervix is completely dilated (Ref. 2, p. 641).

39.28. (B) Shoulder dystocia should be the first thought of the physician when the head is not followed by external rotation and delivery of the body of the infant. It is most common following instrumental delivery and in large babies, as occur with diabetics (Ref. 3, p. 669).

39.29. (D) As soon as the head emerges, the physician should clear the oropharynx of all foreign material. In the presence of meconium, this is important to prevent meconium aspiration (Ref. 2, p. 652).

39.30. (D) Whenever the umbilical cord is compromised, immediate delivery is indicated to protect the viable fetus (Ref. 1, p. 746).

39.31. **(E)** During labor, the best course is little or no medication. However, some patients cannot tolerate the pain of labor and seek pain relief. The best of these methods appears to be epidural block, if it is available (Ref. 1, p. 669).

39.32. **(C)** A latent phase which lasts longer than 8–12 hr is prolonged and may represent dysfunctional labor (Ref. 1, pp. 647–693).

39.33. **(E)** In some pregnancies, the fetal vessels traverse the membranes to reach the placenta, rather than insert directly into the placenta. This can result in fetal hemorrhage if they are damaged during rupture of the membranes. This type of insertion is called a velamentous insertion (Ref. 2, p. 866).

39.34. **(B)** As the fetal lung matures, there is a change in the amniotic fluid phospholipids. The levels of lecithin increase as the fetal lungs mature, whereas the levels of sphingomyelin remain stable. When there is a ratio of 2.0, the lungs are considered functionally mature (Ref. 2, pp. 827–829).

39.35. **(A)** Two or more cell types from the same zygote are called a mosaic (Ref. 2, p. 25).

39.36. **(C)** A chromosome number deviating from the basic number and from an exact multiple is called aneuploidy (Ref. 2, p. 25).

39.37. **(E)** As compared to a mosaic, two or more cell types from different zygotes are called a chimera (Ref. 2, p. 25).

39.38. **(A)** Maternal levels of growth hormone are reduced during pregnancy, whereas other similar hormones are increased (Ref. 2, pp. 351–352).

39.39. **(B)** Evidence now shows that maternal cholesterol is the primary precursor of progesterone in the pregnant woman (Ref. 2, pp. 351–352).

39.40. **(C)** The blood volume increases rapidly in early pregnancy and reaches its peak at the end of the second trimester (Ref. 1, p. 81).

39.41. **(D)** As the uterus enlarges in the third trimester, it puts pressure on the vena cava, thereby reducing venous return and hypotension (Ref. 3, pp. 195–196).

39.42. **(D)** The levels of fibrinogen increase from a normal of 350–500 mg/100 ml during the third trimester (Ref. 3, pp. 193–194).

39.43. **(E)** The narrowest diameter of the pelvic inlet is called the obstetric conjugate (Ref. 3, p. 222).

39.44. **(B)** The smallest distance in the midplane is the distance between the ischial spines (Ref. 3, p. 223).

39.45. **(C)** The distance between the ischial tuberosities measures the pelvic outlet (Ref. 3, p. 223).

39.46. **(A)** Almost all cases of hydatidiform mole will have vaginal bleeding (Ref. 2, pp. 398–399).

39.47. **(D)** As a result of trophoblastic release of large amounts of thyroid-stimulating hormone, some patients may develop hyperthyroidism (Ref. 2, pp. 398–399).

39.48. **(C)** Preeclampsia, especially before 20 weeks, occurs in 15% of patients with hydatidiform mole (Ref. 2, pp. 398–399).

39.49. **(E)** In late pregnancy, bleeding which has fetal hemoglobin is usually due to rupture of a fetal vessel, as may occur with a vasa previa or a velamentous insertion (Ref. 2, p. 453).

39.50. **(A)** External bleeding may be associated with any placental problem, but it is usually associated with placenta previa (Ref. 2, p. 453).

39.51. **(C)** Severe placental separation is frequently associated with maternal coagulation defects (Ref. 2, p. 453).

39.52. **(E)** Eclampsia is frequently associated with renal shutdown and necrosis of the renal cortex (Refs. 2, p. 469; 3, p. 671).

39.53. (C) A characteristic of pheochromocytoma is the paroxysmal nature of the hypertension (Refs. 2, p. 469; 3, p. 671).

39.54. (D) A common finding in lupus nephritis is massive proteinuria (Refs. 2, p. 469; 3, p. 671).

39.55. (A) Any anomaly that prohibits absorption of amniotic fluid by the fetus will result in an elevated volume of amniotic fluid (Ref. 3, pp. 462–463).

39.56. (D) As Rh-immune antibodies destroy fetal red cells, the heart rate increases until cardiac failure ensues (Ref. 3, p. 776).

39.57. (E) Diabetic mothers tend to have large babies (Ref. 3, p. 600).

39.58. (B) When the posterior parietal bone presents, it is referred to as posterior asynclitism. If the anterior parietal bone presents, it is called anterior asynclitism (Ref. 3, p. 325).

39.59. (E) Flexion of the vertex occurs during the second stage immediately prior to or at the time of internal rotation (Ref. 3, p. 326).

39.60. (A) When the posterior parietal bone presents, it is referred to as posterior asynclitism. If the anterior parietal bone presents, it is called anterior asynclitism (Ref. 3, p. 325).

39.61. (D) A persistent, severe pelvic pain immediately postpartum is a sign of a hematoma formation (Ref. 3, p. 738).

39.62. (E) The physician can assist delivery by gentle extension of the fetal head as the biparietal diameter emerges (Ritgen maneuver) (Ref. 3, pp. 339–340).

39.63. (A) During the third stage, the uterus becomes globular and firm as the placenta separates (Ref. 3, p. 342).

39.64. (B) The most frequent cause of postpartum hemorrhage is failure of the uterus to contract, or atony (Ref. 2, pp. 746–797).

39.65. (E) Hemorrhage occurring more than 24 hr after delivery is usually caused by a retained placental fragment (Ref. 2, pp. 796–797).

39.66. (D) Growth of the placenta into the uterine wall usually requires a hysterectomy to prevent hemorrhage (Ref. 2, pp. 796–797).

39.67. (C) During a normal pregnancy, the hCG levels rise rapidly during the first 3 months of pregnancy, then begin to fall. Human placental lactogen levels rise slowly throughout pregnancy to levels of 5–7 μg/ml (Ref. 1, p. 79).

39.68. (B) Placental lactogen stimulates lipolysis and is similar to growth hormone in that it inhibits gluconeogenesis (Ref. 1, pp. 79–80).

39.69. (D) Neither hCG nor hCS suppress lactation; hCS (placental lactogen) stimulates lactation (Ref. 1, pp. 78–79).

39.70. (C)
39.71. (D) Immunologic tests of pregnancy are sensitive at 750–2000 IU of hCG. Proteinuria may give a false positive test (Ref. 2, p. 359).

39.72. (B) Hydatidiform mole is characterized by high levels of hCG (Ref. 1, p. 729).

39.73. (C) The first sign of a spontaneous abortion is vaginal bleeding. The aborted tissue frequently shows hydropic degeneration (Ref. 2, p. 382).

39.74. (C) Choriocarcinoma may be preceded by vaginal bleeding, especially persistent. The tissue may also undergo hydropic degeneration (Ref. 2, p. 382).

39.75. (D) Maternal rubella does not cause vaginal bleeding or placental degeneration. It does affect fetal development (Ref. 2, p. 382).

542 / Obstetrics and Gynecology

39.76. (D)

39.77. (C) After a sensitized Rh negative mother is diagnosed, either initially or previously, she should be followed by amniocentesis and spectrophotometric fluid analysis (Ref. 2, p. 426).

39.78. (D) Patients who are sensitized should not receive Rh immune globulin (Ref. 2, p. 426).

39.79. (C)
39.80. (C)
39.81. (D) The greatest risk of cardiac decompensation occurs with maximum cardiac stress. This occurs at the end of the second trimester and during labor. This is also the time of greatest risk for death (Ref. 2, pp. 507–510).

39.82. (A) A fetal heart rate that is a mirror image of the contraction is a normal finding due to vagal stimulation (Ref. 2, pp. 816–820).

39.83. (B) A fetal scalp pH of less than 7.2 is indicative of acidosis (Ref. 2, pp. 816–820).

39.84. (D) Maternal cardiac decompensation has no effect on the fetal heart rate or scalp pH (Ref. 2, pp. 816–820).

39.85. (A)
39.86. (D)
39.87. (C) Pelvic measurements of the various pelvic types indicate that a gynecoid pelvis has an A–P diameter of over 11 cm; an android pelvis has prominent spines and a narrow sacrosciatic notch; platypelloid measurements have a shortened A–P of the inlet with spines, which are rarely prominent (Ref. 3, pp. 225–226).

39.88. (B) Adrenogenital syndrome in a genetic female is most often caused by 21-hydroxylase or 11-B-hydroxylase deficiency (Ref. 2, p. 41).

39.89. (D) During pregnancy, serum estriol levels are progressively increased, whereas 17-ketosteroids are decreased; estradiol and dehydroepienadosterone levels are increased (Ref. 2, p. 348).

39.90. (B) As pregnancy progresses, the renal plasm flow increases by 25−50% and calcium stores, circulatory WBCs, and the heart rate increase (Ref. 2, p. 339).

39.91. (E) During early pregnancy, almost any systemic infection with virus or similar virulent organism can affect the fetus (Ref. 1, p. 646).

39.92. (A) The classical triad for the diagnosis of ectopic pregancy is pain, abnormal uterine bleeding, and an adnexal mass. The pregnancy test will be positive in 80+% of patients (Ref. 2, p. 414).

39.93. (C) Any woman with a recent or remote history of hydatidiform mole, who has abnormal bleeding or a uterine/pelvic mass should have a β-hCG determination to rule out possible gestational trophoblastic disease (Ref. 2, p. 403).

39.94. (C) Therapy for premature placental separation should include immediate rupture of the membranes and determination of baseline fibrinogen levels. The patient can then be observed unless further problems occur, such as fetal distress (Ref. 2, pp. 450−452).

39.95. (D) In patients with pregnancy-induced hypertension, the hematocrit, BUN, and fibrinogen levels are increased, along with uric acid. Uric acid is diagnostic if diuretics have not been utilized (Ref. 2, pp. 467−469).

39.96. (C) During labor, gastric emptying is delayed and secretions of acids increase. As a result, the patient should be maintained NPO (nothing by mouth) and given antacids. In early labor she should be allowed to ambulate. She should be examined as often as necessary to determine progress (Ref. 2, p. 646).

39.97. (A) An episiotomy helps prevent overdistention and tears of the perineum. It shortens the second stage by reducing perineal resistance and rarely has problems with healing. Although the midline is preferred, an extremely short perineal body is a relative contraindication (Ref. 2, pp. 654−656).

39.98. (D) Uterine involution is painful, especially in the multiparous patient. It begins immediately after delivery and reduces the uterus to about 500 g at the end of the first week. Infection is not a usual accompaniment of involution (Ref. 2, p. 787).

39.99. (C)

39.100. (C) Once the diagnosis of hydatidiform mole is made, the uterus should be promptly evacuated. Suction curettage is the preferred method. Follow-up should then be made by weekly hCG assays until negative or other treatment is indicated (Ref. 2, pp. 398−400).

39.101. (D)

39.102. (B) This patient has a narrow diagonal conjugate and a narrow midplane consistent with an android type of pelvis. She is at risk for cephalopelvic disproportion (Ref. 2, pp. 624−627).

39.103. (D)

39.104. (C) This patient has two of the classical triad of ectopic pregnancy: pain and abnormal menses. Based on these findings, she should have a culdocentesis. If nonclotting blood is obtained, she should have an immediate laparotomy (Ref. 2, pp. 413−432).

39.105. (B) An amniocentesis which revealed bilirubin levels in the high level 2 weeks ago would necessitate an immediate repeat, plus plans for delivery or intrauterine transfusion (Ref. 2, pp. 430−432).

39.106. (A) A patient who has a persistently elevated blood pressure, hemoconcentration, and elevated uric acid has pregnancy-induced hypertension. This disease is more prevalent in primigravidas, especially those over 30 years of age (Ref. 2, pp. 467−469).

39.107. (B) This pattern represents a variable deceleration or cord pattern. Therapy is expectant with careful observation, position change, and oxygen (Ref. 2, pp. 815−816).

39.108. (E)

39.109. (D) The most common cause of postpartum bleeding is uterine atony. Initial therapy is uterine massage, as most patients will respond to this initial treatment (Ref. 2, pp. 796−797).

39.110. (C) This patient shows a repetitive pattern of heart rate dips compatible with uteroplacental insufficiency on a contraction stress test. A carefully controlled and monitored initiation of labor is indicated (Ref. 2, pp. 821−823).

39.111. (B)
39.112. (E) Severe perineal pain postpartum is most likely due to hematoma. Therapy is evacuation as soon as possible (Ref. 2, p. 730).

39.113. (B)
39.114. (D) The Apgar score is based on heart rate, respiratory effort, muscle tone, color, and reflex. This baby received 1 for heart rate, 1 for a weak cry, and 1 for reflex at 1 min. At 5 min the child has 2 for heart rate, 1 for muscle tone, 2 for reflex, 1 for color, and 2 for respiratory effort (Refs. 1, pp. 792−793; 2, pp. 844).

References

1. Benson, R.C.: *Current Obstetric and Gynecologic Diagnosis and Treatment*, 5th Ed., Lange Medical Publications, Los Altos, CA, 1984.

2. Danforth, D.N.: *Obstetrics and Gynecology*, 4th Ed., Harper & Row, Hagerstown, MD, 1982.

3. Pritchard, J. and McDonald, P.C.: *Williams Obstetrics*, 17th Ed., Appleton-Century-Crofts, New York, 1985.

40

Gynecology
Ralph W. Hale, M.D.

DIRECTIONS Each of the questions or incomplete statements below is followed by five suggested answers or completions. Select the **one** that is best in each case.

40.1. The antibiotic of choice in a patient with a suspected *Chlamydia* infection would be
  A. penicillin G
  B. ampicillin
  C. tetracycline
  D. cephalosporin
  E. vancomycin

40.2. Which of the following structures passes out of the pelvis through the greater sciatic notch and reenters through the lesser sciatic notch?
  A. Ureter
  B. Internal pudendal artery
  C. Superior vesical artery
  D. Obturator nerve
  E. Middle rectal artery

40.3. The vagina of the woman is derived from tissue that originates in
- **A.** genital tubercle
- **B.** mesonephric duct
- **C.** primitive urethral groove
- **D.** urogenital fold
- **E.** urogenital sinus

40.4. In the metabolism of progesterone, the principal metabolite measured in the urine is
- **A.** pregnanetriol
- **B.** 17-hydroxypregnenolone
- **C.** pregnenolone
- **D.** pregnanediol
- **E.** dehydroepiandrosterone

40.5. Of the following steroid compounds, which of the following serves as the direct precursor for estradiol?
- **A.** Dehydroepiandrosterone
- **B.** Androstenedione
- **C.** Testosterone
- **D.** 17-Hydroxypregnenolone
- **E.** 17-Hydroxyprogesterone

40.6. Which of the following gynecologic problems is encountered most frequently in the early childhood years (ages 2−8)?
- **A.** Vulvovaginitis
- **B.** Congenital anomalies
- **C.** Bleeding disorders
- **D.** Precocious puberty
- **E.** Ovarian tumors

40.7. The most common cause of precocious puberty is
- **A.** McCune-Albright syndrome
- **B.** feminizing ovarian mesenchymoma
- **C.** adrenal hyperplasia
- **D.** idiopathic or cryptogenic
- **E.** hypothyroidism

40.8. Which of the following is considered a contraindication to the use oral contraceptives in women 35–40 years of age?
A. Two or more prior pregnancies
B. Lactation
C. Obesity
D. History of rheumatic fever
E. Smoking 2 packs of cigarettes per day

40.9. Which of the following conditions appears to have the most significant increase in nulliparous women who use an IUD for contraception?
A. Acute pelvic infection
B. Ectopic pregnancies
C. Venous thrombophlebitis
D. Incompetent cervix
E. Habitual abortion

40.10. The most common gynecologic complaint of women relative to their menstrual cycle is
A. dysmenorrhea
B. migraine headache
C. mastodynia
D. premenstrual tension
E. midcycle pain and bleeding

40.11. In a 34-year-old gravida 4 para 4 patient with a normal pelvic examination who has developed spotting and flow on days 8–9 and days 16–18 of her cycle, the most important initial screening test should be
A. thyroid profile
B. endometrial biopsy
C. serum LH levels
D. serum β subunit of hCG
E. hysterosalpingogram

40.12. In addition to a serum prolactin, which of the following studies should be ordered routinely in a patient with galactorrhea—amenorrhea syndrome?
   A. TSH levels
   B. Urinary 17-ketosteroids
   C. Serum LH levels
   D. Serum β subunit of hCG
   E. Urinary pregnanediol

40.13. In an investigation of the infertile couple, which of the following tests should be performed first?
   A. Endometrial biopsy on day 22−24
   B. Uterotubal CO_2 insufflation (Rubin's)
   C. Sperm penetration assay
   D. Semen analysis
   E. Hysterosalpingography

40.14. The most important diagnostic test to perform in a patient with an indurated, firm, painless vulvar ulcer with non-tender inguinal lymphadenopathy is
   A. treponemal antibody (FTA-ABS)
   B. biopsy the ulcer edge
   C. VDRL
   D. chlamydial trachomatis culture
   E. identification of Donovan's bodies

40.15. The most important risk factor for the development of endomyometritis following delivery is
   A. vaginal delivery
   B. cesarean section
   C. frequent sexual intercourse
   D. prior urinary tract infection
   E. coexistent upper respiratory infection

40.16. In the diagnosis of endometriosis, the most significant historical finding is
   A. acquired dysmenorrhea
   B. infertility
   C. irregular menstruation
   D. dyspareunia
   E. onset after age 32

40.17. A patient with small painful ulcers of the labia minora and introitus would most likely be diagnosed as having
    A. psoriasis
    B. herpes genitalis
    C. pyogenic granuloma
    D. molluscum contagiosum
    E. primary syphilis

40.18. The most likely diagnosis of the lesion shown in Figure 87 is
    A. Bartholin's cyst
    B. hemangioma
    C. Gartner's duct cyst
    D. neurofibroma
    E. sebaceous cyst

Figure 87

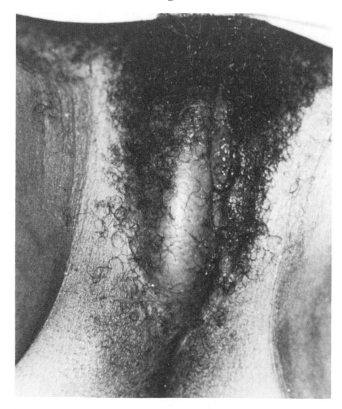

40.19. In a patient who complains of vulvovaginitis, you view the slide of the secretion shown in Figure 88. Your diagnosis would be
    A. *Trichomonas* vaginitis
    B. *Hemophilus* vaginitis
    C. nonspecific vaginitis
    D. candidiasis
    E. herpes genitalis

40.20. The most common benign lesion of the cervix is
    A. endometriosis
    B. cervical stenosis
    C. adenosis
    D. cervical polyps
    E. papilloma

Figure 88

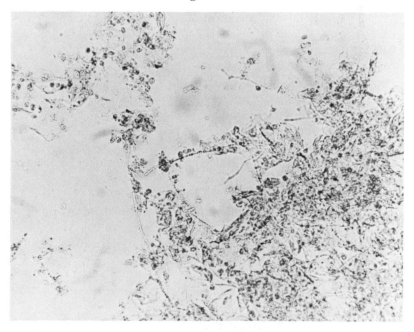

40.21. Death from cervical cancer is most often due to
   A. bowel obstruction
   B. uremia
   C. infection
   D. hemorrhage
   E. hepatic failure

40.22. In a patient with repeated class II Pap smears, the preferred treatment would be
   A. cryocautery
   B. conization
   C. colposcopic directed biopsy
   D. systemic antibiotics
   E. vaginal antibiotics

40.23. Endometrial polyps are most frequently encountered during which of the following periods of time?
   A. 10 years postmenopausal
   B. Following a delivery
   C. Perimenopausal
   D. Concurrent with postmenopausal or perimenopausal estrogen therapy
   E. Following cessation of oral contraceptives

40.24. The most common type of endometrial hyperplasia is
   A. cystic hyperplasia
   B. adenomatous hyperplasia
   C. atypical adenomatous hyperplasia
   D. endometrial polyps
   E. endolymphatic stromal myosis

40.25. Treatment for endometrial carcinoma stage 1B usually involves
   A. radiation alone
   B. total abdominal hysterectomy with bilateral salpingo-oophorectomy
   C. radiation plus total abdominal hysterectomy and bilateral salpingo-oophorectomy
   D. radical hysterectomy
   E. radiation plus radical hysterectomy

40.26. The primary lymph node spread of endometrial carcinoma is to the
   A. paracervical nodes
   B. obturator nodes
   C. inguinal nodes
   D. sacral nodes
   E. hypogastric nodes

40.27. The most common benign ovarian neoplasm is a
   A. dermoid cyst
   B. serous—mucinous cystadenoma
   C. cystadenofibroma
   D. granulosa cell tumor
   E. fibroma

40.28. In a patient with an adnexal mass that is cystic in nature and 20 cm in diameter, your most likely diagnosis would be
   A. serous cystadenoma
   B. theca lutein cyst
   C. endometriosis
   D. mucinous cystadenoma
   E. cystadenofibroma

40.29. Benign cystic teratomas occur most frequently in which age group?
   A. Premenarchal
   B. Menarche to 20 years
   C. 20—35 years
   D. 35—50 years—menopause
   E. Postmenopausal

40.30. The most frequent cause of death in a patient with advanced ovarian carcinoma is
   A. uremia
   B. hemorrhage
   C. intestinal obstruction
   D. hydrothorax
   E. cerebral metastases

40.31. The primary treatment for ovarian malignancy is
   A. immunotherapy
   B. external radiation
   C. chemotherapy
   D. intraperitoneal installation of radioactive materials
   E. surgery

40.32. Screening for early breast cancer is best accomplished by
   A. patient self-examination
   B. physician examination
   C. mammography
   D. Pap smear of nipple secretion
   E. thermography

40.33. The most common benign neoplasm of the breast is
   A. lipoma
   B. fibroadenoma
   C. adenoma
   D. fat necrosis
   E. thrombosis of veins (Mondor's disease)

40.34. The anatomic area of greatest concern in performance of a hysterectomy is
   A. approximation of the ureter to the uterine artery
   B. attachment of the bladder to the cervix
   C. uterine–ovarian artery anastomosis
   D. cervical attachment to the vagina
   E. relationship of the uterosacral ligaments to the rectosigmoid colon

---

DIRECTIONS: Each group of questions below consists of five lettered headings or a diagram with lettered components, followed by a list of numbered words or statements. For each numbered word or statement, select the **one** lettered heading that is most closely associated with it. Each lettered heading may be selected once, more than one, or not at all.

A. Uterine artery
B. Obturator artery
C. Internal pudendal artery
D. Inferior gluteal artery
E. Superior gluteal artery

40.35. A branch of the posterior division of the hypogastric artery

40.36. Supplies the lateral pelvic wall

40.37. Supplies the area inferior to the piriformis muscle

For questions 40.38–40.40, refer to Figure 89.

Figure 89

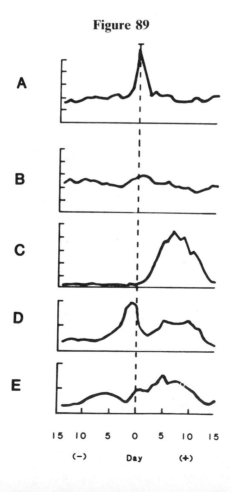

40.38. LH

40.39. Estradiol

40.40. Progesterone

Given a patient with a history of one of the following conditions, choose the form of contraception that would be most contraindicated:

A. Salpingitis
B. Irregular bleeding
C. Diabetes mellitus
D. Hypertension
E. Multiparity

40.41. Oral contraceptives

40.42. Intrauterine device

40.43. Calendar method of rhythm

A. Profuse bleeding at the expected time of a normal menstrual flow (hypermenorrhea)
B. Midcycle staining
C. Irregular bleeding throughout the cycle (metrorrhagia)
D. Frequent menstrual-like episodes (polymenorrhea)
E. Delayed menses followed by heavy bleeding

40.44. Leiomyomata

40.45. Anovulatory cycle

40.46. Endometrial malignancy

A. Clear, mucoid
B. Thick with white, curdlike consistency
C. Yellow-green and frothy
D. Gray, blood-streaked
E. Pink, serous

40.47. Trichomonas vaginitis

40.48. Cervical mucous

40.49. Vaginal mycosis

    A. Chronic cervicitis
    B. Cervical polyps
    C. Cervical adenosis
    D. Mesonephric cysts
    E. Cervical papillomas

40.50. Cryotherapy

40.51. Focal endocervical hyperplasia

40.52. Located on portio vaginalis

In evaluation of cervical carcinoma, the following findings would be expected.

    A. Stage I
    B. Stage II
    C. Stage IIA
    D. Stage III
    E. Stage IV

40.53. Extension to upper one-third of vagina

40.54. Extension into the bladder mucosa

40.55. Extension to the pelvic sidewall

In evaluation of endometrial carcinoma, the following findings would be expected.

    A. Stage IA
    B. Stage IB
    C. Stage II
    D. Stage III
    E. Stage IV

40.56. Involves the cervix

40.57. Involves the lateral pelvic wall

40.58. Confined to the corpus in a 10-cm uterus

In evaluation of ovarian carcinoma, the following findings would be expected.

      A.   Stage IB
      B.   Stage IIA
      C.   Stage IIB
      D.   Stage III
      E.   Stage IV

40.59. Extends to uterus

40.60. Widespread intraperitoneal metastases

40.61. Limited to both ovaries

For questions 40.62–40.64, refer to Figure 90.

Figure 90

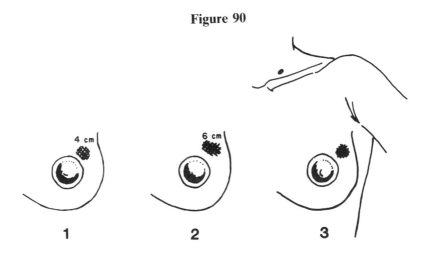

1   2   3

In evaluation of breast cancer, the following findings would be expected.

    A. Stage I
    B. Stage II
    C. Stage IIIA
    D. Stage IIIB
    E. Stage IV

40.62. 1

40.63. 2

40.64. 3

    A. Cystocele
    B. Urethra diverticula
    C. Procidentia
    D. Enterocele
    E. Rectocele

40.65. Postvoiding urine loss

40.66. Urinary incontinence

40.67. Urinary retention

    A. Paramesonephric
    B. Mesonephric
    C. Both
    D. Neither

40.68. Ureter

40.69. Hymen

40.70. Uterine tube

    A. Occurs in adolescence
    B. Occurs in childhood
    C. Both
    D. Neither

40.71. Ovarian tumors are usually benign

40.72. Dysontogenetic tumors occur more frequently

40.73. Vaginal clear-cell adenocarcinoma

    A. Elevated serum FSH levels
    B. Elevated serum LH levels
    C. Both
    D. Neither

40.74. Menopause

40.75. Polycystic ovarian disease

40.76. Anovulatory bleeding

A. Direct spread through the uterine cavity
B. Spreads directly to the parametrium
C. Both
D. Neither

40.77. *Neisseria gonorrhea*

40.78. *Escherichia coli*

40.79. Tuberculosis

    A. Penicillin
    B. Metronidazole
    C. Both
    D. Neither

40.80. *Bacteroides fragilis*

40.81. *Clostridium difficile*

40.82. *Neisseria gonorrhea*

    A. Endometriosis
    B. Adenomyosis
    C. Both
    D. Neither

40.83. Onset before age 30

40.84. Multiparous patient

40.85. Severe dysmenorrhea

    A. Mucinous cystadenoma
    B. Serous cystadenoma
    C. Both
    D. Neither

40.86. 20−50% bilateral

40.87. Rarely malignant

40.88. Occurs in the third to fifth decade of life

DIRECTIONS: For each of the questions or incomplete statements below, **one or more** of the answers or completions given is correct. Select
  (A) if only 1, 2, and 3 are correct
  (B) if only 1 and 3 are correct
  (C) if only 2 and 4 are correct
  (D) if only 4 is correct
  (E) if all are correct

40.89. The levator ani is composed of which of the following portions?
  1. Iliococcygeus
  2. Pubococcygeus
  3. Puborectalis
  4. Coccygeus

40.90. Pubertal development in young girls has which of the following characteristics?
  1. The growth spurt occurs prior to the onset of menses
  2. Axillary hair develops immediately following menses
  3. Breast development reaches secondary mound development (Tanner stage 4) before menses
  4. Pubic hair growth occurs after axillary hair growth

40.91. Indications for removal of an intrauterine device include
  1. persistent uterine bleeding
  2. downward displacement of the device
  3. intrauterine pregnancy
  4. hypertension

40.92. In a patient who is 10 years postmenopausal
  1. vaginal bleeding is indicative of endometrial cancer
  2. osteoporosis is the most serious health hazard
  3. *Candida* vulvovaginitis occurs in a high percentage of women
  4. incidence of heart disease increases

40.93. Abnormal uterine bleeding is
   1. associated with grossly evident pelvic disease in 75% of patients
   2. unrelated to age
   3. associated with histologic evidence of endometrial pathology in 80% of patients
   4. most frequent in women 40–50 years of age

40.94. In a patient with polycystic ovarian disease
   1. obesity is present in 95% of patients
   2. serum LH levels are high
   3. wedge resection of the ovaries is an important initial therapy
   4. three out of four are usually infertile

40.95. Cancer of the vulva
   1. is almost always a postmenopausal disease
   2. rarely requires a biopsy to make the diagnosis
   3. may appear as a chronic vulvar dermatitis
   4. is characterized by lack of pruritus or discomfort

40.96. In treatment of recurrent vaginal candidiasis
   1. diabetes mellitus should be considered
   2. feminine hygiene products should be discontinued
   3. systemic antibiotics should be stopped
   4. no change in sexual intercourse is indicated

40.97. The uterus with leiomyomata shold be removed when
   1. the tumors are larger than a 12-week pregnant uterus
   2. the tumors suddenly increase in size
   3. hypermenorrhea occurs
   4. pregnancy is no longer desired

40.98. Which of the following statistics are associated with benign ovarian neoplasm?
   1. Brenner tumors originate from Walthard's cell rests
   2. Adrenal rest tumors are masculinizing
   3. Dermoid tumors are rarely malignant
   4. Granulosa cell tumors can cause postmenopausal bleeding

DIRECTIONS SUMMARIZED

A	B	C	D	E
1,2,3	1,3	2,4	4	All are
only	only	only	only	correct

40.99. Women at high risk for breast cancer are associated with which of the following?
1. Menopause after age 50
2. Mother or sister with breast cancer
3. Nulliparity
4. First-term pregnancy before age 30

DIRECTIONS: This section of the test consists of situations, each followed by a series of questions. Study each situation and select the **one** best answer to each question following it.

Questions 40.100–40.101: A 3-year-old girl is brought to your office for examination. She was the product of a normal second pregnancy and an uncomplicated labor and delivery. She was noted at birth to have an enlarged clitoris and this has continued to grow. Your examination reveals a normal 3-year-old child who, on genital examination, has a clitoris that is 5 cm in length and a posterior labial fusion. A chromosomal analysis of the patient is shown in Figure 91.

40.100. Based on this finding, the most important laboratory test you could order to confirm the diagnosis would be
A. urinary estrogens
B. serum testosterone
C. urinary pregnanetriol
D. urinary 19-nortestosterone
E. serum cortisone

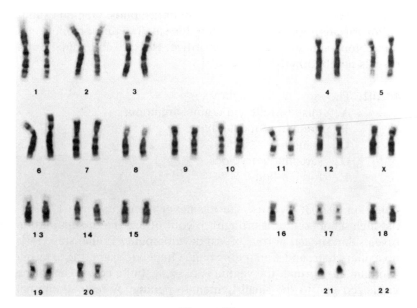

Figure 91

40.101. Based on the finding, the most likely etiology would be
  A. an adrenal tumor
  B. an ovarian tumor
  C. maternal drug ingestion
  D. nondysjunction of the sex chromosomes
  E. 21-hydroxylase enzyme deficiency

Question 40.102: A 7-year, 4-month-old girl is brought to your office by her mother with a chief complaint of vaginal bleeding. The mother's prenatal course had been uneventful for this, her first child, and she had an uneventful delivery. The girl was last examined by her pediatrician 5 months ago. She has had normal growth and development and is in the 65th percentile for her age. The mother noted the appearance of bloody discharge on the girl's pajamas 3 days ago. Since that time she has noted streaks of blood on both her underpants and pajamas. This morning the mother noted spots of red blood. The child denies any pain or discomfort.

On examination the patient is found to be a normal 7-year-old without axillary or pubic hair and with breast buds. Genital examination reveals normal external genitalia, small vaginal opening, and some blood-stained mucus in the orifice. Rectal—abdominal exam reveals no abnormalities.

40.102. The most likely diagnosis is
  A. mixed Müllerian adenocarcinoma
  B. premature menarche
  C. trauma
  D. sarcoma botryoides
  E. foreign body

Question 40.103: Because she has never menstruated, a 17-year-old high school senior is brought to your office. Your examination reveals that she has normal breast development (Tanner stage IV), no axillary hair, and scant pubic hair. On pelvic exam, the external genitalia are normal, the vagina is present, but a cervix cannot be visualized due to the small hymenal opening. A rectoabdominal examination reveals no abdominal masses and the uterus and ovaries are nonpalpable.

40.103. In your evaluation of the patient, the working diagnosis should be
  A. idiopathic delayed pubertal development
  B. Turner's (gonadal dysgenesis) syndrome
  C. androgen insensitivity syndrome
  D. failure of Müllerian development (Rokitansky-Kuster-Hauser-Mayer syndrome)
  E. hypogonadotropic amenorrhea

Questions 40.104–40.105: A 46-year-old gravida 2 para 1 ab 1 woman comes to your office with a 2-month history of irregular uterine bleeding. She had a normal pelvic examination with a class I Pap smear by you 4 months ago. She has an otherwise uneventful history and has been in good health. Further questioning reveals that the bleeding begins with spotting on approximately day 10 of the cycle and that she will spot or bleed enough to require a pad on almost every day of the cycle until her menses begins on day 24. Her menstrual flow is described as light; she has no other positive findings. An endometrial biopsy is performed which reveals the pattern shown in Figure 92.

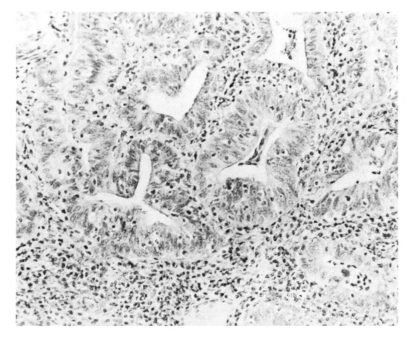

Figure 92

40.104. Based on this histologic finding, your most likely diagnosis would be
  A. endometrial carcinoma
  B. squamous cell carcinoma
  C. cystic hyperplasia of the endometrium
  D. endometrial adenomatous hyperplasia
  E. endometriosis

40.105. Based on the diagnosis, your initially recommended treatment would be
  A. radiation therapy
  B. triple-regimen chemotherapy
  C. progesterone therapy
  D. estrogen therapy
  E. reassurance and observation

Questions 40.106—40.107: A 22-year-old woman gravida 0 para 0 is seen in the hospital emergency room with a history of gradual onset of acute lower abdominal pain. She has never had a similar episode and has no significant past history. She is sexually active but not using birth control. Her last normal menstrual period was 5 days ago. Examination reveals a young female in obvious distress. Her temperature is 101.4°F, pulse 98, and respirations 22. The physical examination is negative except for the abdomen and pelvis. Abdominal examination reveals diffuse tenderness in all quadrants, with more pain in the right lower quadrant than the others. There is positive rebound tenderness and bowel sounds are absent. Pelvic examination reveals an acutely tender cervix on motion with bilateral adnexal tenderness and a 3- × 4-cm tender mass on the right side. Initial laboratory studies are as follows:

Urine		CBC	
Sp. gr.	1.026	Hgb	10.9
Protein	trace	Hct	34
Ketones	neg	RBC	4.8×10^6
Sugar	neg	WBC	18,200
Micro		Diff	
WBC	0–2	Seg	78
RBC	0	Bands	12
Epithelial	1–4	Stabs	1
Bact	0–1	Lymph	6
		Eos	1
		Mono	2

40.106. Based on your initial assessment, the most likely diagnosis is
  A. ectopic pregnancy
  B. acute appendicitis
  C. torsion of an ovarian cyst
  D. Meckel's diverticulitis
  E. salpingo-oophoritis

40.107. Your initial treatment plan should be based around
  A. immediate surgery (laparotomy)
  B. culdocentesis
  C. intravenous antibiotics
  D. ultrasonography
  E. immediate surgery (laparoscopy)

Questions 40.108–40.109: A 24-year-old gravida 0 para 0 patient is seen by you with a complaint of gradually increasing pain with her periods. Past history reveals that she was on oral contraceptives until age 21. She has used no contraceptives since that time, although she has remained sexually active. Her last normal menstrual period was 1 week ago and she has a normal menstrual cycle (29 days with 4 days' flow) and has noted gradually increasing pain over the last 14 months. At present, she is debilitated for 2–3 days with pain and receives relief only with codeine. Examination is normal, except for the pelvis, where the uterus is retroflexed, nonmobile, and tender. The right ovary is 3 × 4 × 4 cm. On rectal examination, thickening is palpated in the uterosacral areas.

40.108. Your most likely diagnosis would be
  A. adenomyosis
  B. dermoid cyst
  C. polycystic ovarian disease
  D. endometriosis
  E. adenomatous hyperplasia

40.109. Assuming your diagnosis is correct, you should recommend
  A. ovarian resection
  B. hysterectomy
  C. cyclic progesterone
  D. clomiphene citrate
  E. danazol

Questions 40.110–40.111: A 63-year-old woman is seen in your office for a routine pelvic examination. Examination of the vulva reveals the finding shown in Figure 93. A colposcopic-directed biopsy reveals the lesion to be an intraepithelial cancer (Bowen's disease).

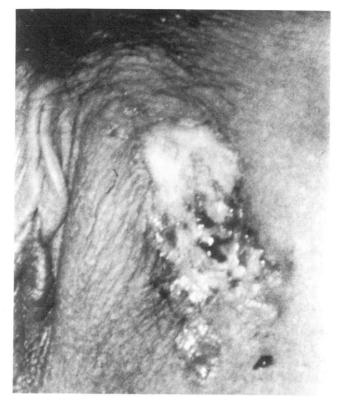

Figure 93

40.110. Your best course of therapy would be
- **A.** topical 5-fluorouracil
- **B.** radical vulvectomy
- **C.** wide lacal excision
- **D.** vulvar irradiation
- **E.** systemic chemotherapy

40.111. As part of the evalution, the patient should be carefully screened for coexistent
- **A.** rectal carcinoma
- **B.** intraductal breast carcinoma
- **C.** vulvar melanoma
- **D.** cervical carcinoma
- **E.** large intestine carcinoma

Question 40.112: A 32-year-old gravida 3 para 0 who is asymptomatic is seen by you for a routine gynecologic examination. No pathology is found, but the Pap smear is reported as class III−IV. A colposcopic examination reveals the findings shown in Figure 94, and a colposcopic-directed biopsy of the suspected lesion is shown in Figure 95.

Figure 94

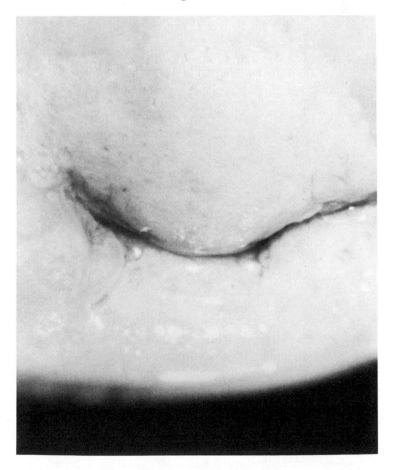

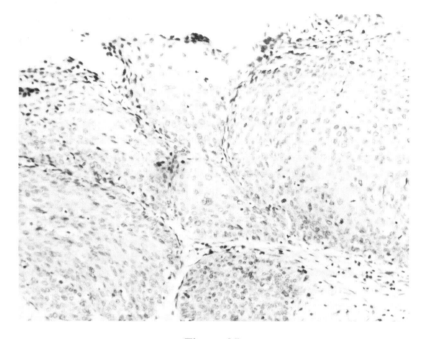

Figure 95

40.112. Based on the pathologist's report of intraepithelial squa-
mous cell carcinoma extending to the limits of the biopsy,
you should
  A. observe and repeat the biopsy in 3 months
  B. perform a hysterectomy with wide-cuff excision
  C. cone biopsy
  D. perform a hysterectomy with lymph node dissection
  E. perform cryocautery

Question 40.113: A 34-year-old gravida 5 para 4 ab 1 has come to
your office complaining of severe dysmenorrhea. She relates that
following the birth of her last child 4 years ago she had a surgical
sterilization. She further states that she has had a normal cycle until
6 months ago. At that time she noted the onset of sharp, crampy
abdominal pains at the time of her menses. She states these pains
have been gradually increasing in intensity over the past 6 months.
For the past 2 months, she has noticed increased flow with her

menses and deep dyspareunia. On pelvic examination, the uterus is found to be the size and consistency of an 8-week pregnancy and it is tender to palpation.

40.113. Your most likely diagnosis is
  A. endometriosis
  B. intrauterine pregnancy
  C. adenocarcinoma
  D. adenomyosis
  E. posttubal ligation syndrome

Questions 40.114–40.115: An 18-year-old gravida 0 para 0 is seen in the hospital emergency room complaining of severe abdominal pain. She is using a diaphragm for contraception and had her last normal menstrual period 2 weeks ago. The pain had its onset approximately 3 hr before admission and is described as colicky in nature and localized in the right lower quadrant. Examination reveals hypoactive bowel sounds and right lower quadrant tenderness. On pelvic examination, the uterus is tender to motion and an acutely tender 6 cm right adnexal mass is palpated. Laboratory data includes the following:

Urine		CBC	
Sp. gr.	1.016	Hgb	11.4
Protein	neg	Hct	34
Sugar	neg	RBC	4.2×10^6
Ketones	1+	WBC	12,750
Micro		Diff	
WBC	0–2	Seg	64
RBC	0–1	Bands	4
Bact	few	Lymph	23
Pregnancy test	neg	Mono	5
		Eos	3
		Baso	1

A flat plate of the abdomen shows the following (Figure 96).

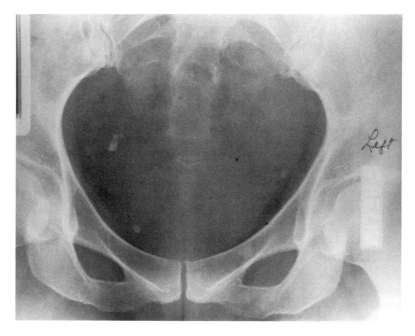

Figure 96

40.114. Based on these findings, your most likely diagnosis is
   A. acute appendicitis
   B. tuboovarian abscess
   C. ectopic pregnancy
   D. benign teratoma with torsion
   E. hemorrhagic corpus luteum

40.115. The appropriate therapy would be
   A. intravenous antibiotics
   B. ultrasonography
   C. immediate laparotomy
   D. observation for 24 hr
   E. progesterone suppression

Question 40.116: A 49-year-old gravida 0 para 0 is seen in your office for a complaint of heavy vaginal discharge. She has no history of any menstrual bleeding abnormality; her last menstrual period was 3 years ago. She does relate that she had had a lower pelvic discomfort for the past 3 months, with occasional episodes of sharp pain on the right side. She describes her discharge as yellow and slightly blood-tinged on occasion, whereas at other times it is clear. She describes the amount as enought to cause her to wear a pad. On examination the only positive finding is a 3 × 3 cm right adnexal mass that is mildly tender.

40.116. Your initial diagnosis would be
   A. Postmenopausal ovary syndrome
   B. mucinous cystadenoma
   C. tuboovarian abcess
   D. fallopian tube carcinoma
   E. ovarian neoplasm

Answers and Comments

40.1. (C) Tetracyclines are still the drug of choice in *Chlamydia* infections. Penicillins and cephalosporins have not been shown to be effective (Ref. 1, p. 1030).

40.2. (B) The pudendal artery and nerve exit the pelvic cavity through the greater sciatic foramen; it courses under the ischial spine and then reenters the pelvic cavity through the lesser foramen (Ref. 2, p. 64).

40.3. (E) The urogenital sinus invaginates to create the vagina in women (Ref. 2, pp. 119–120).

40.4. (D) The principal metabolic product of progesterone is pregnanediol. This occurs by reduction of the A ring and the keto groups. Although it only represents 20% of the metabolites, it is an excellent measure of progesterone metabolism (Ref. 2, p. 137).

40.5. (C) Testosterone, which is converted from androstenedione, is the direct precursor of estradiol (Ref. 2, p. 138).

40.6. (A) The inflammatory disorders of vulvovaginitis are the most common gynecologic complaints of young children after the second year of life (Ref. 1, p. 413).

40.7. **(D)** Although specific etiologies can be found in a few individuals, 80–90% of all cases of precocious puberty have no demonstrable etiology (Ref. 2, pp. 416–418).

40.8. **(E)** Newer studies of women over the age of 35 have found that the greatest negative variable is cigarette smoking. When these women are identified separately, they account for most of the complications reported (Ref. 1, p. 531).

40.9. **(A)** Although there may be a slight increase in the incidence of ectopic pregnancy, this is more relative than real. Evidence is mounting, however, that pelvic infections may occur in as many as 1–2% of IUD users (Ref. 1, pp. 536–537).

40.10. **(A)** The most common gynecologic complaint of women is painful menstruation (dysmenorrhea) (Ref. 1, pp. 113–146).

40.11. **(B)** Any woman who develops an abnormal bleeding pattern should have a tissue diagnosis of the endometrium (Ref. 2, p. 910).

40.12. **(A)** In patients with galactorrhea, TSH levels are ordered, because primary hypothyroidism may also be a cause (Ref. 2, p. 922).

40.13. **(D)** The initial evaluation of the infertile couple should include a male factor investigation. The only readily available test is the semen analysis (Ref. 1, p. 995).

40.14. **(A)** Primary syphilitic chancres are painless, firm, and indurated. Inguinal nodes are likewise nontender and the most widely used treponemal test is the fluorescent treponemal antibody absorption test (FTA-ABS) (Ref. 1, pp. 368–369).

40.15. **(B)** The rate of endomyometritis is greater following cesarean section than vaginal delivery (Ref. 2, p. 243).

40.16. **(A)** The classical finding in a patient with endometriosis is acquired dysmenorrhea (Ref. 2, p. 1009).

40.17. **(B)** Small painful ulcers or vesicles of the genitalia will usually be the result of a Herpes infection, type II. This is a sexually transmitted, recurring disease (Ref. 1, p. 207).

40.18. (A) An enlarged cystic mass located at the vaginal introitus is usually a Bartholin's gland cyst (Ref. 1, p. 213).

40.19. (D) Pseudohyphae are characteristic of *Candida albicans* infection (Ref. 1, p. 199).

40.20. (D) Polyps are second only to inflammation in occurrence as the most common cervical disease (Ref. 2, p. 1049).

40.21. (B) Death from cervical cancer usually follows blockage of the ureters and subsequent uremia (Ref. 2, p. 1057).

40.22. (C) When a suspicious Pap smear is repeated and the repeat smear is also suspicious, the physician should schedule a colposcopic evaluation immediately. Only after colposcopy should treatment be recommended (Ref. 2, p. 1059).

40.23. (C) Endometrial polyps occur most frequently around the menopause (Ref. 2, p. 1079).

40.24. (A) The initial and most common stage of endometrial hyperplasia is cystic hyperplasia (Ref. 2, pp. 1076–1077).

40.25. (C) Early endometrial carcinoma is most frequently treated by radiation, followed by hysterectomy and removal of the ovaries (Ref. 2, p. 1102).

40.26. (E) Endometrial cancer spreads first to the lateral pelvic wall and internal iliac (hypogastric) lymph nodes (Ref. 1, pp. 273–274).

40.27. (B) Serous or mucinous cystadenomas comprise about one-fourth of all benign ovarian tumors (Ref. 2, p. 1126).

40.28. (D) Mucinous cystadenomas are the largest occurring ovarian tumors (Ref. 1, p. 320).

40.29. (C) Benign cystic teratomas have their peak incidence in young adult women. They may occur, however, at any age (Ref. 2, p. 1135).

40.30. **(C)** Most patients with advanced ovarian carcinoma develop intraabdominal adhesions, ascites, and ultimately bowel obstruction, which leads to death (Ref. 2, p. 1164).

40.31. **(E)** Surgery is still the first and main treatment for ovarian malignancy (Ref. 2, pp. 1161–1162).

40.32. **(C)** Although 70% of breast cancers are found on self-examination, the best diagnostic tool available is mammography. If all women were screened we could detect most cases of breast cancer early (Ref. 2, pp. 120–123).

40.33. **(B)** The most common benign neoplasm of the breast is a fibroadenoma (Ref. 2, p. 1196).

40.34. **(A)** During performance of a hysterectomy, the surgeon must be aware of the course of the ureter under the uterine artery. This is the site of most injuries to the ureter (Ref. 2, p. 1246).

40.35. **(E)** The internal iliac (hypogastric) artery branches into an anterior and posterior division. The superior gluteal originates in the posterior division (Ref. 2, pp. 63–64).

40.36. **(B)** The obturator artery of the anterior division of the hypogastric artery supplies the lateral pelvic wall (Ref. 2, pp. 63–64).

40.37. **(D)** The inferior gluteal artery dips into the pelvis to supply the piriformis muscle (Ref. 2, pp. 63–64).

40.38. **(A)** LH has its peak at midcycle (Ref. 2, p. 130).

40.39. **(D)** Estradiol is elevated at midcycle and then has a second but smaller elevation in the secretory phase (Ref. 2, p. 130).

40.40. **(C)** Progesterone is elevated during the secretory phase (Ref. 2, p. 130).

40.41. **(D)** Preexisting hypertension is a contraindication to use of the oral contraceptives (Ref. 3, pp. 816–817).

40.42. **(A)** Intrauterine devices are contraindicated with salpingitis (Ref. 1, p. 537).

40.43. **(B)** A regular bleeding cycle is essential to success in the rhythm method (Ref. 1, pp. 528−529).

40.44. **(A)** A characteristic of leiomyomata is profuse menses (Ref. 2, p. 907).

40.45. **(D)** Anovulatory cycles are often associated with frequent menses (Ref. 2, p. 907).

40.46. **(C)** Irregular bleeding throughout the cycle is characteristic of malignancy (Ref. 2, p. 907).

40.47. **(C)** Trichomonas infection results in a yellow or green frothy discharge (Ref. 1, p. 199).

40.48. **(A)** The cervical mucus is primarily responsible for fluid in the vagina. The fluid is clear and mucoid. It may at times be profuse but is without symptoms (Ref. 1, p. 9).

40.49. **(B)** Vaginal mycosis is characterized by a thick, cottage cheese-like discharge (Ref. 2, p. 994).

40.50. **(A)** The therapy of chronic cervicitis is cryotherapy (Ref. 1, p. 233).

40.51. **(B)** Cervical polyps are associated with focal endocervical hyperplasia (Ref. 1, pp. 236−237).

40.52. **(E)** Fibrous tissue papillomas originate on the portio vaginalis of the cervic (Ref. 1, p. 239).

40.53. **(C)** Cervical malignancy extending into the upper one-third of the vagina is classified as stage IIA (Ref. 1, p. 246).

40.54. **(E)** Extension of cervical carcinoma into the bladder mucosa is classified as stage IV (Ref. 1, p. 246).

40.55. **(D)** When cervical carcinoma reaches the pelvic sidewall, the lesion is classified as stage III (Ref. 1, p. 246).

40.56. (C) Extension of endometrial carcinoma to the cervix is classified as stage II (Ref. 1, p. 272).

40.57. (D) Involvement of the lateral pelvic wall occurs in stage III (Ref. 1, p. 272).

40.58. (B) A 10-cm corpus is found with endometrial carcinoma, stage IB (Ref. 1, p. 272).

40.59. (B) Ovarian carcinoma extending to the uterus is classified as stage IIA (Ref. 1, p. 310).

40.60. (D) Widespread peritoneal metastases occur in stage III ovarian carcinoma (Ref. 1, p. 310).

40.61. (A) Ovarian caracinoma limited to both ovaries is classified as stage IB (Ref. 1, p. 310).

40.62. (B) A breast cancer less than 5 cm in diameter is a stage II lesion (Ref. 2, pp. 1205–1207).

40.63. (C) A breast cancer over 5 cm in diameter is a stage IIIA lesion (Ref. 2, pp. 1205–1207).

40.64. (D) When a supraclavicular node is found in breast cancer, the lesion is classified stage IIIB (ref. 2, pp. 1205–1207).

40.65. (B) Loss of urine postvoiding occurs with a urethral diverticula (Ref. 1, p. 288).

40.66. (A) Involuntary loss of urine is the most common symptom of cystocele (Ref. 1, p. 288).

40.67. (C) Procidentia can cause acute angulation of the urethra and result in retention (Ref. 1, p. 296–297).

40.68. (B) The ureter is derived from the mesonephric duct (Ref. 1, pp. 7–12).

40.69. (D) The hymen is a derivative of the Müllerian tubercle (Ref. 1, pp. 7–12).

40.70. (A) The fallopian tube is derived from the paramesonephric (Müllerian) duct (Ref. 1, pp. 7–12).

40.71. (A) Ovarian tumors that occur in childhood are more likely to be malignant than those that occur in adolescence (Ref. 1, p. 466).

40.72. (B) The incidence of dysontogenetic tumors is much higher in childhood than in adolescents (Ref. 1, p. 466).

40.73. (A) Clear-cell adenocarcinoma arising from Müllerian remnants, and often associated with maternal ingestion of diethylstilbestrol, occurs most frequently in postmenarchal girls of the teenage years (Ref. 1, p. 466).

40.74. (C) During menopause, serum FSH and LH levels are elevated (Ref. 1, p. 573).

40.75. (B) A characteristic of polycystic ovarian disease is elevated LH levels (Ref. 1, p. 315).

40.76. (D) Anovulatory bleeding is not associated with any changes in FSH and LH levels (Ref. 1, p. 141).

40.77. (A) Gonorrhea spreads directly through the uterine cavity to the tubes (Ref. 1, p. 352).

40.78. (B) *E. coli* spreads directly through the uterine wall to cause parametritis (Ref. 1, p. 352).

40.79. (D) Tuberculosis infects the pelvis by hematogenous spread (Ref. 1, p. 353).

40.80. (B) The most bactericidal drug to *B. fragilis* is metronidazole (Ref. 2, pp. 247–250).

40.81. (D) Vancomycin is the drug of choice for *C. difficile* (Ref. 2, pp. 247–250).

40.82. (A) Penicillin is still the drug of choice for *N. gonorrhea* (Ref. 2, pp. 247–250).

40.83. (A) Endometriosis is a disease of young women, usually less than age 30 (Ref. 1, p. 382).

40.84. (B) Adenomyosis is a disease of multiparous patients (Ref. 1, p. 269).

40.85. (C) Dysmenorrhea occurs in both endometriosis and adenomyosis (Ref. 1, pp. 269, 382).

40.86. (B) Of serous cystadenomas, 20−50% are bilateral (Ref. 2, pp. 1126−1129).

40.87. (A) Mucinous cystadenomas are rarely malignant (Ref. 2, pp. 1126−1129).

40.88. (C) Mucinous and serous cystadenomas occur most frequently during ages 30−50 (Ref. 2, pp. 1126−1129).

40.89. (A) The levator ani muscle is composed of three components: iliococcygeus, puborectalis, and pubococcygeus (Ref. 1, p. 58).

40.90. (B) The pubertal process begins with axillary hair growth and breast development. Menses is the last event of puberty (Ref. 2, p. 164).

40.91. (A) An intrauterine device should be removed when there is persistent bleeding, displacement, or pregnancy (Ref. 2, pp. 272−274).

40.92. (C) During menopause the reduced levels of estrogen facilitate bone (calcium) reabsorption and susceptibility to heart disease (Ref. 1, pp. 576−579).

40.93. (D) Abnormal uterine bleeding is associated with pelvic disease in only 35% of patients, whereas histologic evidence is present in 45%. The most frequent age group for bleeding is 40−50 years (ref. 2, p. 907).

40.94. (C) Polycystic ovarian disease is associated with elevated LH levels. Seventy-five percent of these patients have a history of infertility (Ref. 2, p. 919).

40.95. (B) Vulvar carcinoma occurs in the postmenopausal age group and usually presents as a chronic dermatitis (Ref. 2, p. 174).

40.96. (A) Vaginal mycosis frequently follows systemic antibiotics and occurs in diabetics. Feminine hygiene products can cause irritation and treatment of the sexual partner may be necessary (Ref. 1, p. 193).

40.97. (A) Removal of the uterus is indicated when the size of the uterus exceeds 12 weeks, the size suddenly increases, or heavy bleeding occurs (Ref. 2, p. 1088).

40.98. (E) Brenner tumors are fibroepithelial tumors which originate in inclusions of germinal cell epithelium (Walthard's cell rests). Adrenal rest tumors are masculinizing, whereas granulosa cell tumors secrete estrogens and may cause postmenopausal bleeding. Benign teratomas are rarely malignant (Ref. 2, pp. 1131–1139).

40.99. (A) Women who have a prologed period of menstruation, a strong family history, or nulliparity are at a greater risk for development of breast cancer (Ref. 2, p. 1192).

40.100. (C)
40.101. (E) In a patient with congenital adrenal hyperplasia and a normal karyotype, a pregnanetriol is diagnostic. The most frequent defect is a 21-hydroxylase deficiency (Ref. 1, 2, pp. 174–175).

40.102. (E) The most likely diagnosis in a young girl with vulvovaginitis is foreign body (Ref. 2, p. 892).

40.103. (C) In evaluation of primary amenorrhea in a patient who has normal breasts and scanty or absent axillary or pubic hair, testicular feminization should be considered first (Ref. 1, pp. 155, 468).

40.104. (D)
40.105. (C) This histologic pattern is that of benign adenomatous hyperplasia. The glands are back to back. Initial therapy would be progesterone (Ref. 1, pp. 272–273).

40.106. (E)
40.107. (C) A patient with an elevated WBC count who is febrile

and has abdominal pain should be suspected of having pelvic inflammatory disease (PID). With an adnexal mass, salpingo-oophoritis should be suspected. The initial treatment is high doses of antibiotics (Ref. 2, pp. 239–242).

40.108. (D)
40.109. (E) Acquired dysmenorrhea in a young woman is usually due to endometriosis. Once the diagnosis is established, the best treatment is danazol (antigonadotropin) (Ref. 2, pp. 1009–1012).

40.110. (C)
40.111. (D) A carcinoma in situ of the vulva in a 60-year-old woman should be treated with wide local excision. About 20% will have a second primary and 75% of these are cervical (Ref. 1, pp. 220–222).

40.112. (C) A patient who has a carcinoma in situ extending to the edge of the biopsy should have a conization performed to rule out invasion (Ref. 1, pp. 241–243).

40.113. (D) Acquired dysmenorrhea in a multiparous patient with an enlarged soft uterus is usually due to adenomyosis (Ref. 1, p. 270).

40.114. (D)
40.115. (C) In a young girl with a benign teratoma shown on x-ray and an acute abdomen, torsion should be suspected. The immediate treatment is removal of the cyst without releasing the torsion (Ref. 2, pp. 1116–1117).

40.116. (D) Yellow or honey-colored clear fluid in large amounts in a perimenopausal woman with pain and an adnexal mass is indicative of fallopian tube carcinoma (Ref. 2, p. 1110).

References

1. Benson, R.C.: *Current Obstetric and Gynecologic Diagnosis and Treatment*, 5th Ed., Lange Medical Publications, Los Altos, CA, 1984.

2. Danforth, D.N. *Obstetrics and Gynecology*, 4th Ed., Harper & Row, Hagerstown, MD, 1982.

SURGERY

41

General Surgery (Abdominal, Gastrointestinal, Endocrinology, Basic Surgical Sciences, Neoplasms)

**M. D. Ram, B.Sc., M.D., M.S. (Surg.), Ph.D.,
F.R.C.S. (Eng.), F.R.C.S. (Ed.),
F.R.C.S. (Can.), F.A.C.S.**

DIRECTIONS: Each of the questions or incomplete statements below is followed by five suggested answers or completions. Select the **one** that is best in each case.

41.1. Transfusion reaction in an anesthetized patient is usually evidenced by
   A. excessive bleeding
   B. renal failure
   C. skin rashes
   D. fever
   E. respiratory insufficiency

41.2. The nerve most likely to be injured in fractures of the humeral shaft is the
   A. radial
   B. median
   C. ulnar
   D. axillary
   E. musculocutaneous

41.3. Effects of a large arteriovenous fistula include all of the following EXCEPT
   A. tachycardia
   B. high cardiac output
   C. increased blood volume
   D. increased collateral vessels
   E. diastolic hypertension

41.4. The inferior mesenteric vein drains into the
   A. superior mesenteric vein
   B. portal vein
   C. splenic vein
   D. left common iliac vein
   E. inferior vena cava

41.5. The most common presenting feature of postoperative pulmonary embolism is
   A. edema of legs
   B. congestive heart failure
   C. significant hemoptysis
   D. dyspnea
   E. stridor and wheezing

41.6. Antibiotic-induced colitis is frequently associated with
   A. neomycin
   B. chloramphenicol
   C. gentamicin
   D. clindamycin
   E. vancomycin

41.7. A 5-cm breast lump, which was freely movable, was found to be malignant on histologic examination. The best prognosis is if the lesion is a/an
  A. infiltrating duct carcinoma
  B. infiltrating papillary carcinoma
  C. colloid carcinoma
  D. medullary cancer
  E. lobular carcinoma

41.8. All of the following statements regarding malignant melanoma are correct EXCEPT
  A. there is an increasing incidence of cutaneous melanoma
  B. repeated trauma induces malignant change in a benign mole
  C. most malignant melanomas arise from a junctional nevus or as part of a compound nevus
  D. melanomas occur most often in the palms and soles in the black race
  E. superficial spreading melanoma accounts for approximately two-thirds of all cutaneous melanomas and has an equal distribution in both sexes

41.9. The incidence of which of the following cancers has decreased in the last 40 years?
  A. Pancreas
  B. Lung
  C. Stomach
  D. Colon
  E. Prostate

41.10. The drug of choice for treatment of intraabdominal abscess due to *Bacteriodes fragilis* is
  A. penicillin
  B. gentamicin
  C. ampicillin
  D. cephalothin
  E. clindamycin

41.11. Creeping fat from mesentery onto bowel wall is a feature of
  A. Crohn's disease
  B. ulcerative colitis
  C. ischemic colitis
  D. amebic colitis
  E. bacterial enteritis

41.12. The most frequent diaphragmatic hernia in the newborn is
  A. sliding hiatal hernia
  B. paraesophageal hernia
  C. hernia of foramen of Bochdalek
  D. hernia of foramen of Morgagni
  E. agenesis of diaphragm

41.13. Which of the following indications for splenectomy is an autoimmune disease?
  A. Thalassemia
  B. Hypersplenism
  C. Thrombocytopenic purpura
  D. Gaucher's disease
  E. Spherocytic anemia

41.14. Malignant ascites is frequently due to
  A. carcinoma of pancreas
  B. malignant hepatoma
  C. carcinoma of ovary
  D. carcinoma of bladder
  E. carcinoma of breast

41.15. Desmoid tumors of the abdominal wall
  A. spread by venous invasion
  B. spread through lymphatics
  C. have a high incidence of local recurrence
  D. invade peritoneal cavity
  E. arise from remnants of cartilage

41.16. Rupture of which of the following visceral arterial aneurysms is more likely in association with pregnancy?
   A. Hepatic
   B. Ovarian
   C. Splenic
   D. Renal
   E. Uterine

41.17. The most serious complication of hepatic adenomas induced by oral contraceptive pills is
   A. malignant transformation
   B. rupture and hemorrhage
   C. invasion into inferior vena cava through the hepatic veins
   D. jaundice due to ductal obstruction
   E. pseudomyxoma peritonei

41.18. Metabolic changes associated with pyloric stenosis include all of the following EXCEPT
   A. hypokalemia
   B. hypochloremia
   C. respiratory acidosis
   D. dehydration
   E. hemoconcentration

41.19. Hepatic adenomas are associated with
   A. vinyl chloride
   B. cirrhosis
   C. oral contraceptives
   D. infectious hepatitis
   E. aflatoxin

41.20. The most common cause of chronic pancreatitis is
   A. chronic alcoholism
   B. gallstone disease
   C. hyperparathyroidism
   D. familial
   E. recurrent trauma

41.21. The most useful method to diagnose cause of upper gastro-
intestinal hemorrhage is
   A. barium study
   B. celiac angiography
   C. hepatic wedge pressures
   D. gastric biopsy
   E. endoscopy

41.22. Four days following appendectomy for a perforated appen-
dicitis, a 20-year-old patient develops fever, despite antibi-
otics. The most likely cause is
   A. atelectasis and pneumonia
   B. venous thrombosis
   C. wound infection
   D. urinary infection
   E. phlebitis due to IV fluids

41.23. The most common type of lesion in congenital esophageal
atresia is
   A. blind proximal pouch and a distal tracheal or bronchial
      fistula
   B. esophageal stenosis without fistula
   C. proximal pouch fistula to trachea, blind distal pouch
   D. esophagus in continuity with tracheal fistula
   E. both pouches blind and no fistula

41.24. Liver metastases of carcinoid tumor most frequently arise
from a primary in the
   A. jejunum
   B. ileum
   C. appendix
   D. colon
   E. rectum

41.25. Choice of treatment of a pseudocyst of pancreas located in
the lesser sac is
   A. external drainage
   B. observation and antibiotics
   C. transductal drainage
   D. excision
   E. cyst-gastrostomy or cyst-jejunostomy

41.26. The incidence of thyroid cancer is increased in patients with a history of
    A. antithyroid drug treatment
    B. iodine-deficient diet
    C. childhood irradiation to neck
    D. autoimmune thyroiditis
    E. thyrotoxicosis

41.27. The most common cause of adrenogenital syndrome in infancy is
    A. pituitary basophil adenoma
    B. adrenal cortical adenoma
    C. adrenal cortical carcinoma
    D. deficiency of C-21 hydroxylation
    E. ovarian tumor

41.28. Which of the following complications is most likely to be life threatening in the immediate phase following total thyroidectomy?
    A. Thyroid storm
    B. Hypercalcemic crisis
    C. Tetany
    D. Shock
    E. Airway obstruction

DIRECTIONS: Each group of questions below consists of five lettered headings followed by a list of numbered words or statements. For each numbered word or statement, select the **one** lettered heading that is most closely associated with it. Each lettered heading may be selected once, more than once, or not at all.

    A. Superior laryngeal nerve
    B. Recurrent laryngeal nerve
    C. Spinal accessory nerve
    D. Facial Nerve
    E. External laryngeal nerve

41.29. Parathyroidectomy

41.30. Parotidectomy

41.31. Radical neck dissection

    A. Osteomas
    B. Metastatic carcinoids
    C. Hypokalemia, hypochloremia
    D. Very high incidence of cancer
    E. Melanin spots on oral mucosa

41.32. Gardner's syndrome

41.33. Villous adenomas

41.34. Familial polyposis

    A. Digitalis
    B. Norepinephrine
    C. Dopamine
    D. Phenylephrine (Neo-Synephrine)
    E. Metaraminol (Aramine)

41.35. Enhances renal blood flow

41.36. Least efficient inotropic effect

41.37. Hypokalemia and hypercalcemia should be avoided

    A. Gastrin
    B. Secretin
    C. Insulin
    D. Glucagon
    E. VIP (vasoactive intestinal polypeptide)

41.38. Normally produced by the antrum

41.39. Zollinger-Ellison syndrome is usually produced by pancreatic tumor's secretion

41.40. Beta cell tumors of pancreas produce large amounts

A. Pheochromocytoma
B. Insulinoma
C. Parathyroid adenoma
D. Thyroid cancer
E. Carcinoid tumor

41.41. Urinary VMA levels

41.42. Urinary 5-HIAA levels

41.43. Urinary hydroxyproline level

DIRECTIONS: Each set of lettered headings below is followed by a list of numbered words or phrases. For each numbered word or phrase select

(A) if the item is associated with A only
(B) if the item is associated with B only
(C) if the item is associated with both A and B
(D) if the item is associated with neither A nor B

A. *Clostridium perfringes*
B. *Clostridium sporogenes*
C. Both
D. Neither

41.44. Infection results with gas in wound

41.45. Breaks down muscle

41.46. Methicillin is the drug of choice for treatment

A. Cancer of colon
B. Cancer of pancreas
C. Both
D. Neither

41.47. Elevated serum carcinoembryonic antigen (CEA) levels

41.48. Elevated α-fetoprotein levels

41.49. Elevated serum CEA levels correlate with extent of disease

    A. Gastric ulcer
    B. Duodenal ulcer
    C. Both
    D. Neither

41.50. Associated with high gastric acid levels

41.51. Could be induced by drugs

41.52. Undergoes malignant change

    A. Crohn's disease
    B. Ulcerative colitis
    C. Both
    D. Neither

41.53. Disease essentially mucosal

41.54. Disease involves both large and small bowel

41.55. Therapy with corticosteroids

DIRECTIONS: For each of the questions or incomplete statements below, **one or more** of the answers or completions given is correct. Select
    A. if only 1, 2, and 3 are correct
    B. if only 1 and 3 are correct
    C. if only 2 and 4 are correct
    D. if only 4 is correct
    E. if all are correct

41.56. The anterior vagus branches into which of the following?
    1. Stomach
    2. Pancreas
    3. Liver
    4. Celiac plexus

41.57. Delayed hypersensitivity is mediated by
1. B cells
2. T cells
3. mast cells
4. macrophage products

41.58. Treatment of hemophilia involves which of the following?
1. Cryoprecipitate with Factor VIII
2. Whole blood
3. Fresh frozen plasma
4. Platelet packs

41.59. Features of carcinoma of the lower lip include which of the following?
1. Occurs most often in blacks
2. Is related to pipe smoking
3. Has a high incidence in women
4. Spreads to regional lymph nodes

41.60. Treatment of a 0.5-cm superficial melanoma of the forearm without palpable axillary nodes includes
1. local excision and skin grafting
2. prophylactic axillary dissection
3. no chemotherapy
4. adjuvant treatment with BCG

41.61. Structures removed in a modified radical mastectomy are which of the following?
1. Breast
2. Axillary lymph nodes
3. Pectoralis minor muscle
4. Internal mammary lymph nodes

41.62. Features of abdominal aortic aneurysms include which of the following?
1. Usually infrarenal
2. Risk of rupture low unless larger than 8 cm or more
3. Inferior mesenteric artery usually occluded
4. Associated with tertiary syphilis

DIRECTIONS SUMMARIZED				
A	B	C	D	E
1,2,3	1,3	2,4	4	All are
only	only	only	only	correct

41.63. Preferred treatment of traumatic transection of the tail of the pancreas includes
  1. drains—sump, penrose
  2. anastomosis to a Roux-en-Y loop
  3. distal pancreatectomy
  4. direct end-to-end anastomosis

41.64. Abdominal wound dehiscence is associated with
  1. old age
  2. malignancy
  3. malnutrition
  4. anemia

41.65. Features of acute cholangitis include
  1. fever with chills
  2. pain in right upper quadrant
  3. jaundice
  4. positive Murphy's sign

41.66. Treatment of a 15-year-old boy with familial polyposis includes
  1. frequent evaluation
  2. ileostomy
  3. resection of involved small bowel
  4. subtotal colectomy and ileoproctostomy

41.67. Obstructive jaundice due to cancer is associated with
  1. increased direct bilirubin in serum
  2. prolonged prothrombin time
  3. elevated serum alkaline phosphate
  4. increased urinary urobilinogen

41.68. The disease type and treatment of Hashimoto's thyroiditis are which of the following?
  1. Viral infection
  2. Autoimmune disease
  3. Total thyroidectomy
  4. Thyroid suppression

41.69. Papillary carcinoma of the thyroid
  1. is the most common thyroid cancer
  2. is more common in females than males
  3. is indicated by psammoma bodies
  4. spreads through venous invasion

DIRECTIONS: This section of the test consists of situations, each followed by a series of questions. Study each situation and select the **one** best answer to each question following it.

Questions 41.70–41.72: A 40-year-old obese woman underwent cholecystectomy and operative cholangiography. On the fourth postoperative day, she developed dyspnea, along with substernal and left chest pain. Vital signs: temp. 99°F, BP 110/70, pulse 100/min, resp. 30/min.

41.70. The most likely cause is
  A. myocardial infarction
  B. aspiration pneumonia
  C. pulmonary embolism
  D. subphrenic abscess
  E. cholangitis due to retained stone

41.71. A lung scan was performed (Figure 97); the diagnosis based on the scan is
  A. pulmonary embolus
  B. bronchopneumonia
  C. left lower lobe collapse due to mucus plug
  D. acute pulmonary congestion due to massive coronary occlusion
  E. subphrenic abscess

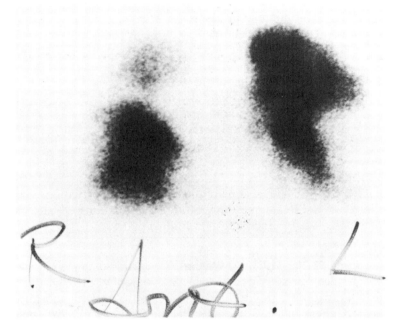

Figure 97

41.72. Treatment of choice is
    A. antibiotics
    B. coumadin by mouth
    C. IV heparin
    D. vena caval interruption
    E. pulmonary embolectomy

Questions 41.73—41.75: A 55-year-old man presented with a history of blood per rectum, weight loss, and occasional mucous diarrhea. A barium enema is shown in Figure 98.

41.73. The diagnosis is
    A. villous adenoma
    B. diverticulitis
    C. cancer of sigmoid/descending colon
    D. stricture due to ulcerative colitis
    E. granulomatous colitis

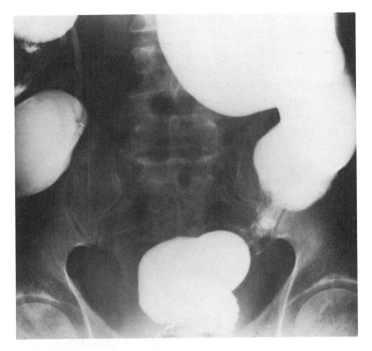

Figure 98

41.74. The preparation of bowel of this patient prior to resection is best performed by
    A. proximal colostomy
    B. mechanical cleanout
    C. systemic antibiotics alone
    D. mechanical washout and oral nonabsorbable antibiotics
    E. oral and systemic antibiotics

41.75. Of the follow-up care of this patient, which of the following measurements would be most useful?
    A. Serial α-fetoprotein
    B. Serial carcinoembryonic antigen
    C. Serial liver function tests
    D. Fecal fats
    E. Immunoglobulin levels

Questions 41.76–41.78: A 20-year-old white man was involved in an auto accident and was brought to the emergency room. During initial evaluation, he was found to be conscious and breathing but pale. BP 90/60, pulse 120/min.

41.76. The next step in management of this patient is
    A. IV Ringer's lactate
    B. nasogastric tube
    C. Foley catheter
    D. diagnostic peritoneal lavage
    E. Swan-Ganz catheter

41.77. In the subsequent management of this patient, arteriography was performed (Figure 99). The x-ray shows
    A. traumatic renal artery stenosis
    B. no excretion on left
    C. extravasation of dye due to renal pelvic injury
    D. ruptured spleen
    E. A-V fistula

Figure 99

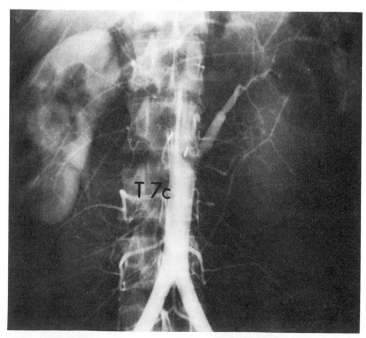

41.78. At operation, the left kidney was found to have been avulsed from its pedicle and had a stellate tear. Treatment includes
   A. aortorenal bypass with dacron graft
   B. reimplantation of kidney
   C. partial nephrectomy
   D. nephrectomy
   E. suture the tear and give antibiotics

Questions 41.79−41.81.: A 64-year-old man is admitted with a history of passing a large quantity (estimated 1500 cc) of bright red blood from rectum. There was no pain and this was his first episode. Admitting vital signs were BP 140/90, pulse 90/min, resp. 20/min. No obvious fresh blood in rectum.

41.79. Which of the following is the investigation of choice?
   A. Upper gastrointestinal barium series
   B. Barium enema
   C. Proctosigmoidoscopy and colonoscopy
   D. Arteriography
   E. Upper endoscopy

41.80. Later a barium enema was obtained (Figure 100). Based on this study, the diagnosis is
   A. ulcerative colitis
   B. diverticular disease
   C. cancer of colon
   D. granulomatous colitis
   E. ischemic colitis

41.81. Treatment of choice is
   A. colonoscopic fulguration
   B. subtotal colectomy and ileoproctostomy
   C. total proctocolectomy
   D. sigmoid colectomy
   E. IV infusion of vasopressin (Pitressin)

Questions 41.82−41.83: A 30-year-old woman presents with a history of paroxysmal hypertension, weight loss, and diabetes. Two years prior to this admission she underwent "thyroidectomy" for a nodule.

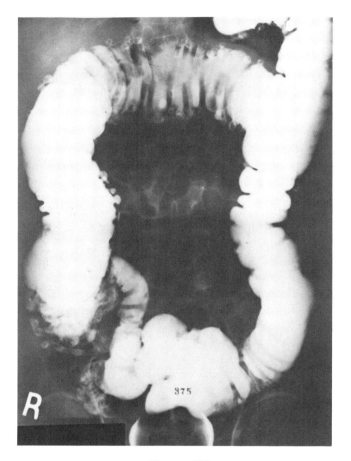

Figure 100

41.82. Workup includes all of the following EXCEPT
  A. serum calcitonin
  B. thyroid scan
  C. angiogram
  D. urinary vanilylmandelic acid levels
  E. urinary 5-hydroxyindoleacetic acid levels

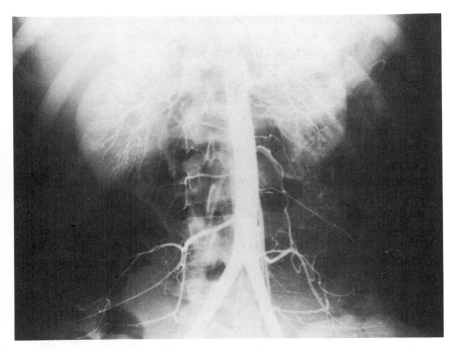

Figure 101

41.83. The angiogram is shown in Figure 101; the cause of the hypertension is
   A. aldosteronoma
   B. renal artery stenosis
   C. hypernephroma
   D. pheochromocytoma
   E. bilateral adrenal hyperplasia (Cushing's disease)

Answers and Comments

41.1. (A) In the anesthetized patient who is being operated on, the most significant features that indicate transfusion reaction are excessive bleeding from the wound and continued hypotension. On the other hand, in the awake patient the most common symptoms are a sensation of fever, pain along the site of the transfusion, skin reactions, and, much later, renal failure (Ref. 1, p. 109).

41.2. (A) The radial nerve is most likely to be injured in fractures of the shaft of the humerus as it winds around the middle third of the humerus. The result would then be a paralysis of all of the extensors of the wrist (Ref. 1, p. 1968).

41.3. (E) The immediate effects of an arteriovenous fistula are increases in the heart rate and cardiac output. Both the systolic and diastolic pressures decrease, but the subsequent compensatory changes result in an increase in systolic blood pressure. The diastolic blood pressure, however, is not increased. There is an increase in blood volume (Ref. 1, p. 932).

41.4. (C) The inferior mesenteric vein drains into the splenic vein. The portal vein is a continuation of the superior mesenteric vein (Ref. 1, p. 1430).

41.5. (D) Dyspnea is usually the first and maybe the only symptom of pulmonary embolism. Some patients also complain of chest pain and have hemoptysis (Ref. 1, p. 983).

41.6. (D) Clindamycin-associated pseudomembranous colitis has been described often enough to be a serious risk. The treatment of pseudomembranous colitis of clindamycin origin is the administration of vancomycin (Ref. 1, p. 1183).

41.7. (D) The best prognosis of carcinoma of the breast, based on histologic diagnosis, is that of medullary cancer. The overall survival rate is 85−90%. The most common variety of breast cancer is an infiltrating duct cancer. It accounts for about 80% of all breast cancers. The incidence of medullary carcinoma is only 5% of all breast cancers (Ref. 1, pp. 538−539).

41.8. (B) There is no evidence that repeated trauma induces malignant change in benign lesion. All other statements regarding malignant melanoma are correct (Ref. 1, 516−517).

41.9. (C) During the last 30 years, there has been a significant decrease in the incidence of cancer of the stomach. This decrease is in both sexes and its cause is not known. On the other hand, the incidence of cancer of the pancreas and lung has increased in the last 40 years (Ref. 1, p. 314−315).

41.10. (E) The drug of choice for treatment of infections due to *B. fragilis* is clindamycin. Other drugs useful in this situation are chloramphenicol, metronidazole, and erythromycin. The cephalosporins and the aminoglycosides are not particularly effective against *B. fragilis* (Ref. 1, pp. 191, 1402).

41.11. (A) In Crohn's disease, mesenteric fat tends to grow over the serosa so that it nearly encompasses the wall of the bowel. This is a feature specific for Crohn's disease and does not occur in the other forms of enteritis or colitis (Ref. 1, p. 1148).

41.12. (C) Hernia of the foramen of Bochdalek is the most common diaphragmatic hernia in the newborn and is a failure of the development of the diaphragm. The result is that the pleural and peritoneal cavities remain in continuity. This type of defect is much more common on the left side (Ref. 1, p. 1641).

41.13. (C) Of the conditions listed, idiopathic thrombocytopenic purpura is considered to be an autoimmune process. The initial treatment is with steroids, but when the response decreases, splenectomy is indicated. Thalassemia and spherocytic anemias are congenital varieties. The causes of hypersplenism are numerous. Gaucher's disease is a metabolic disease involving the reticuloendothelial system (Ref. 1, p. 1381).

41.14. (C) Malignant ascites is most often due to carcinoma of the ovary. The cancers of the GI tract also could result in malignant ascites, but this is not quite as common. Ovarian tumors could seed through the entire peritoneal cavity, producing ascites without involving or blocking the intestinal tract (Ref. 1, pp. 330, 1769–1770).

41.15. (C) Desmoid tumors of the abdominal wall have a high risk of local recurrence. On the other hand, they do not spread through the lymphatics or venous system. Invasion of the posterior peritoneum behind the tumor is seen occasionally, but they do not invade the peritoneal cavity (Ref. 1, p. 1423).

41.16. (C) Splenic artery aneurysms are generally asymptomatic. They have a high risk of rupture during pregnancy and evidence of massive hemorrhage should lead one to suspicion of rupture of splenic artery aneurysm. Aneurysms of the rest of the vessels are not very common and are not associated with rupture during pregnancy (Ref. 1, p. 958).

41.17. (B) Rupture into the peritoneal cavity and massive hemorrhage from the tumor are a dreaded complication of hepatic adenomas produced by ingestion of oral contraceptive pills. They generally do not produce ductal obstruction. Pseudomyxoma is a mucus-producing tumor usually from the appendix or the stomach and involves the peritoneal cavity diffusely. Recent evidence indicates that these adenomas regress after the discontinuation of contraceptive pills (Ref. 1, p. 1271).

41.18. (C) Respiratory acidosis is not a feature of pyloric stenosis. The significant metabolic abnormality is a metabolic alkalosis from hypokalemia and hypochloremia. The loss of gastric juice by vomiting results in dehydration and hemoconcentration (Ref. 1, p. 1125).

41.19. (C) As noted earlier, oral contraceptives have been known to produce hepatic adenomas and focal nodular hypoplasia. On the other hand, the other causes listed (e.g., vinyl chloride, cirrhosis, infectious hepatitis, and aflatoxin) have been implicated in the development of malignant tumors of the liver, specifically primary carcinoma of the liver (Ref. 1, p. 1271).

41.20. (A) The most common cause of chronic pancreatitis is chronic alcoholism. Gallstone disease tends to produce recurrent attacks and usually these attacks decrease after cholecystectomy. Hyperparathyroidism, trauma, and familial types produce recurrent pancreatitis but are not the common cause of chronic pancreatitis (Ref. 1, p. 1354).

41.21. (E) Upper endoscopy, using one of the fiberoptic flexible scopes, is the most useful method to diagnose the source of upper gastrointestinal bleeding. In patients who are actively bleeding, angiography may be useful by demonstrating the site of the leak. Barium studies should only be done after the other two are completed, because once barium is instilled into the stomach, it is not possible to do an adequte endoscopy or angiography. Hepatic wedge pressures are only indicated when the patient is known to have portal hypertension and is to undergo a shunt procedure.

Gastric biopsy will indicate the nature of the lesion but requires endoscopy (Ref. 1, p. 1048).

41.22. (C) The most serious early complications of operation for appendicitis are septic in nature and include abscesses and wound infections. The other conditions listed might produce some fever but are not as common as wound infections. The wound infection is usually confined to subcutaneous tissues and is much more common when there is a rupture of the appendix (Ref. 1, p. 1254).

41.23. (A) The most common type of lesion in congenital esophageal atresia is a blind proximal pouch with the distal part of the esophagus having a fistula to the trachea or the left bronchus. Other varieties are much less common (Ref. 1, pp. 1643–1644).

41.24. (B) The ileum is the most common primary site for liver metastases of carcinoid tumor. About 35% of all ileal carcinoids metastasize, whereas the appendix, which is the most common site for a carcinoid tumor, metastasizes to the liver in only about 3% of the cases. An interesting hormonal syndrome associated with liver metastases of carcinoid tumor is the carcinoid syndrome (Ref. 1, p. 1156).

41.25. (E) When the pseudocyst of the pancreas is in the lesser sac, the preferred treatment is a cyst-gastrostomy. When this for some reason is not feasible, drainage through a Roux-en-Y loop is the next choice. Excision is only possible for small cysts which are attached to the tail of the pancreas. External drainage is not preferred because of persistent fistula. Transductal drainage was successful in a few patients but is not the usual method of management. Observation and antibiotics are short-term maneuvers and surgery is recommended because of complications (Ref. 1, p. 1360).

41.26. (C) Irradiation of the neck during childhood for treatment of thymic disorders or of cervical lymph node disorders is carcinogenic to the thyroid. None of the other conditions listed are associated with an increase of thyroid cancer (Ref. 1, p. 1568).

41.27. (D) In the congenital varieties of adrenogenital syndrome, the most common cause is a deficiency of C-21 hydroxylation. The next most common variety is C-11 hydroxylation block. Pituitary

adenomas and adrenal adenomas are not very common causes in
infancy (Ref. 1, p. 1503).

41.28. (E) Airway obstruction due to hemorrhage in the wound
is a life-threatening complication following total thyroidectomy.
Small amounts of blood in the wound may produce tracheal obstruction and are due to inadequate hemostasis of the inferior
thyroid or superior thyroid artery. Thyroid storm is rarely seen
these days. Tetany following total thyroidectomy occurs if all the
parathyroids have been accidently removed, but it takes a couple of
days to manifest (Ref. 1, p. 1576).

41.29. (B) Recurrent laryngeal nerve is likely to be damaged during a parathyroidectomy. The problem is to be avoided by identifying and separating the nerve from the parathyroids and the inferior
thyroid artery. If there is a bilateral laryngeal nerve injury, severe
respiratory problems will occur in the postoperative period (Ref. 1,
p. 1616).

41.30. (D) During a superficial parotidectomy, the plane of dissection is marked by the facial nerve. Dissection should start with
either the trunk of the facial nerve posteriorly or the branches in the
front. If the nerve or its branches are not identified early in the
procedure, it is liable to be damaged during the operation (Ref. 1,
p. 592).

41.31. (C) The spinal accessory nerve, which supplies the sternomastoid and trapezius, is normally removed during a radical neck
dissection. The sternomastoid muscle itself is removed so that there
is no major problem there and the trapezius receives partial nerve
supply from C-3, 4 roots (Ref. 1, p. 590–591).

41.32. (A) Gardner's syndrome is an inherited disease characterized by polyps in the colon and other lesions, such as osteomas,
epidermoid or sebaceous cysts, or dermoid tumors of the abdominal
wall. This is one variety of inherited polypoid disease of the colon
(Ref. 1, p. 1194).

41.33. (C) In patients with villous adenomas, there is an interesting syndrome consisting of passage of watery stools and a large
amount of fluid loss rich in potassium and chloride. Therefore, the

patient would demonstrate hypokalemia and hypochloremia. Therapy of this metabolic abnormality should be undertaken before the patient is subjected to operative treatment (Ref. 1, p. 1192−1193).

41.34. (D) Familial polyposis is a rare hereditary disese resulting in multiple polyps of the colon. Unless this disease is treated surgically early in life, almost all the patients develop cancer of the colon or rectum (Ref. 1, p. 1194).

41.35. (C) Dopamine is a precursor of norepinephrine and like other vasopressors it acts by both positive inotropic and chronotropic effects on the heart. It has a lower potential for causing tachyarrhythmias. It increases renal blood flow and maintains urine flow and for this reason, dopamine is often chosen in the treatment in hypovolemic shock (Ref. 1, p. 149).

41.36. (D) Phenylephrine (Neo-Synephrine) has the least effective inotropic action and is predominately a peripheral vascular pressor and hence is not used too often (Ref. 1, p. 149).

41.37. (A) Digitalis is, of course, the most effective drug to improve myocardial ability. However, it is important to note that hypokalemia tends to increase the sensitivity of the heart to digitalis and the levels of potassium and calcium should be carefully monitored (Ref. 1, p. 151).

41.38. (A) Gastrin is normally produced by the antral mucosa, both in humans and animals. The principal action of gastrin is a stimulation of secretion of water, electrolytes, and the intrinsic factor by the stomach (Ref. 1, p. 1118).

41.39. (A) Zollinger-Ellison syndrome is produced by a non-β cell tumor of the pancreas secreting large amounts of gastrin. Normally the pancreas does not secrete gastrin; however, in this particular syndrome, there is an enormous production of gastrin. This results in fulminant peptic ulcer disease, not only in the stomach and duodenum but even in the small bowel. Treatment is total gastrectomy and/or removal of the tumor when this can be identified (Ref. 1, pp. 1125, 1367)

41.40. (C) Another endocrine tumor of the pancreas is the insulinoma. This tumor arises from the β cells of the pancreatic islets and secretes large amounts of insulin. The treatment of this condition is identification of this pancreatic tumor or a distal pancreatectomy when no tumor can be identified (Ref. 1, p. 1365).

41.41. (A) A simple useful test to screen for pheochromocytoma is measurement of urinary VMA levels. VMA is a metabolic end product of catecholamines secreted by these tumors. The test is nonspecific and requires strict dietary control. False positives have been reported in other similar tumors such as ganglioneuromas and neuroblastomas (Ref. 1, p. 1525).

41.42. (E) Carcinoid tumors, particularly of the ileum or when they have metastasized to the liver, produce large amounts of serotonin. The metabolic end product of serotonin is 5-HIAA. The diagnosis of malignant carcinoid tumor or carcinoid syndrome is helped by the measurement of urinary HIAA levels (Ref. 1, p. 1158).

41.43. (C) Urinary hydroxyproline measurement is a useful test in the diagnosis of hyperparathyroidism. The levels are elevated because of collagen breakdown and, since most of the collagen is in bone, the test is helpful in determining hyperparathyroidism (Ref. 1, pp. 1599).

41.44. (C) Infections with both *C. perfringens* and *C. sporogenes* result in gas in the wound or in the subcutaneous tissues. *Perfringens* predominantly produces muscle necrosis, whereas *sporogenes* breaks down subcutaneous tissue and does not invade the muscle (Ref. 1, pp. 184–185).

41.45. (A) *C. perfringens* breaks down muscle. This is the classic gas gangrene of wounds (Ref. 1, p. 185).

41.46. (D) Methicillin is not the drug of choice for clostridial infections. The most useful antibiotic to treat clostridial infection is penicillin. Tetracycline also has been used. Other useful therapeutic measures include antitoxin and hyperbaric oxygen (Ref. 1, p. 185).

41.47. (C) Elevated carcinoembryonic antigen levels have been found originally in colon cancers and more recently in pancreatic cancers. Other adenocarcinomas of the gastrointestinal tract also occasionally produce elevated CEA levels. In addition, a number of nonmalignant conditions have been known to increase CEA levels in the serum, but the cancers which produce significant elevations are colon and pancreas (Ref. 1, p. 326).

41.48. (D) Alpha fetoprotein is a fetal antigen found in about 70% of patients with primary hepatomas and is useful in the diagnosis of hepatomas (Ref. 1, p. 326).

41.49. (A) In cancer of the colon, the serum levels of CEA do correlate with the extent of known disease. This is particulary useful in the postoperative management of patients with colon cancer, and an elevated CEA level will strongly indicate recurrence or metastatic disease somewhere in the body (Ref. 1, p. 326).

41.50. (B) Duodenal ulcers are associated with high gastric acid secretion. In contrast, gastric ulcers are not associated with high-acid secretion (Ref. 1, pp. 1124, 1131).

41.51. (A) Gastric ulcers are known to be induced by a number of drugs, including steroids, indomethacin, phenylbutazone, and aspirin. Duodenal ulcers are not induced by any drugs (Ref. 1, pp. 1131, 1132).

41.52. (D) Neither gastric nor duodenal ulcers undergo malignant change. In the past it was believed that peptic gastric ulcers underwent malignant change. It is now no longer believed that this is true. Ulcerated gastric cancers are probably de novo lesions (Ref. 1, p. 1131).

41.53. (B) Ulcerative colitis is essentially a mucosal disease, whereas Crohn's disease is a transmural disease (Ref. 1, p. 1172).

41.54. (A) Crohn's disease may involve both large bowel and small bowel, producing strictures. On the other hand, ulcerative colitis never involves the small bowel. Occasionally one might see some ulcerated lesions in the terminal ileum in ulcerative colitis but these are superficial and not like those of Crohn's disease (Ref. 1, p. 1172).

41.55. (C) Both conditions are examples of the group of inflammatory bowel disease and respond to corticosteroid treatment. Steroids might be given as oral preparations or by retention enemas as needed. The response is usually good although the long-term outlook is not changed (Ref. 1, pp. 1151, 1174).

41.56. (B) The anterior vagus, which is derived from the left vagus, gives off branches to the stomach and liver. The posterior vagus gives branches to the stomach and through the celiac plexus to the pancreas (Ref. 1, p. 1114).

41.57. (C) Delayed hypersensitivity of the nature of graft rejection is mediated by the T cells and by a number of cellular mediators such as macrophages and platelets. The macrophages seem to act through production of two important factors, namely, the migration inhibitory and the chemotactic factors. The B cells are responsible for the humoral response (Ref. 1, pp. 372–374).

41.58. (B) The treatment of hemophilia involves replacement of Factor VIII deficiency. Cryoprecipitates of plasma containing a high concentration of Factor VIII are usually used both prophylactically and in actively bleeding hemophiliacs. Fresh frozen plasma also works in the same manner, except it is less concentrated. Whole blood is generally not used in hemophiliacs because of the risk of sensitization and hemolytic reactions (Ref. 1, p. 92).

41.59. (C) Cancer of the lower lip is perhaps related to pipe smoking, particularly clay pipes and wood pipes. The relationship to cigarette smoking, on the other hand, is not quite as close and is only seen in people who smoke the cigarettes all the way to the end. These lesions are slow growing but with progress they do involve the lymph nodes on the same side. The lesions seldom occur in black people and there is no increased incidence in women (Ref. 1, pp. 564–565).

41.60. (B) The treatment of a superficial melanoma of the forearm without palpable axillary nodes is local excision and, if necessary, skin grafting. Chemotherapy is only used when there is recurrence or metastatic disease. Prophylactic axillary dissection is recommended when there is evidence of deep invasion but is not necessary in superficial lesions. Adjuvant treatment with BCG is only considered when there is recurrent or metastatic disease (Ref. 1, pp. 517–518).

41.61. **(A)** In the modified radical mastectomy described by Patey (the type that is performed most often), the structures that are removed are the breast, the axillary lymph nodes, and the pectoralis minor muscle. The pectoralis major is removed in the standard radical mastectomy and the internal mammary lymph nodes are sampled in a supraradical or extended radical mastectomy (Ref. 1, p. 541).

41.62. **(B)** The usual abdominal aortic aneurysms are infrarenal in location. The inferior mesenteric artery is usually occluded. The blood supply to the left colon comes from the marginal artery, which is supplied by the superior mesenteric artery and additionally from the internal iliac vessels. These aneurysms are usually arteriosclerotic and not syphilitic in origin. The risk of rupture is high even at 5 or 6 cm in diameter and, hence, operation is recommended electively in all individuals with aneurysms greater than 5 cm in size (Ref. 1, pp. 948, 950).

41.63. **(B)** When there is a transection of the tail of the pancreas with ductal disruption, the treatment would be distal pancreatectomy with closure of the stump. The area should be drained by both sump and penrose drains. It is not worthwhile to do an anastomosis to a loop of bowel, and direct end-to-end anastomosis is not recommended because of the risk of leak (Ref. 1, p. 1356).

41.64. **(A)** Abdominal wound dehiscence is associated with old age, malignancy, and malnutrition. Postoperative abdominal distention and coughing also contribute. There is no relationship to anemia (Ref. 1, p. 456).

41.65. **(A)** The classic features of acute cholangitis, which were described by Charcot, are fever with chills, pain in the right upper quadrant, and jaundice. These are referred to as Charcot's triad. A positive Murphy's sign is a feature of acute cholecystitis. Other features of cholangitis are central nervous system depression, septic shock, and renal failure (Ref. 1, p. 1329).

41.66. **(D)** Patients with familial polyposis have a high risk of developing cancer, and untreated, almost all of them develop cancer before age 40 and die. Therefore, the colon has to be removed. The operation of choice is a subtotal colectomy and ileoproctostomy. The retained rectum should be examined frequently to see if there are any recurring polyps or cancer. Ileostomy alone does not do any good and frequent evaluation is not very helpful in prevention of cancer. Because the disease involves the large bowel, resection of the small bowel has no place in the management (Ref. 1, p. 1194).

41.67. **(A)** In obstructive jaundice, the laboratory studies would show an elevated direct bilirubin in the serum. There is also an elevated serum alkaline phosphatase. The prothrombin time is prolonged because of failure of the intestines to absorb the fat-soluble vitamins, such as A, D, E, K, in the absence of bile salts. On the other hand, urobilinogen is not increased. In fact, because the bile does not reach the intestinal tract, urobilinogen is absent in the urine. There may be bilirubin in the urine (Ref. 1, pp. 1056–1057).

41.68. **(C)** Hashimoto's thyroiditis is an autoimmune disease and is usually treated by thyroid suppression. Surgical treatment is not required because the patients do become hypothyroid and surgical removal worsens the situation. It is not a viral infection. The subacute thyroiditis, also called de Quervain's thyroiditis, is viral in origin (Ref. 1, p. 1562).

41.69. **(A)** Papillary carcinoma is the most common variety of thyroid cancer and occurs more often in women than men. The tumor shows punctate calcification, which is referred to as psammoma bodies. The spread of this cancer is predominantly through the lymphatic channels and venous invasion is uncommon. On the other hand, follicular cancers spread through the venous system (Ref. 1, pp. 1568–1569).

41.70. **(C)** Pulmonary embolism is the most likely complication to be suspected because of the early onset of dyspnea along with substernal and left-sided chest pain. This is much more common in obese women, who probably do not get out of bed. In the absence of significantly elevated temperature, the diagnosis of pneumonia and abscess are low in priority. Cholangitis due to retained stones would show some jaundice and if operative cholangiography was satisfactory, the possibility of retained stones is low. Myocardial infarction would be something that should be excluded but is usually associated with older age group patients; the first finding is usually left chest pain radiating to the arm (Ref. 1, pp. 466, 983).

41.71. (A) The lung scan shows significant defects, one in the right upper lobe and a large one in the left lower lobe. Such a situation is most likely due to multiple pulmonary emboli. Bronchopneumonia would not produce that finding. Because the lesion is bilateral, singular lobular collapse does not explain the findings (Ref. 1, p. 984).

41.72. (C) The immediate treatment of patients with pulmonary emboli is adequate heparinization. This is supplemented by oxygen by mask and general supportive measures. There is no need for antibiotic usage in patients with pulmonary emboli. Coumadin would be considered once the acute phase is over and anticoagulation can then be carried by oral route. Vena caval interruption is considered in patients who are having pulmonary emboli in spite of adequate anticoagulation, and pulmonary embolectomy is occasionally attempted when there is a massive occlusion. This should be performed within a very short period after the onset (Ref. 1, pp. 984–985).

41.73. (C) The barium enema shows a constricting lesion at the rectosigmoid junction. This is the most common site for cancer of the colon. The examination does not show any diverticular disease. Strictures are not commonly due to ulcerative colitis. Granulomatous colitis could also give a stricture but it is not common to have the patient present with the history as noted (Ref. 1, p. 1199).

41.74. (D) The ideal method of preparation of the colon prior to elective resection is a mechanical washout and oral nonabsorbable antibiotics. The mechanical washout includes laxatives by mouth and also irrigation from the anus. The nonabsorbable antibiotics that are commonly used are neomycin- and erythromycin-base. Systemic antibiotics alone cannot prevent infections and, similarly, mechanical cleanouts by themselves are not adequate. The proximal colostomy is only performed when there is an emergency obstruction and is not necessary in elective colonic resections provided the bowel has been prepared as previously outlined (Ref. 1, p. 1200).

41.75. **(B)** In the follow-up care of this patient, serial measurements of serum carcinoembryonic antigen are useful in predicting recurrence of metastatic disease. Liver function tests do not indicate specific problems due to the cancer. Alpha fetoprotein is useful in the study of patients with malignant hepatomas (Ref. 1, p. 1205).

41.76. **(A)** In the initial resuscitation of a trauma victim, the most important step is to use one or two 18-gauge needles or catheters and restore fluid volume with Ringer's lactate. This patient is hypotensive and has a tachycardia. Before further evaluation for specific lesions is pursued, the initial steps would be maintaining the airway, checking the breathing, and restoring the circulating blood volume. The other procedures will come lower in priority (Ref. 1, p. 200).

41.77. **(B)** The arteriogram shows only the right kidney functioning. There is no function on the left side and that should strongly raise the suspicion of either a congenital absence or, much more likely, an avulsion of the renal pedicle and thrombosis of the renal artery on that side (Ref. 1, p. 202).

41.78. **(D)** Although nephrectomy is not undertaken lightly, in this particular patient the kidney has been avulsed from the pedicle and also has a stellate tear. Such a kidney is not worth salvaging either by bench surgery or by reimplantation of the kidney. Hence, nephrectomy is the procedure of choice. If the kidney has not had major trauma, it is possible to do either reimplantation or restore blood flow through aortorenal bypass (Ref. 1, pp. 202, 1721).

41.79. **(C)** The most common cause of massive bleeding from the rectum in elderly men is diverticular disease. The first procedure of choice in the investigation is proctosigmoidoscopy and colonoscopy. The bowel should be washed so that adequate examination can be obtained. Arteriography is useful if there is massive bleeding. Barium enema should not be attempted unless colonoscopy and arteriography are either unavailable or have not been successful. If the bleeding is massive and bright red, it is unlikely that the cause is in the upper intestinal tract and therefore upper endoscopy and upper gastrointestinal series are low in priority (Ref. 1, p. 1051).

41.80. (B) The barium enema shows diverticular disease involving large parts of the colon even all the way up to the cecum. Because there is no single lesion, it is unlikely that cancer of the colon is the cause. Ischemic and granulamatous colitis produce narrowing in segmental areas. Ulcerative colitis would have a pipe stem or smooth colonic wall on the outside. The picture is one of pandiverticular disease (Ref. 1, pp. 1051, 1188).

41.81. (B) In a patient with massive bleeding and diffuse diverticular disease, treatment of choice is subtotal colectomy and ileoproctostomy. Total proctocolectomy is not necessary because diverticular disease does not involve the rectum where the longitudinal wall is no longer limited by the tenia but includes the circumference. Because the lesions are multiple, colonoscopy and fulguration have no place. In the past, sigmoid colectomy was done as the sigmoid is the most common site of diverticular disease. This has resulted in a number of failures of the operation because the bleeding could be from the right side. In travenous infusion of vasopressin (Pitressin) is a temporary measure and is not particularly advantageous in diverticular disease (Ref. 1, p. 1187).

41.82. (E) Urinary hydroxyindoleacetic acid levels are useful in the diagnosis of carcinoid syndrome. This patient has had a history of thyroid surgery and has a present history of paroxysmal hypertension, weight loss, and diabetes. The last three were indicative or suspicious of a pheochromocytoma. In the presence of previous history of thyroid surgery one should consider Sipple's syndrome; therefore, workup includes studies on medullary cancer of the thyroid by thyroid scan and serum calcitonin, an angiogram, and urinary vanillyl mandelic acid level to exclude pheochromocytoma (Ref. 1, pp. 1523–1525, 1528).

41.83. (D) The angiogram shows a lesion located above the right kidney. The renal perfusion on both sides appears satisfactory and there is no evidence of renal arterial stenosis. Hypernephromas do not produce hypertension except in a small number of instances and the angiogram does not show a renal tumor. Because the lesion is unilateral and is located on the right side, the question of bilateral adrenal hypoplasia does not arise. Aldosteronomas are very small tumors and are seldom visualized by angiography (Ref. 1, p. 1527).

References

1. Schwartz, S.I. (ed.): *Principles of Surgery*, 4th Ed., McGraw-Hill, New York, 1984.

42

Neurologic Surgery
James G. McMurtry III, M.D.

DIRECTIONS: Each of the questions or incomplete statements below is followed by five suggested answers or completions. Select the **one** that is best in each case.

42.1. Intracranial meningiomas
- **A.** became malignant in 42% of cases
- **B.** are most commonly located in the cerebellopontine angle
- **C.** may be diagnosed on plain skull x-rays by the presence of hyperostoses, increased vascularity, tumor classification
- **D.** should be treated by radiation prior to operative removal
- **E.** constitute the majority of intracranial tumors in most large series

42.2. Trigeminal neuralgia

    A. is caused most commonly by adjacent intracranial meningiomas

    B. is associated with the gradual paralysis of the facial nerve

    C. is probably due to compression of the fifth cranial nerve by a branch of the middle cerebral artery

    D. is diagnosed by pain of a continuous nature which is relieved by washing the face

    E. symptoms may be relieved by alcohol block, percutaneous rhizotomy, or intraoperative decompression

42.3. Brain abscess

    A. is associated with a markedly elevated cerebrospinal fluid white count (when incapsulated)

    B. may occur as metastases from infection elsewhere in the body

    C. is no longer seen from direct extension from the mastoid region

    D. has a high percentage of pneumococci and meningococci when cultured

    E. none of the above

DIRECTIONS: Each group of questions below consists of five lettered headings followed by a list of numbered words or statements. For each numbered word or statement, select the **one** lettered heading that is most closely associated with it. Each lettered heading may be selected once, more than once, or not at all.

    A. Subdural hematoma in infants
    B. Epidural hematoma
    C. Cerebral concussion
    D. Postconcussion syndrome
    E. Basilar skull fracture

42.4. "Lucid interval"

42.5. Failure to thrive

42.6. Headaches, dizziness, insomnia, irritability, restlessness, depression

42.7. Brief loss of consciousness

42.8. Otorrhea and a "battle's sign"

    A. Medulloblastoma
    B. Optic neuroma
    C. Acoustic neuroma
    D. Subfrontal meningioma
    E. Cystic cerebellar astrocytoma of childhood

42.9. May be associated with von Recklinghausen's disease, predominantly in childhood, enlarged optic canal

42.10. Dense interlacing fibrous tissue and loose reticular tissue, numbness about the face, gait unsteadiness

42.11. Mural nodule, predominantly in childhood or young adults, high percentage of cure

42.12. Most primitive glial cell, tumor of the vermis, rapidly growing, tends to metastasize

    A. L4−L5 herniated disc
    B. L5−S1 herniated disc
    C. Ulnar neuropathy
    D. Median neuropathy
    E. Long thoracic neuropathy

42.14. Winging of the scapula, seen in men who do heavy work

42.15. Weakness of dorsiflexion of the great toe, numbness of the dorsum of the foot, normal ankle jerks

42.16. Absent ankle jerk, numbness of the small toe

42.17. Atrophy of the hypothenar and interosseous muscles, weakness of flexion and adduction of the wrist, paralysis of adduction and abduction of the fingers

42.18. Paralysis and atrophy of the thenar muscles, paralysis of the oppenens pollicis muscle

DIRECTIONS: For each of the questions or incomplete statements below, **one or more** of the answers or completions given is correct. Select
(A) if only 1, 2, and 3 are correct
(B) if only 1 and 3 are correct
(C) if only 2 and 4 are correct
(D) if only 4 is correct
(E) if all are correct

42.19. Subdural hematomas
1. may occur with blood dyscrasias
2. are almost always of venous origin
3. are usually on the convexity of the hemisphere
4. may be associated with clear spinal fluid

42.20. Congenital hydrocephalus
1. is described as an excess of fluid in the cranial cavity
2. may be divided into communicating and noncommunicating
3. in infants is associated with thin cranial bones, bulging fontanel, and widened sutures
4. progresses in an unrelenting fashion in all cases unless surgically treated

DIRECTIONS: Each of the questions or incomplete statements below is followed by five suggested answers or completions. Select the **one** that is best in each case.

Questions 42.21–42.23: A 45-year-old woman developed headaches, often occurring in the early morning hours, approximately 4 weeks prior to being examined by the physician. For 1 week, she had difficulty expressing herself, numbness and tingling in the right hand, and then a change in her handwriting. She became somewhat dull and apathetic. While walking, she would often stumble into objects on the right side. Examination showed normal vital signs. There was a drift of the outstretched right arm and right hyperreflexia with a Babinski. She searched for and substituted inappropriate words in her talk.

42.21. The most likely cause of her illness is
   A. an acute cerebrovascular insufficiency
   B. severe migraine headache syndrome
   C. a cerebral neoplasm, such as a glioma
   D. brain abscess
   E. a cerebral neoplasm, such as a meningioma

42.22. Visual field examinations would most likely reveal
   A. left optic atrophy
   B. a left homonymous hemianopsia
   C. bitemporal hemianopsia
   D. a right homonymous hemianopsia
   E. tunnel vision

42.23. The most informative initial examination would be
   A. an electroencephalogram
   B. a cerebral angiogram
   C. computerized axial tomography (CAT)
   D. a pneumoencephalogram
   E. electromyograms of the right upper extremity

Questions 42.24–42.26: A 55-year-old woman was awakened at 4:00 A.M. with sudden, excruciating, right temporal head pain. She then developed neck pain and, according to her husband, fell in the bathroom, striking her head against the tub. Upon arrival at a nearby hospital, she regained consciousness and complained of severe head and neck pain. Examination showed the pulse to be 52/min. Photophobia was present. The right pupil was 4.0 mm and the left was 2.0 mm. There was ptosis on the right side. The remainder of the neurologic examination was normal.

42.24. The most likely cause of the symptoms is
   A. extracranial carotid atherosclerotic disease with embolization of the middle cerebral artery
   B. intracranial bleed from a right temporal arteriovenous malformation
   C. acute rupture of a mycotic aneurysm
   D. rupture of a right internal carotid artery aneurysm arising near the posterior communicating artery
   E. intracranial bleeding from an oligodendroglioma

42.25. The definitive test to localize the pathology is a/an
    A. electroencephalogram with nasopharyngeal leads
    B. lumbar puncture
    C. four vessel cerebral angiogram
    D. brain scan
    E. CAT scan without contrast

42.26. Cerebrovasospasm
    A. is a benign condition occurring after subarachnoid hemorrhage
    B. is present in a high percentage of subarachnoid hemorrhage patients secondary to cerebral aneurysms
    C. is not affected by early operation on cerebral aneurysms
    D. is a radiologic diagnosis
    E. is more common in cases of arteriovenous malformation than after aneurysm bleed

Answers and Comments

42.1. (C) Intracranial meningiomas are the principal benign intracranial tumors. They occur in the minority of intracranial tumor cases. They do not metastasize or turn to malignancy. They exert their symptoms by local pressure. They often are of long-standing nature and produce erosion of bone, tumor calcification, or increased vascularity to the region of the tumor. Their most common location is over the parasaggital region of the convexity of the brain (Refs. 1, pp. 29−36; 2, p. 213).

42.2. (E) Trigeminal neuralgia is a problem of unknown etiology. It is characterized by sharp lancinating pain occurring commonly in colder weather and made worse by washing the face, cold wind, eating, chewing, or talking. Efforts to treat this include injection of nerve with Novocain or alcohol, production of a radiofrequency lesion of the nerve, or actual moving of an artery near the nerve via microvascular dissection (Ref. 3, pp. 35−54).

42.3. (B) Brain abscesses when incapsulated act as mass lesions and are not associated with elevated white counts. They may be spread from direct extensions, such as from the infected mastoid region, or from metastasis from another part of the body, such as an infection in the lungs or heart. Staphylococcus and streptococcus are most commonly cultured from this (Ref. 2, p. 46).

42.4. (B)
42.5. (A)
42.6. (D)
42.7. (C)
42.8. (E) Subdural hematomas in infants are commonly associated with a failure to thrive. Children are very sickly and do not gain weight. The diagnosis is at times difficult to make. Epidural hematoma patients very commonly are unconscious, caused by the cerebral concussion. They then have a lucid interval, at which time they become awake and then become comatose secondary to the pressure of the epidural blood clot. Cerebral concussion is most commonly associated with a brief loss of consciousness. Postconcussion syndrome may occur weeks after a severe concussion and be associated with numerous and various symptomatology, such as listed. Basilar skull fractures are often associated with a leak at the base of the skull, causing spinal fluid to come into the ear or blood to go about the base of the skull and produce discoloration of the skin (Ref. 2, p. 321).

42.9. (B)
42.10. (C)
42.11. (E)
42.12. (A)
42.13. (D) Tumors of the optic nerve tend to enlarge the optic canal; they are commonly slow growing and occur usually in childhood. Acoustic neuromas are very slow growing and have two types of cell tissue as outlined. They produce pressure on the fifth cranial nerve, producing some numbness of the face, and as they enlarge and produce pressure on the brainstem, they produce unsteadiness when walking. Cystic cerebellar astrocytomas are one of the few gliomas that can be cured. They very commonly have a nodule tumor in the cyst, and this can be removed. Medulloblastomas are high malignant tumors, in general, of the posterior fossa in childhood. They occur in the vermis, which is the midline, and they may tend to spread by seeding down the spinal canal. Subfrontal tumors are commonly benign, such as meningiomas. They may compro-

mise both auditory nerves, producing the loss of the sense of smell. They may irritate the brain cortex, producing seizures. They produce ipsilateral optic atrophy and contralateral papilledema because of the nature of their location (Ref. 1, pp. 2733, 2759, 2936).

42.14. (E)
42.15. (D)
42.16. (B)
42.17. (C)
42.18. (A) Lumbar herniated discs may produce pressure on different parts of the nerve, causing weakness in different parts of the muscle and loss of different reflexes. The ulnar knee and nerve have different structures, and their dysfunction can be shown appropriately (Ref. 2, pp. 363, 395).

42.19. (E) Subdural hematomas are often either acute or chronic. Acute ones are often related to trauma. They are nearly always due to a sheering of the veins bridging between the cerebral hemisphere and the dura. The bleeding may occur into this space in bleeding dyscrasias. The bleeding is nearly always in the convexity of the hemisphere. Lumbar puncture usually shows bloody fluid, but it may in chronic cases show clear fluid (Ref. 2, p. 321).

42.20. (A) Congenital hydrocephalus is described as an excess of fluid and produces very slowly enlarging head size. It does not produce papilledema because the fontanel is usually open. It is associated with thinning of the cranial bone, widening of the sutures, and bulging of the fontanel. It does not progress in an unrelenting fashion. Many cases are either arrested or progress slowly. It has been divided into communicating and noncommunicating (Ref. 2, p. 428).

42.21. (C) This woman most likely has a very rapidly growing malignant tumor producing signs of pressure, signs of weakness of the right arm and leg secondary to involvement of the left side of the brain, and signs of a right homonymous hemianopsia secondary to involvement of the visual fibers (Ref. 1, p. 2759).

42.22. (D) The lesion is most likely in the left temporal or partietal lobe and affects the visual fibers in this area (Ref. 1, p. 2759).

42.23. (C) Very often people who have rapidly developing tumors awaken early in the morning because of increased intracranial pressure at that time. The CAT scan now is the major test to diagnose these lesions, and this can be done as an outpatient (Ref. 1, p. 2759).

42.24. (D)
42.25. (C)
42.26. (B, D) Approximately 50% of cerebral aneurysms bleed during the night. They are associated with severe and excruciating head and neck pain and may be associated with a brief period of unconsciousness. A large percentage are associated with vasospasm. Early operation during the period of vasospasm may result in catastrophe. The diagnosis of vasospasm is made on repeated angiograms. Aneurysms that are near the third cranial nerve arising from the internal carotid artery and posterior communicating artery may produce ptosis and dilatation of the pupil. Other possibilities in the differential diagnosis include bleed from a brain tumor or arteriovenous malformation (Ref. 4, p. 1627).

References

1. Youmans, J.R.: *Neurological Surgery*, Vol. 5, W.B. Saunders, Philadelphia, 1982.

2. Meritt, H.H.: *A Textbook of Neurology*, 6th Ed., Lea & Febiger, Philadelphia, 1979.

3. Youmans, J.R.: *Neurological Surgery*, Vol. 6, W.B. Saunders, Philadelphia, 1982.

4. Youmans, J.R.: *Neurological Surgery*, Vol. 3, W.B. Saunders, Philadelphia, 1982.

43

Orthopedic Surgery
James R. Ryan, M.D.

DIRECTIONS: Each of the questions or incomplete statements below is followed by five suggested answers or completions. Select the **one** that is best in each case.

43.1. Congenital dislocation of the hip in the newborn may best be diagnosed on physical examination by
  A. abduction and internal rotation of the hips
  B. flexion and abduction of the hips
  C. adduction and external rotation of the hips
  D. extension and external rotation of the hips
  E. extension and internal rotation of the hips

43.2. In the posterior surgical approach to the shoulder, care must be taken not to injure the following nerve:
  A. suprascapular nerve
  B. axillary nerve
  C. median nerve
  D. infrascapular nerve
  E. ulnar nerve

43.3. The radial nerve may be damaged in fractures of the humerus. The most common fracture location to cause radial nerve injury is the
  A. humeral neck
  B. humeral shaft where the nerve is injured in the musculospiral groove
  C. supracondylar fracture of the humerus
  D. spiral distal third fracture of the humerus
  E. none of the above

DIRECTIONS: The group of questions below consists of five lettered headings followed by a list of numbered words or statements. For each numbered word or statement, select the **one** lettered heading that is most closely associated with it. Each lettered heading may be selected once, more than once, or not at all.

  A. Epiphysis
  B. Metaphysis
  C. Diaphysis
  D. Periosteal
  E. Epiphyseal plate

43.4. Osteogenic sarcoma

43.5. Adamantinoma

43.6. Chondroblastoma

DIRECTIONS: For each of the questions or incomplete statements below, **one or more** of the answers or completions given is correct.

    (A) if only 1, 2, and 3 are correct
    (B) if only 1 and 3 are correct
    (C) if only 2 and 4 are correct
    (D) if only 4 is correct
    (E) if all are correct.

43.7. Angular bony deformities secondary to fractures in children will tend to correct with growth. The amount of spontaneous correction of an angular deformity will depend upon the
    1. age of the child
    2. location of the fracture
    3. degree of angulation
    4. amount of comminution

43.8. Which of the following statements are true regarding this radiograph of both hips (Figure 102)?
    1. It represents avascular necrosis of the left proximal femoral epiphysis
    2. It is typical of acute septic arthritis of the hip
    3. It usually occurs between 4 and 8 years of age
    4. Elevated temperature, WBC, and sedimentation rate are usual

DIRECTIONS: This section of the test consists of a situation, followed by a series of questions. Study the situation and select the **one** best answer to each question following it.

Questions 43.9–43.10: A 27-year-old man is brought to the emergency room after being hit by an automobile as a pedestrian. Initial evaluation reveals the patient to be semicomatose with labored respirations at 30/min. BP 80/60; pulse 100/min. The skin is cool and clammy with a grayish discoloration. There is a 3-cm laceration over the anterior forehead; three teeth are noted to be missing, apparently avulsed. There is an open fracture of both bones of the left forearm with the proximal bone ends of the radius and ulna protruding through the wound. The abdomen is tense; however, bowel sounds are present.

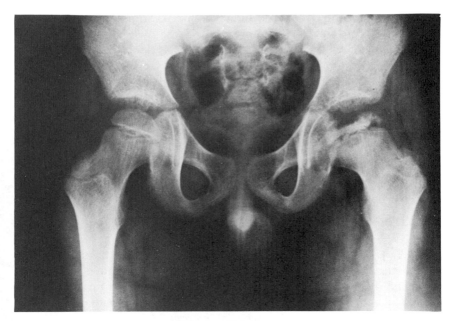

Figure 102

43.9. The initial management of this patient should be
   A. start an IV drip in the right arm and leg
   B. control hemorrhage
   C. obtain an adequate airway
   D. reduce the open fracture of the forearm and place a sterile dressing over the wound
   E. tap the abdomen

Figure 103

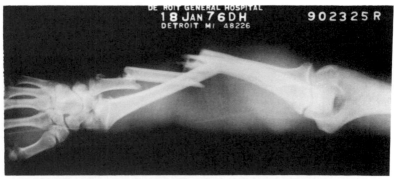

43.10. After the patient has been stabilized, attention is directed toward the open fracture of the forearm (Figure 103). The recommended initial treatment of this open fracture would be

    A. immediate open reduction and fixation with compression plates

    B. immediate open reduction and fixation with intramedullary rods

    C. splinting with sterile dressings in situ

    D. closed reduction and cast immobilization

    E. adequate debridement and copious irrigation

Answers and Comments

43.1. (B) Because of the shortening of the extremity, the adductor muscles are tight and, consequently, the infant's involved hip cannot be placed in the "frog-leg position." (In doing this maneuver, the hips and knees are flexed $90°$ and then both hips are abducted fully.) Normally, when this procedure is done in a newborn, the knee rests comfortably on the examining table. On the involved side, because of the tight adductor muscles, the hip will not abduct fully and the knee will not touch the examining table. With this maneuver, if the index finger is kept over the greater trochanter and pressure is applied while abducting the extremity, the dislocation may be reduced. As the femoral head slides over the posterior rim of the acetabulum, a palpable or audible click may be heard. This is termed Ortolani's sign (Ref. 1, p. 140).

43.2. (B) The axillary nerve is a branch of the posterior cord of the brachial plexus. It runs down along the posterior wall of the axilla on the surface of the scapularis, far from the incision made in the muscle during the anterior approach to the shoulder. The nerve then runs through the quadrangular space, where it touches the surgical neck of the humerus. At that point, it can be easily damaged by surgery (Ref. 2, p. 41).

43.3. (D) In our experience, when paralysis of the radial nerve complicates fractures of the shaft of the humerus, a specific situation exists. The fracture is in the distal third of the humerus, it is spiral in type, the distal bone fragment is always displaced proximally with its proximal end deviated radialward, the radial nerve is caught in the fracture site, and if there is a comminuted fragment, it is the oblique surface of the distal end of the proximal fragment that damages the nerve (Ref. 3).

43.4. (B) In a long bone, it is usually the end of the shaft and part of the adjacent epiphyseal area that are involved, but occasionally the tumor may develop more toward the midshaft region (Ref. 4, p. 222).

43.5. (C) The strongly predilective involvement of the tibia (for adamantinoma) has already been noted. In that bone, and in the few other long bones found affected, the lesion is nearly always in the shaft (Ref. 5, p. 213).

43.6. (A) Typically, chondroblastomas form within the epiphyseal region of a long bone with occasional extension into the adjacent metaphysis (Ref. 6, p. 172).

43.7. (A) Greater angulation is acceptable when the child is young and the deformity is near the end of the bone. The reduction must be more nearly perfect if the child is near the end of the growth period of if the fracture is near the middle of the bone (Ref. 7, p. 533).

43.8. (B) Legg-Calve-Perthes disease (avascular necrosis of the proximal femoral epiphysis) is common in children. Its clinical onset occurs within a narrow age range, usually between 4 and 8 years of age. There is a marked predominance in boys, its incidence being 1 in 750 in boys as compared to only 1 in 3700 girls (Ref. 8, p. 385).

43.9. (C) It is important to recognize that in the patient with multiple injuries, the osseous component is seldom the most urgent. Unfortunately, severe deformities of the extremity are often so striking that they tend to receive much of the initial attention with consequent neglect of other often more serious injuries. Obtaining and maintaining an adequate airway, control of hemorrhage, and correction of hypovolemia and shock take precedence, in that order (Ref. 9, p. 251).

43.10. (E) Open fractures require emergency treatment, including adequate debridement and copious irrigation. Internal fixation by plates or intramedullary rods should not be used. External skeletal fixation by skeletal traction, pins above and below the fracture site incorporated in a plaster cast, or such devices as the Roger Anderson or Müller apparatus is recommended (Ref. 10).

References

1. Ryan, J.R.: *Orthopedic Surgery*, 2nd Ed., Medical Examination Publishing, New York, 1981.

2. Hoppenfeld, S. and deBoer, P.: *Surgical Exposures in Orthopaedics—The Anatomic Approach*, J.G. Lippincott, Philadelphia, 1984, p. 41.

3. Holstein, A. and Lewis, G.B.: Fractures of the humerus with radial nerve paralysis. J. Bone Joint Surg. 65-A:1382, 1963.

4. Lichtenstein, L.: *Bone Tumors*, 6th Ed., C.V. Mosby, St. Louis, Mo, 1982.

5. Jaffe, H.L.: *Tumors and Tumorous Conditions of the Bones and Joints*, Lea & Febiger, Philadelphia, 1961.

6. Huvos, A.G.: *Bone Tumors: Diagnosis, Treatment and Prognosis*, W.B. Saunders, Philadelphia, 1979.

7. Edmonson, A.S. and Crenshaw, A.H. (eds.): *Campbell's Operative Orthopaedics*, 6th Ed., C.V. Mosby, St. Louis, MO, 1980.

8. Tachdjian, M.O.: *Pediatric Orthopedics*, W.B. Saunders, Philadelphia, 1972.

9. Walt, A.J. and Wilson, R.F.: *Management of Trauma: Pitfalls and Practice*, Lea & Febiger, Philadelphia, 1975.

10. Gustilo, R.B. and Anderson, J.T.: Prevention of infection in the treatment of 1,025 open fractures of long bones. J. Bone Joint Surg. 58-A:458, 1976.

44

Pediatric Surgery
Frederick M. Karrer, M.D.,
John R. Lilly, M.D., and
Jorge E. Uceda, M.D.

DIRECTIONS: Each of the questions or incomplete statements below is followed by five suggested answers or completions. Select the **one** that is best in each case.

44.1. In the diagnosis and management of necrotizing entero-colitis
  A. the intestine is frequently malrotated
  B. 35% of the infants are full term
  C. portal gas is a uniformly fatal sign
  D. persistent metabolic acidosis and thrombocytopenia are accepted indications for surgical intervention
  E. 50% of the patients require surgical treatment

44.2. In congenital aganglionic megacolon
  A. total colonic aganglionosis occurs in about 8% of the patients
  B. the dilated bowel seen on barium enema represents the aganglionic segment
  C. females are more commonly affected
  D. "skip" aganglionic areas are not uncommon
  E. diagnosis by rectal manometry is usually unreliable

637

44.3. An omphalocele is characterized by which of the following?

   A. An abdominal wall defect without a covering membrane

   B. A low incidence of associated congenital defects

   C. The cord elements insert in the abdomen to the left of the defect

   D. Prematurity occurs in 70%

   E. A relatively small abdominal cavity

DIRECTIONS: Each group of questions below consists of lettered headings followed by a list of numbered words or statements. For each numbered word or statement, select the **one** lettered heading that is most closely associated with it. Each lettered heading may be selected once, more than once, or not at all.

Relate the following conditions causing obstructive jaundice in children to the subsequent statements.

   A. Choledochal cyst

   B. Noncorrectable biliary atresia

   C. Idiopathic perforation of the bile duct

   D. Common duct stones

   E. Caroli's disease

44.4. May involve one or both lobes of the liver

44.5. Drainage alone is usually sufficient therapy

44.6. Drainage alone results in increased incidence of bile duct malignancy

44.7. Frequently occur(s) in association with biliary tract malformation

44.8. Must be surgically treated in the first months of life

Match the following childhood tumors with the subsequent features.

   A. Wilm's tumor
   B. Neuroblastoma
   C. Hepatoblastoma
   D. Sacrococcygeal teratoma
   E. Rhabdomyosarcoma

44.9. Sarcoma botryoides

44.10. Alpha-fetoprotein

44.11. Vanillylmandelic acid (VMA)

44.12. Aniridia

44.13. Female greater than male

The following relates to childhood hernias.

   A. Umbilical hernia
   B. Female inguinal hernia
   C. Male inguinal hernia

44.14. The most frequent inguinal hernia

44.15. May be the presenting feature of the testicular feminization syndrome

44.16. Rarely incarcerates

44.17. Nuck's canal

44.18. Higher incidence of incarceration

DIRECTIONS: For each of the questions or incomplete statements below, **one or more** of the answers or completions given is correct. Select

(A) if only 1, 2, and 3 are correct
(B) if only 1 and 3 are correct
(C) if only 2 and 4 are correct
(D) if only 4 is correct
(E) if all are correct

44.19. In congenital pulmonary malformations,
1. bronchogenic cysts are best treated by simple aspiration
2. congenital cystic adenomatoid malformation may present as a cystic or solid lung lesion
3. extralobar sequestrations differ from intralobar sequestrations by having a communication with the tracheobronchial tree
4. congenital lobar emphysema usually involves the upper lobes

44.20. For gastrointestinal obstruction in infants and children,
1. intussusception under 1 year of age is usually not associated with a pathologic lead point
2. children with pyloric stenosis usually present between 2 and 6 weeks of age with bilious vomiting
3. patients with meconium ileus usually have cystic fibrosis
4. duodenal, jejunal, and ileal atresias are always accompanied by microcolon

DIRECTIONS: This section of the test consists of a situation, followed by a series of questions. Study the situation and select the **one** best answer to each question following it.

Questions 44.21–44.22: A 48-hr-old male is admitted from another institution. He has moderately severe respiratory distress with abundant salivation, mild peripheral cyanosis, and a radiologic examination as shown in Figure 104.

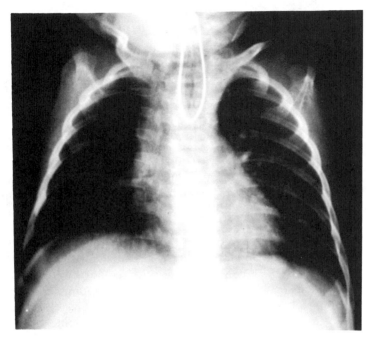

Figure 104

44.21. The most likely diagnosis is
   A. isolated tracheoesophageal fistula
   B. distal tracheoesophageal fistula with esophageal atresia
   C. esophageal foreign body with aspiration pneumonia
   D. pure esophageal atresia
   E. gastroesophageal reflux with esophageal stricture

44.22. The next step in the surgical management should be
   A. Nissen fundoplication
   B. bronchoscopy
   C. gastrostomy
   D. thoracotomy
   E. cervical division of the fistula

Answers and Comments

44.1. **(D)** Pneumoperitoneum is the usual indication for operation. However, nonresponsive metabolic acidosis in spite of adequate therapy and a persistently low platelet count are highly suggestive of bowel necrosis and the need for operation (Ref. 1, pp. 1013–1022).

44.2. **(A)** In 75% of the patients, the aganglionosis involves the rectum and sigmoid, and total involvement of the colon occurs in only 8% of the patients. The aganglionic segment is narrower than the dilated normal bowel above the transition zone. Males outnumber females, 4 to 1. Rectal manometry is a useful diagnostic tool (Ref. 2, pp. 399–411).

44.3. **(E)** The small abdominal cavity in patients with an omphalocele is responsible for today's use of a temporary prosthesis. About one-half of the patients have associated anomalies. In patients with omphalocele, the cord elements enter separately into the abdomen; in patients with gastroschisis the cord elements enter together, to the left of the defect. Prematurity is characteristic of gastroschisis, although 30% of omphalocele patients are premature (Ref. 1, pp. 1037–1049).

44.4. **(E)** True Caroli's disease can be cured (by resection) only in those patients in whom the condition is confirmed to one lobe of the liver (Ref. 3, pp. 155–165).

44.5. **(C)** Most instances of idiopathic bile duct perforation are self-limited and will seal, so treatment by simple drainage is preferred (Ref. 3, pp. 155–165).

44.6. **(A)** The incidence of bile duct malignancy is 20 times higher than normal in patients with a retained choledochal cyst; thus, excision is the treatment of choice (Ref. 3, pp. 155–165).

44.7. **(D)** Choledochal cyst, gallbladder duplication, bifid gallbladder, and anomalies of the extrahepatic bile ducts may be associated choledocholithiasis (Ref. 3, pp. 155–165).

44.8. **(B)** Because of progressive obliteration of the extrahepatic biliary system, corrective surgery is rarely successful in patients with noncorrectable biliary atresia after 4 months of age (Ref. 3, pp. 155–165).

44.9. **(E)** Sarcoma botryoides, a subtype of rhabdomyosarcoma, is the most common primary malignant tumor involving the vagina in childhood (Ref. 4, p. 279).

44.10. **(C)** Alpha-fetoprotein is found in the serum of over two-thirds of children with hepatoblastoma (Ref. 4, p. 306).

44.11. **(B)** Vanillylmandelic acid (VMA) and homovanillic acid (HVA), breakdown products of catecholamines, are elevated in many patients with neuroblastoma (Ref. 4, p. 286).

44.12. **(A)** Wilm's tumors may be associated with genitourinary anomalies, aniridia (absence of the iris), hemihypertrophy, or Beckwith's syndrome (visceromegaly) (Ref. 4, p. 293).

44.13. **(D)** Seventy-five percent of patients with sacrococcygeal teratoma are female (Ref. 4, p. 268).

44.14. **(C)** Eighty-five percent of pediatric inguinal hernias occur in males (Ref. 5, pp. 107–120).

44.15. **(B)** Of "female" inguinal hernias, 1–2% may actually be phenotypic males with testicular feminization (Ref. 5, pp. 107–120).

44.16. **(A)** Umbilical hernias are not operated upon in the first few years of life because they usually regress spontaneously and rarely incarcerate (Ref. 5, 173–175).

44.17. **(B)** Nuck's canal is the female equivalent of the processus vaginalis of males (Ref. 5, pp. 107–120).

44.18. **(C)** Of all inguinal hernias, 10–15% incarcerate during the first year of life (Ref. 5, pp. 107–120, 173–175).

44.19. **(C)** Bronchogenic cysts frequently present with air trapping and are best treated by operative excision. Cystic adenomatoid malformations may present as a solid mass (primarily adenomatous) or as multiple cysts. Extralobar sequestrations do not communicate with the bronchial tree but occasionally communicate with the foregut (esophagus, stomach). Congenital lobar emphysema nearly always involves the upper lobes or right middle lobe (Ref. 6, pp. 33–43).

44.20. **(B)** Intussusception in infancy is nearly always idiopathic. Pyloric stenosis is accompanied by *non*-bilious vomiting. Meconium ileus is a form of intraluminal intestinal obstruction seen in the early newborn period in infants with cystic fibrosis. Usually distal small bowel obstructions are associated with microcolon (Ref. 7, pp. 1648–1656).

44.21. **(D)** Isolated tracheoesophageal fistula usually presents later in the neonatal period, and there is no excessive salivation but choking with feedings. Fewer than 2% of infants with esophageal atresia with distal tracheoestrophageal fistula will have no gas in the abdomen because of a very stenotic lumen or mucous plug in the fistula. Foreign bodies in the esophagus occur in the 1–4-year-old child. Pure esophageal atresia shows a gasless abdomen. Patients with gastroesophageal reflux do not show excess salivation, but regurgitate after feedings and strictures are a late complication (Ref. 3, pp. 115–153).

44.22. **(C)** A gastrostomy is the next best step for a patient with pure esophageal atresia, to allow contrast studies, calibration of the "gap" between esophageal ends, and enteral feeding. Suction of the upper pouch, parenteral antibiotics, and intravenous fluids are applied before definitive repair (or cervical esophagostomy and delayed esophageal substitution) (Ref. 3, pp. 115–153).

References

1. Grosfeld, J.L. (ed.): Pediatric surgery. Surg. Clin. North Am. 61(5), 1981.

2. Silverman, A. and Roy, C.C.: *Pediatric Clinical Gastroenterology*, C.V. Mosby, St. Louis, 1983.

3. deVries, P.A. and Shapiro, S.R.: *Complications of Pediatric Surgery*, Wiley Medical, New York, 1982.

4. Welch, K.J., Randolph, J.G., Ravitch, M.M., et al. (eds.): *Pediatric Surgery*, 4th Ed. Year Book Medical, Chicago, 1986.

5. Raffensperger, J.G.: *Swenson's Pediatric Surgery*, 4th Ed., Appleton-Century-Croft, New York, 1980.

6. Haller, J.A., Golladay, E.S., Pickard, L.R. et al.: Surgical management of lung bud anomalies: Lobar emphysema, bronchogenic cyst, cystic adenomatoid malformation and intralobar pulmonary sequestration. Ann. Thorac. Surg. 28: 33–43, 1978.

7. Schwartz, S.I., Shires, G.T., and Spencer, F.C.: *Principles of Surgery*, 4th Ed., McGraw-Hill, New York, 1984.

45

Plastic, Head, and Neck Surgery

Michael I. Kulick, D.D.S., M.D.

DIRECTIONS Each of the questions or incomplete statements below is followed by five suggested answers or completions. Select the **one** that is best in each case.

45.1. Which of the following does NOT decrease the quality of a surgically created and closed wound?
   A. Local infection
   B. Increase in tension
   C. Size of the suture material
   D. Length of time sutures are left in
   E. Type of closure

45.2. The most common location of mandibular fractures is the
   A. body
   B. angle
   C. symphysis
   D. condyle
   E. alveolar ridge

45.3. The patient shown in Figure 105 has lost the middle one-third of her lower lip as a result of a cut by a clean, sharp knife. Best treatment would be

A. close the defect primarily

B. use part of the upper lip as a rotation flap to replace part of the actual lower lip tissue loss

C. allow the wound to granulate in

D. place a split-thickness skin graft over the defect and repair it later

E. none of the above

Figure 105

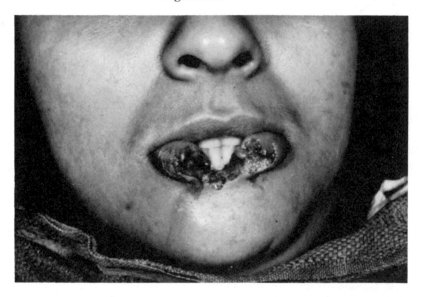

DIRECTIONS: The group of questions below consists of five lettered headings followed by a list of numbered words or statements. For each numbered word or statement, select the **one** lettered heading that is most closely associated with it. Each lettered heading may be selected once, more than once, or not at all.

   A. Palate
   B. Submandibular gland (submaxillary)
   C. Parotid
   D. Sublingual gland
   E. Mucosal portion of the lower lip

45.4. Most common site of minor salivary gland tumors

45.5. Approximately one-half of the tumors in this location are malignant

45.6. The least favorable site for any malignant tumor of the salivary glands

DIRECTIONS: For each of the questions or incomplete statements below, **one or more** of the answers or completions given is correct. Select
   (A) if only 1, 2, and 3 are correct
   (B) if only 1 and 3 are correct
   (C) if only 2 and 4 are correct
   (D) if only 4 is correct
   (E) if all are correct

45.7. True statements regarding hand function is (are):
   1. The prime flexors of the metacarpal phalangeal joint are the superficialis (sublimis) musculotendinous units.
   2. There are 20 intrinsic muscles in the hand.
   3. Isolated paralysis of the entire extensor digitorum communis muscle group will eliminate complete extension of the index, middle, ring, and little fingers.
   4. The thumb adductor is the largest and most powerful intrinsic muscle.

45.8. When performing a "Z" plasty on a linear scar
   1. the limbs of the "Z" plasty must equal the length of the central member
   2. a 60° angle is the largest angle that will permit transposition of the flaps while obtaining maximal increase in length in human tissues
   3. the greater the length of the central member, the greater the actual gain performed by the "Z" plasty
   4. the actual gain in length performed by the "Z" plasty is equal to the theoretical gain in length as determined by the angles of the "Z" plasty

---

DIRECTIONS: This section of the test consists of situations, each followed by a series of questions. Study each situation and select the **one** best answer to each question following it.

Question 45.9: The patient shown in Figure 106 had boiling water spilled on his leg. He was able to pull his clothing off after 2–3 min. After 2 hr the local pain was severe. The patient came to the emergency room and was examined by you.

Figure 106

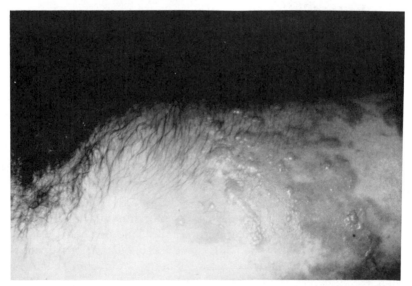

45.9. The leg burn most likely represents
   A. first-degree burn (superficial)
   B. first-degree burn (deep)
   C. second-degree burn
   D. second-degree burn with underlying muscle involvement
   E. third-degree burn

Question 45.10: A patient comes in to see you with a scar created by the removal of a nevus on her arm 4 weeks after excision. The patient tells you that she does not like the color and that the scar has increase in redness as compared to its appearance at the time of suture removal, which was 1 week after excision. She now requests that it be revised.

45.10. You should do which of the following?
   A. Schedule the patient for reexcision
   B. Treat the patient with antibiotics for possible infection
   C. Treat the patient with antibiotics for 7 days and, if not effective, reexcise the scar
   D. Reassure the patient and wait at least 6 months
   E. None of the above

Answers and Comments

45.1. (C) The size of the suture material does not worsen the quality of a scar as long as the suture material is taken out in 3−7 days. On the face, the sutures should be removed within 3−5 days and steristrips placed; anterior trunk and extremities in 7−10 days, and back and feet in 10−14 days. Local infections hinder the healing process and often increase scar tissue. Tension produces ischemia and possible loss of tissue. The type of closure is important, for it is imperative to evert the skin edges to get the best possible results. In certain situations, the "mattress" type of closures is necessary to create wound edge eversion (Ref. 1, pp. 10−15).

45.2. (D) The most common location of mandibular fractures in order of the frequency of occurrence is: condyle, body, angle, symphysis, ramus/alveolar ridge, and coronoid. Approximately 60% of the mandibular fractures are bilateral. Most often, mandibular fractures are treated by closed intermaxillary fixation, provided the occlusion is stable. Radiographs used to diagnose mandibular fractures are: right and left lateral obliques, P-A view of the mandible, a modified Townes view, or a panorex (Ref. 2, p. 2142).

45.3. (A) There is so much excess tissue in the lower lip that approximately one-third of its length can be removed and the wound closed primarily. The upper lip is not as full as the lower, but primary closure is still possible when one-fourth or less has been excised. Since the wound was created with a clean sharp knife, and contamination was minimal or nonexistent other than that caused by the patient's own oral flora, primary closure would be the best form of treatment for this patient (Ref. 1, p. 7).

45.4. (A)
45.5. (A)
45.6. (B) The least favorable site for any malignant tumor of the salivary glands is in the submandibular gland, followed by the parotid, followed by the palate. The palate is the most common site of minor salivary gland tumors. Approximately one-half of the palatal tumors are malignant, but they have the most favorable prognosis (Ref. 3, pp. 16–17).

45.7. (C) There are 20 intrinsic muscles of the hand which, by definition, originate distal to the wrist. Fifteen are innervated by the ulnar nerve and 5 by the median nerve. The prime flexors of the metacarpal phalangeal joint are the intrinsic not the superficialis muscle groups. Of all the intrinsic muslces, the thumb adductor is the largest and most powerful muscle. Finger extension is provided by a combination of forces from both the intrinsic and extrinsic extensor groups of muscles. The index and little fingers are unique in that they have a second extrinsic extensor tendon group, the extensor indicis proprius and extensor digiti minimi, which prevent full extension with complete loss of extensor digitorum communis function. When all the extrinsic extensors of the hand are functioning, these two musculotendinous units permit independent extension of the index and little fingers (Ref. 4, pp. 26–30).

45.8. (A) When performing a "Z" plasty, the limbs of the "Z" must equal the length of the central member. The potential range of the angles of the limbs to the central axis is from 30–90°, but 60° is the largest angle that will permit transposition of the flaps while obtaining the maximal increase in length in the direction of the central member. The greater the length of the central member, the greater the actual gain performed by the "Z" plasty. The length gained by the "Z" plasty is in the direction of the central member. In most instances, the theoretical gain exceeds the actual gain expected, as determined by the angle of the limbs to the central member (Ref. 1, pp. 58–66).

45.9. (C) This patient has a typical picture of a second-degree burn. Because of the type of injury, scalding water, and the fact that the area is painful, this burn is a partial versus a full thickness injury. Therefore, deep tissue involvement is unlikely. A first-degree burn is one in which only the epidermis is involved and is characterized by erythema and edema. Second-degree burns go into the dermis and blistering is present. Third-degree burns go through the dermis. These third-degree burns are usually nontender and the skin is of leathery consistency. When determining the depth of the burn, the manner and cause of the burn, the appearance of the wound, and the presence or absence of sensation should all be considered (Ref. 1, pp. 457–459).

45.10. (D) In this situation, the best choice would be to wait at least 6 months. Often, the appearance of a linear scar is worse at 3–5 weeks after closure when compared to its appearance at the time of suture removal. It is unwise to reoperate on a scar in less than 6 months and often improvement continues through 12 months. This allows the natural process of scar maturation to occur. Even after 12 months, it is not advisable to reoperate on a scar because the color is disliked (Ref. 2, pp. 2101–2104).

References

1. Grab, W. C. and Smith, J. W.: *Plastic Surgery, A Concise Guide to Clinical Practice*, 3rd Ed., Little, Brown, Boston, 1980.

2. Schwartz, S. I.: *Principles of Surgery*, 4th Ed., McGraw-Hill, New York, 1984.

3. Batsakis, J. G.: *Tumors of the Head and Neck, Clinical and Pathological Considerations*, 2nd Ed., Williams and Wilkins, Baltimore, 1979.

4. Kilgore, E. S. and Graham, W. P. III. (eds.): The hand. In *Surgical and Non-Surgical Management*, Lea & Febiger, Philadelphia, 1977, pp. 26−30.

46

Thoracic and Cardiovascular Surgery

Richard J. Thurer, M.D.

DIRECTIONS: Each of the questions or incomplete statements below is followed by five suggested answers or completions. Select the **one** that is best in each case.

46.1. The most common congenital abnormality of the trachea is
   A. stenosis
   B. fistula to the esophagus
   C. atresia
   D. duplication
   E. diverticulum

46.2. Blood supply to a portion of the lung via anomalous systemic artery defines the congenital anomaly as
   A. pulmonary agenesis
   B. pulmonary sequestration
   C. pulmonic atresia
   D. congenital lobar emphysema
   E. none of the above

46.3. The best indication of alveolar ventilation is provided by measurement of
  A. blood pH
  B. forced expiratory volume
  C. blood P_{CO_2}
  D. blood P_{O_2}
  E. tidal volume

46.4. The major advantage of a homograft or heterograft valve prosthesis over a mechanical prosthesis is
  A. hemodynamic superiority
  B. ready availability
  C. the low incidence of thromboembolic complications
  D. long-term durability
  E. the ease with which it can be implanted

46.5. The most common neoplasms of the posterior mediastinum are
  A. teratomas
  B. thymomas
  C. neurogenic tumors
  D. cardiogenic in origin
  E. bronchogenic cysts

46.6. Epidermoid carcinoma of the lung
  A. is the most common cell type of bronchogenic carcinoma
  B. usually arises as a solitary peripheral pulmonary nodule
  C. is less aggressive than small-cell carcinoma
  D. should not be resected in the presence of pulmonary osteoarthropathy
  E. is more common in women than in men

46.7. The most common cardiac malformation present at birth is
  A. aortic stenosis
  B. tetralogy of Fallot
  C. atrial septal defect
  D. transposition of the great arteries
  E. ventricular septal defect

46.8. Which of the following is NOT a feature of tetralogy of Fallot?
  A. Ventricular septal defect
  B. Patent ductus arteriosus
  C. Overriding of the aorta
  D. Right ventricular hypertrophy
  E. Right ventricular outflow obstruction

DIRECTIONS: The group of questions below consists of five lettered headings followed by a list of numbered words or statements. For each numbered word or statement, select the **one** lettered heading that is most closely associated with it. Each lettered heading may be selected once, more than once, or not at all.

  A. Tuberculosis
  B. Carcinoma of the lung
  C. Syphilis
  D. Rheumatic heart disease
  E. Lymphoma

46.9. Superior vena caval syndrome

46.10. Pancoast's syndrome

46.11. Spontaneous chylothorax

DIRECTIONS: The set of lettered headings below is followed by a list of numbered words or phrases. For each numbered word or phrase select
  (A) if the item is associated with A only
  (B) if the item is associated with B only
  (C) if the item is associated with both A and B
  (D) if the item is associated with neither A nor B

  A. Atrial septal defect, uncomplicated
  B. Ventricular septal defect, uncomplicated
  C. Both
  D. Neither

46.12. Right-to-left shunt

46.13. Asymptomatic during first year of life

46.14. Spontaneous closure in 40% of cases by age 3

DIRECTIONS: For each of the questions or incomplete statements below, **one or more** of the answers or completions given is correct. Select

 (A) if only 1, 2, and 3 are correct
 (B) if only 1 and 3 are correct
 (C) if only 2 and 4 are correct
 (D) if only 4 is correct
 (E) if all are correct

46.15. Complications of myocardial infarction amenable to surgical therapy include
 1. ventricular septal defect
 2. papillary muscle rupture
 3. ventricular aneurysm
 4. myocardial rupture

46.16. Permanent transvenous pacemaker implantation may be used in the treatment of
 1. complete heart block
 2. sick sinus syndrome
 3. postsurgical heart block
 4. hypersensitive carotid sinus

46.17. Pyogenic lung abscess
 1. rarely requires surgical therapy
 2. is usually related to aspiration
 3. may have an x-ray appearance similar to cavitating bronchogenic carcinoma
 4. usually harbors anaerobic organisms

DIRECTIONS: This section of the test consists of a situation, followed by a series of questions. Study the situation and select the **one** best answer to each question following it.

Questions 46.18–46.20: A 55-year-old man in previous good health was involved in an auto accident. When brought to the emergency room, he was awake and alert with normal vital signs. On examination, he complained of precordial chest pain and precordial ecchymosis was present. A chest x-ray was done (Figure 107).

Figure 107

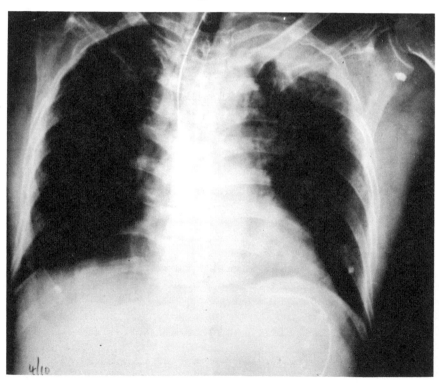

46.18. The finding of most immediate concern is
   A. widened mediastinum
   B. fractured ribs
   C. pneumothorax
   D. pulmonary infiltrate
   E. the level of the left diaphragm

46.19. Evaluation of the aorta is best accomplished in this patient by
   A. immediate left thoracotomy
   B. aortography
   C. close follow of pulses in upper extremities
   D. sequential chest x-rays
   E. exploration via a sternal splitting incision

Figure 108

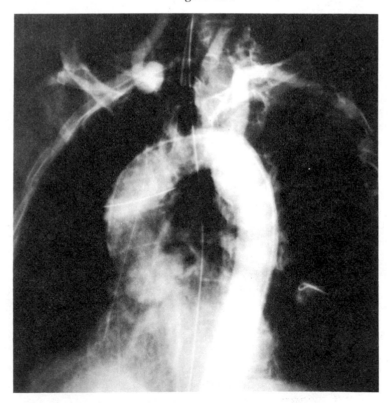

46.20. An aortogram done on this patient reveals (Figure 108)
A. no pathology
B. transection of the aorta
C. aortic insufficiency
D. avulsion of the left subclavian artery
E. evidence of major venous injury

Answers and Comments

46.1. **(B)** Tracheoesophageal fistula is an abnormality of both the trachea and the esophagus and as such is the most common developmental anomaly of the trachea (Ref. 1, p. 674).

46.2. **(B)** Although two forms of sequestration, intralobar and extralobar, are described, this malformation is characterized by an area of lung tissue which derives its bloody supply from a systemic vessel, usually an aberrant branch of the aorta (Ref. 1, p. 685).

46.3. **(C)** Because CO_2 is so readily diffusible, measurement of PCO_2 in the arterial blood is the best measure of alveolar ventilation (Ref. 1, p. 11).

46.4. **(C)** Tissue valves have a lower incidence of thromboembolism than mechanical prostheses, even when anticoagulants are not employed (Ref. 1, p. 1293).

46.5. **(C)** Of all mediastinal tumors, the most common are of neurogenic origin. These usually occur in the posterior mediastinum. Accurate localization of a mediastinal mass narrows the diagnostic possibilities considerably, because certain tumors or cysts commonly occur in certain mediastinal locations (Ref. 1, pp. 413–424).

46.6. **(A)** The four major histologic types of bronchogenic carcinoma as defined by the World Health Organization are epidermoid, adenocarcinoma, small-cell, and large-cell carcinoma. In most reported series, the epidermoid cell type is most common (Ref. 2, p. 369).

46.7. **(E)** Precise data as to the frequency of specific malformations are in general lacking, with analyses of different population groups and a differing definition of malformations contributing to the likely underestimation of the true incidence. Despite this, ventricular septal defect seems to be the most common anomaly recognizable at birth (Ref. 3, p. 942).

46.8. (B) The definition of tetralogy of Fallot is precise, although the severity of each component is variable. The features of tetralogy of Fallot are all those listed except patent ductus arteriosus, which may, however, also be present in children with the anomaly (Ref. 3, p. 990).

46.9. (B) There are a great many causes of the superior vena caval syndrome, including fungal infections, trauma, and septic phlebitis. Malignant neoplasms are the most common cause, with carcinoma of the lung the most common among that group. Obstruction to the cava may occur by direct invasion of the primary neoplasm or be due to impingement on the cava by lymph nodes containing metastatic deposits (Ref. 2, pp. 198−201).

46.10. (B) Pancoast's syndrome is a distinct clinical entity which includes pain in the eighth cervical, first and second thoracic dermatome distributions. This is caused by tumors of the superior pulmonary sulcus which may be of any cell type (Ref. 1, pp. 506−515).

46.11. (E) Accumulation of chyle in the pleural space may occur secondary to trauma, benign neoplasms, or lesions of the thoracic duct itself. Most commonly, a primary malignancy of the lymphoma group is the cause (Ref. 2, pp. 201−204).

46.12. (D) Intracardiac communications between the right and left sides of the heart (ASD and VSD) are among the most commonly recognized anomalies. Increase in pulmonary vascular resistance may occur, causing reversal of shunt flow. In these cases, operative repair should not be undertaken (Ref. 3, p. 961).

46.13. (A) Atrial septal defect is often not recognized until late childhood or early adult life. It rarely results in disability in childhood (Ref. 3, p. 959).

46.14. (B) While ventricular septal defect is the most common congenital cardiac anomaly present at birth, an estimated 40% of these defects will spontaneously close by 3 years of age. In some children, spontaneous closure may occur at an even older age (Ref. 3, pp. 963–965).

46.15. (E) All of the listed complications of myocardial infarction can be surgically treated. Prognosis varies considerably among these complications and relates both to the diagnosis and time following infarction that surgery is undertaken (Ref. 2, pp. 1425–1427).

46.16. (E) Permanent pacing in adult patients is most often accomplished by the transvenous method. Although complete heart block was the most common reason for pacing in the past, the indications have steadily broadened. They now include all those indicated, as well as other conduction system disorders (Ref. 3, pp. 744–748).

46.17. (E) Lung abscess has all the characteristics listed. Antibiotic therapy is usually effective, therefore surgical therapy is not required. Anaerobic organisms are commonly present although mixed infection is not unusual. Cavitating carcinoma of the lung with air–fluid level has a radiographic appearance similar to lung abscess (Ref. 1, pp. 543–550).

46.18. (A)
46.19. (B)
46.20. (B) Traumatic transection of the aorta is a common cause of death following road accidents. The region of the aorta just distal to the left subclavian artery is the usual site of injury. Although often lethal, this injury may be compatible with survival for a period of time sufficient to allow prompt diagnosis and treatment. A high index of suspicion, liberal use of aortography, and prompt surgical repair results in survival of many patients who would otherwise die (Ref. 2, pp. 1489–1492).

References

1. Sabiston, D. C. and Spencer, F. C.: *Gibbon's Surgery of the Chest*, 4th Ed., W. B. Saunders, Philadelphia, 1983.

2. Glenn, W. W. L., Baue, A. E., Geha, A. S., Hammond, G. L. and Laks, H.: *Thoracic and Cardiovascular Surgery*, 4th Ed., Appleton-Century-Crofts, Norwalk, 1983.

3. Braunwald, E.: *Heart Disease—A Textbook of Cardiovascular Medicine*, 2nd Ed., W. B. Saunders, Philadelphia, 1984.

47

Trauma Surgery
Kimball I. Maull, M.D.

DIRECTIONS: Each of the questions or incomplete statements below is followed by five suggested answers or completions. Select the **one** that is best in each case.

47.1. In normovolemic patients, the most significant hemodynamic effect of military antishock trousers (MAST) is related to
   A. autotransfusion
   B. tamponade
   C. reduced distal blood blow
   D. splinting of underlying fractures
   E. increased systemic afterload

47.2. The risk of transfusion reaction to administration of type-specific uncrossmatched blood in an injured patient is
   A. 1%
   B. 5%
   C. 10%
   D. 15%
   E. 25%

47.3. The major pitfall in the nonoperative management of splenic trauma is
   A. delayed splenic hemorrhage
   B. increased susceptibility to secondary splenic injury
   C. missing other serious intraabdominal injuries
   D. increased hospitalization time and costs
   E. disseminated intravascular coagulation (DIC)

DIRECTIONS: The group of questions below consists of five lettered headings followed by a list of numbered words or statements. For each numbered word or statement, select the **one** lettered heading that is most closely associated with it. Each lettered heading may be selected once, more than once, or not at all.

For each injury, indicate the most appropriate diagnostic modality.

   A. Plain roentgenographs
   B. Contrast radiography
   C. Ultrasonography
   D. Computed tomography (CT)
   E. Arteriography

47.4. Mediastinal widening

47.5. Head injury

47.6. Critically injured patient with unstable vital signs

DIRECTIONS: The set of lettered headings below is followed by a list of numbered words or phrases. For each numbered word or phrase select
   (A) if the item is associated with A only
   (B) if the item is associated with B only
   (C) if the item is associated with both A and B
   (D) if the item is associated with neither A nor B

A. Routine exploration of penetrating neck wounds
B. Selective exploration of penetrating neck wounds
C. Both
D. Neither

47.7. Superficial wound not penetrating platysma muscle

47.8. Wound causing major vascular, visceral, or airway injury

47.9. Results in statistically significant decrease in mortality, morbidity, and length of hospital stay

---

DIRECTIONS: This section of the test consists of situations, each followed by a series of questions. Study each situation and select the **one** best answer to each question following it.

Questions 47.10 – 47.12: An 18-year-old man was involved in a motorcycle mishap 30 min before arrival in the emergency unit. On presentation, his vital signs showed BP 90/60, HR 130, RR 26. He did not follow commands but demonstrated a tender lower abdomen and deformity of his right thigh.

47.10. Following initial resuscitation, the first roentgenograph ordered should be
   A. supine chest
   B. upright chest
   C. lateral cervical spine
   D. skull
   E. thigh

47.11. X-ray of the pelvis was taken (Figure 109) and demonstrates
   A. normal pelvis
   B. comminuted pelvis
   C. diametric fractures (unstable)
   D. isolated pubic rami fractures (stable)
   E. fractured acetabulum

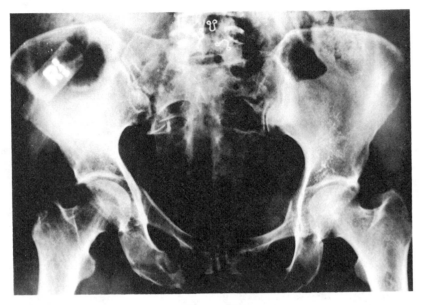

Figure 109

47.12. Diagnostic peritoneal lavage
  A. is contraindicated
  B. is unnecessary because the patient is in shock and will require celiotomy anyway
  C. should be performed by the standard closed technique
  D. should be performed by the standard open technique
  E. may be performed by either technique with supraumbilical placement of the catheter

Questions 47.13–47.15: A 27-year-old unrestrained woman driver was thrown from the vehicle during an automobile crash and brought to the emergency unit 1 hr later, fully alert and conscious. Aside from a nasal fracture and fracture of the tibial plateau, her examination was normal. Admission serum amylase was 180 Somogyi units (nl 50–180). Twelve hours later, she developed mild epigastric tenderness and the following abdominal film was taken (Figure 110).

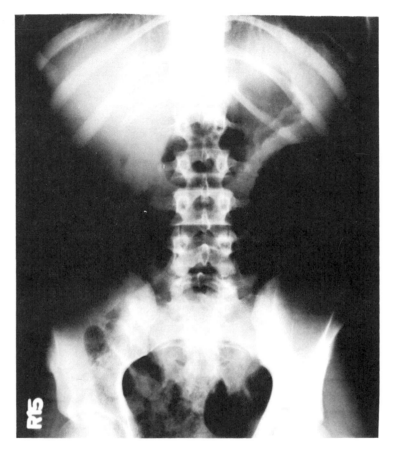

Figure 110

47.13. On the basis of this film, you suspect
  A. ruptured viscus
  B. pancreatic injury
  C. disruption, lumbosacral spine
  D. perinephric hematoma
  E. normal study

47.14. Repeat serum amylase is drawn and returns 840 Somogyi units. The abdominal examination demonstrates increased abdominal tenderness. You advise
A. continued observation
B. diagnostic peritoneal lavage
C. abdominal ultrasound
D. computed tomography
E. exploratory celiotomy

47.15. At operation, the pancreas is transected at the junction of middle and distal thirds. You perform
A. external drainage only
B. internal drainage only
C. pancreaticoduodenectomy
D. pancreaticojejunostomy (Puestow)
E. distal pancreatectomy, external drainage

Answers and Comments

47.1. (E) In the supine position, MAST produces no net auto-transfusion but raises blood pressure by increasing peripheral resistance. (Ref. 2, pp. 931–937).

47.2. (A) In men, the risk of transfusion reaction is less than 1%. In multiparous women, it rises to 2% but, in either sex, the risk is low and justifies the use of type-specific uncross-matched blood in an emergency (Ref. 4, p. 13).

47.3. (C) In this study of 241 patients with splenic trauma, associated intraabdominal injury occurred in 36%. Diagnostic peritoneal lavage is recommended to define patients requiring celiotomy (Ref. 7, pp. 840–849).

47.4. (E)
47.5. (D)
47.6. (A) CT remains the most rapid and accurate method to detect intracranial injury. Mediastinal widening suggests intrathoracic bleeding and arteriography is needed to detect aortic rupture. If the patient's condition is unstable, plain films by portable technique are safest (Ref. 4, p. 16).

47.7. (D)

47.8. (C)

47.9. (D) Regardless of exploration policy, wounds that do not penetrate the platysma do not require exploration, whereas major vascular, visceral, and airway injury are accepted indications for operative management. In a recent prospective study, neither mandatory nor selective exploration offered a clear advantage (Ref. 3, p. 24).

47.10. (C) This patient's impaired sensorium must be assumed to be on the basis of head injury. Any injury above the clavicles increases the chance of cervical spine injury (Ref. 10, p. 131).

47.11. (B) A comminuted pelvic fracture (also known as crushed pelvis, Trunkey type I) involves at least three interruptions in the pelvic ring, has a high incidence of major visceral and vascular injury, and is very unstable (Ref. 10, pp. 203–205).

47.12. (E) Diagnostic peritoneal lavage is indicated to exclude associated intraperitoneal bleeding. A supraumbilical approach is essential to avoid a rising pelvic hematoma. Both techniques are acceptable. (Ref. 11, p. 143).

47.13. (B) Ileus developing 12 hr following blunt injury in a patient with epigastric pain suggests pancreatic injury (Ref. 11, p. 173).

47.14. (E) Rising serum amylase in a patient with abdominal pain following blunt trauma is an indication for exploration. CT and/or ultrasound may confirm the diagnosis, but studies should not prevent operation (Ref. 11, p. 173).

47.15. (E) Distal pancreatectomy is the procedure of choice for major injuries to body and tail of pancreas (Ref. 11, p. 174).

References

1. De Camara, D.L., Raine, T., and Robson, M.C.: Ultrastructured aspects of cooled thermal injury. J. Trauma 21, 1981.

2. Gaffney, F.A., Thal, E.R., et al.: Hemodynamic effects of medical antishock trousers (MAST garment). J. Trauma 21, 1981.

3. Golueke, P.J., Goldstein, A.S., et al.: Routine versus selective exploration of penetrating neck injuries: A randomized prospective study. J. Trauma 24, 1984.

4. Levison, M. and Trunkey, D.D.: Initial assessment and resuscitation. Surg. Clin. N. Amer. 62, 1982.

5. Lewis, F.R.: Thoracic trauma. Surg. Clin. N. Amer. 62, 1982.

6. Meyer, H.A. and Crass, R.A.: Abdominal trauma. Surg. Clin. N. Amer. 62, 1982.

7. Traub, A.C. and Perry, J.F.: Injuries associated with splenic trauma. J. Trauma 21, 1981.

8. Bone, L.L., Seibel, R.W., and Border, J. R.: Primary open reduction and internal fixation of open fractures. J. Trauma 20, 1980.

9. Blaisdell, F.W. and Trunkey, D.D.: *Abdominal Trauma*, Theime-Stratton, New York, 1982.

10. Advanced Trauma Life Support Course. Committee on Trauma, American College of Surgeons, Chicago, 1984.

11. Cowley, R.A. and Dunham, C.M.: *Shock Trauma/Critical Care Manual*, Univ. Park Press, Baltimore, 1982.

48

Urologic Surgery
J. David Moorhead, M.D.

DIRECTIONS: Each of the questions or incomplete statements below is followed by five suggested answers or completions. Select the **one** that is best in each case.

48.1. The most common testicular tumor in children is
  - **A.** seminoma
  - **B.** choriocarcinoma
  - **C.** embryonal carcinoma
  - **D.** Leydig cell tumor
  - **E.** none of the above

48.2. The intercostal nerve is found between what layers of the abdominal wall when the kidney is exposed in the classic lumbar approach?
  - **A.** Superficial to the external oblique fascia
  - **B.** External oblique and internal oblique fascias
  - **C.** Internal oblique and transversalis muscle
  - **D.** Under the transversalis muscle
  - **E.** None of the above

48.3. Retroperitoneal fibrosis is a disease that has been associated with which of the following drugs?
  A. Propranolol hydrochloride (Inderal)
  B. Hydrochlorothiazide
  C. Methysergide (Sansert)
  D. Digoxin
  E. Valium

DIRECTIONS: The group of questions below consists of five lettered headings followed by a list of numbered words or statements. For each numbered word or statement, select the **one** lettered heading that is most closely associated with it. Each lettered heading may be selected once, more than once, or not at all.

  A. Transitional cell carcinoma of bladder
  B. Squamous cell carcinoma of bladder
  C. Adenocarcinoma of prostate
  D. Adenocarcinoma of kidney
  E. Choriocarcinoma of the testes

48.4. Associated with schistosomiasis

48.5. Associated with bony metastasis and increased acid phosphatase

48.6. Associated with increased β subunit HCG

DIRECTIONS: For each of the questions or incomplete statements below, **one or more** of the answers or completions given is correct. Select

- **(A)** if only 1, 2, and 3 are correct
- **(B)** if only 1 and 3 are correct
- **(C)** if only 2 and 4 are correct
- **(D)** if only 4 is correct
- **(E)** if all are correct

48.7. Standard indications for prostatectomy in a 60-year-old man include
1. microhematuria
2. urinary retention
3. perineal pain
4. hydronephrosis 2° to bladder outlet obstruction

48.8. Which of the following statements regarding undescended testes are true?
1. Undescended testes have an increased incidence of malignancy when compared to normally descended testes
2. Orchiopexy should be done after puberty
3. The undescended testis shows decreased spermatogenesis in most pubertal males
4. The administration of hCG is equally effective in effecting the descent of unilateral and bilateral undescended testes

DIRECTIONS: This section of the test consists of a situation, followed by a series of questions. Study the situation and select the **one** best answer to each question following it.

Questions 48.9−48.10: A 14-year-old boy presents to the emergency room 3 hr after having the acute onset of right scrotal pain. He is afebrile, the UA is clear, and there is no history of previous urinary tract infection. Physical examination reveals an erythematous right hemiscrotum and an elevated right testis that is acutely tender.

48.9. The most likely diagnosis is
  A. epididymitis
  B. scrotal trauma
  C. testicular torsion
  D. incarcerated inguinal hernia
  E. none of the above

48.10. The most appropriate treatment is
  A. ampicillin for 10 days
  B. transcrotal exploration, detorsion, and fixation of the contralateral testes
  C. transcrotal exploration and detorsion
  D. drainage of the scrotal hematoma
  E. inguinal exploration and herniorrhaphy

Answers and Comments

48.1. (C) Embryonal carcinoma is by far the most common. A significant percentage of these are the infantile types or "yolk sac" tumors. In adults, seminoma is the most common (Ref. 3, p. 939).

48.2. (C) These nerves are the motor supply to the anterior abdominal wall. Their compromise can lead to herniation or a localized "bulge" (Ref. 1, p. 9).

48.3. (C) Retroperitoneal fibrosis is a disease of the retroperitoneum manifesting as a fibrous investiture of the ureter, great vessels, psoas muscle, etc. It has been strongly linked with Sansert, which is prescribed for treatment of headaches (Ref. 1, p. 429).

48.4. (B) Squamous carcinoma of the bladder is uncommon in the United States. In Egypt, schistosomiasis is endemic in the Nile River delta, and squamous carcinoma is seen in 40% of bladder cancers (Ref. 2, p. 1036).

48.5. (C) Carcinoma of the prostate is well known to metastasize to bone and lymph nodes. Bony involvement is manifested by increased acid phosphatase (Ref. 2, p. 1084).

48.6. (E) Choriocarcinoma is the testicular tumor with the highest mortality rate. The syncytial cells element produce HCG, which can be detected and is an important diagnostic marker (Ref.2, p. 1130).

48.7. (C) Prostatectomy's goals are the preservation of renal function, eradication of infection secondary to urinary retention, and symptomatic relief of voiding symptoms. It is difficult to predict the progression of symptoms, but those patients with definite urinary retention secondary to outlet obstruction deserve treatment (Ref. 2, p. 961).

48.8. (B) Undescended testes have an increased incidence of malignancy of greater than 40 times that of normally descended testes. Cryptorchid tests also show significant abnormalities of spermatogenesis. Orchiopexies should be done before age 3 in an effort to minimize histologic changes. HCG is approximately twice as successful in helping to bring down bilateral undescended testes as it is in unilateral testes (Refs. 2, p. 1561; 3, p. 659).

48.9. (C) The acute onset of unilateral scrotal pain in men under 30 must be considered to be testicular torsion until proven otherwise. The absence of evidence of UTI, trauma, or inguinal mass in this patient makes the other diagnoses unlikely (Ref. 3, p. 652).

48.10. (B) The appropriate treatment is a scrotal exploration with detorsion and contralateral testicular fixation, because the congenital abnormality allowing the torsion is present bilaterally (Ref. 3, p. 652).

References

1. Harrison, J.H., et al (eds.): *Campbell's Urology*, Vol. 1, 4th Ed., W.B. Saunders, Philadelphia, 1978.

2. Harrison, J.H., et al (eds.): *Campbell's Urology*, Vol. 2, 4th Ed., W.B. Saunders, Philadelphia, 1978.

3. Kelalis, P.P., et al (eds.): *Clinical Pediatric Urology*, Vols. 1 and 2, W.B. Saunders, Philadelphia, 1976.

PSYCHIATRY

49

Psychiatry

Barbara Ann Allen, M.S.W., Ph.D. and James R. Allen, M.D.

DIRECTIONS: Each of the questions or incomplete statements below is followed by five suggested answers or completions. Select the **one** that is best in each case.

49.1. The psychosocial task of the oral period, according to Erikson, involves the achievement of
- **A.** basic trust/basic mistrust
- **B.** intimacy/self-absorption
- **C.** generativity/stagnation
- **D.** initiative/shame
- **E.** integrity/despair

49.2. The defense mechanism most characteristic of the obsessive/compulsive disorder is
- **A.** denial
- **B.** reaction−formation
- **C.** conversion
- **D.** sublimation
- **E.** regression

49.3. Splitting refers to
   A. perception of people as "all good" or "all bad"
   B. identification
   C. reaction–formation
   D. primitive idealization
   E. repression

49.4. Which of the following is NOT an ego function?
   A. Reality testing
   B. Defense mechanisms
   C. Interpersonal relationships
   D. Self- and object representations
   E. Instinctual drives

49.5. Which of the following is NOT true?
   A. Normal persons have relatively large and segmented social networks
   B. The social networks of schizophrenics are smaller than those of normal people
   C. Social support systems buffer the individual from external stressors
   D. Normal individuals have more kin in their networks than schizophrenics
   E. The social networks of schizophrenics are more dense than those of normal people

49.6. The WAIS
   A. is a projective test
   B. includes only verbal tests
   C. tests only innate intellectual ability
   D. is of little value in differentiating various types of psychopathology
   E. is an individual IQ test

49.7. Which of the following is NOT a test for assessing neurologic or perceptual defects?
   A. TAT
   B. Nebraska-Luria
   C. Halstead-Reitan
   D. Goldstein-Scheer
   E. ITPA

49.8. Which of the following is NOT a symptom of melancholia?
  A. Anorexia and weight loss
  B. Early morning insomnia
  C. Psychomotor agitation or retardation
  D. Quality of mood distinct from mourning
  E. Initial insomnia

49.9. For a diagnosis of schizophrenic disorder, the person must be ill for
  A. 2 weeks
  B. 1 week
  C. more than 6 months
  D. less than 6 months
  E. more than 2 years

49.10. Which of the following does not produce a secondary depression (organic affective syndrome)?
  A. Talwin
  B. Clonidine (Catapres)
  C. Hydralazine (Apresoline)
  D. Propranolol (Inderal)
  E. Incubus

49.11. Which of the following symptoms is NOT suggestive of organic pathology?
  A. Fluctuating level of consciousness
  B. Disorientation in time
  C. Impaired recent memory
  D. Auditory hallucinations
  E. Visual hallucinations

49.12. Which of the following statements is NOT true?
  A. Competence is a legal, not a medical, term
  B. Testamentary capacity refers to competence to make a will
  C. Privileged communication is limited to things revealed within a particular relationship
  D. Confidentiality is an important responsibility owed to patients
  E. Commitment automatically includes adjudication of incompetence and loss of civil rights

DIRECTIONS: The group of questions below consists of five lettered headings followed by a list of numbered words or statements. For each numbered word or statement, select the **one** lettered heading that is most closely associated with it. Each lettered heading may be selected once, more than once, or not at all.

  A. Splitting
  B. Regression
  C. Repression
  D. Reaction–formation
  E. Rationalization

49.13. A mechanism whereby a person reverts to an earlier level of personality development

49.14. A mechanism that is prominent in people who have not resolved the rapprochement phase of separation–individuation

49.15. A form of forgetting

49.16. A person is indefatigably benevolent because of guilt of which he is unaware

49.17. A person formulates presentable reasons after he has responded to unrecognized motives

DIRECTIONS: The set of lettered headings below is followed by a list of numbered words or phrases. For each numbered word or phrase select
  (A) if the item is associated with A only
  (B) if the item is associated with B only
  (C) if the item is associated with both A and B
  (D) if the item is associated with neither A nor B

  A. Low urinary levels of 3, 4 MHPG
  B. Low levels of 5 HIAA in CSF
  C. Both
  D. Neither

49.18. Major affective disorder, single episode

49.19. Major affective disorder, recurrent

49.20. Bipolar disorder, manic

DIRECTIONS: For each of the questions or incomplete statements below, **one or more** of the answers or completions given is correct. Select

    (A)   if only 1, 2, and 3 are correct
    (B)   if only 1 and 3 are correct
    (C)   if only 2 and 4 are correct
    (D)   if only 4 is correct
    (E)   if all are correct

49.21. Which of the following are true of the antisocial personality disorder?
    1. History of at least three antisocial activities before age 15
    2. No period of 5 years without antisocial activity
    3. Current age of 18 or more
    4. Overidealization

49.22. The significant impairment of reading skills in developmental reading disorder is NOT due to
    1. chronological age
    2. inadequate schooling
    3. hyperactivity
    4. mental age

49.23. Which of the following group(s) of neuroleptics is(are) now in clinical use?
    1. Phenothiazines
    2. Thioxanthenes
    3. Butyrophenones
    4. Rauwolfia alkaloids

DIRECTIONS SUMMARIZED

A	B	C	D	E
1,2,3	1,3	2,4	4	All are
only	only	only	only	correct

49.24. Tardive dyskinesia
  1. is characterized by involuntary movement, especially of the lips and tongue
  2. is usually reversible
  3. may appear after the antipsychotic has been reduced or discontinued
  4. responds to treatment and antiparkinsonian medication

49.25. The anticholinergic action of tricyclic medications can lead to
  1. aggravation of narrow-angle glaucoma
  2. urinary retention
  3. dry mouth
  4. delirium

49.26. Which of the following are characteristic of hallucinations in schizophrenic disorders?
  1. Voices that argue
  2. Voice or voices that comment(s) on the person's behavior
  3. Voice or voices that talk(s) at length
  4. Visual hallucinations

DIRECTIONS: This section of the test consists of situations, each followed by a series of questions. Study each situation and select the **one** best answer to each question following it.

Question 49.27–49.29: A 39-year-old man comes to his physician because he is afraid his wife will leave him. He moved into a friend's apartment the previous day. He states that his wife claims that he suffers from premature ejaculation and does not satisfy her. He drinks a couple of ounces of scotch on coming home from work, and two or three after dinner. For the past several weeks, he has had trouble sleeping, awakening about 4 AM. He is not hungry and has lost at least 5 lb in the last two weeks. Saying that he finds no pleasure in anything, he sighs deeply and pauses.

49.27. At this point, it would be most helpful to say
   A. "What is wrong at work?"
   B. "Tell me about moving out."
   C. "Tell me about your sexual problems."
   D. "What about your drinking problem?"
   E. "Things just not looking good?"

49.28. Which of the following disorders is the LEAST likely diagnosis for this man?
   A. Major depression with melancholia
   B. Schizophrenic disorder
   C. Dysthymic disorder
   D. Adjustment disorder
   E. Dependent personality disorder

49.29. Which of the following symptoms would you NOT expect to respond to tricyclic medication?
   A. Early morning awakening
   B. Anorexia and weight loss
   C. Psychomotor agitation
   D. Psychomotor retardation
   E. Mourning

Question 49.30: A 36-year-old woman has a 15-year history of multiple somatic complaints. She has been worked-up and treated by a number of physicians, but all these diagnoses and all their treatments have made little, if any, impact on her chronic but fluctuating symptoms. She complains, at present, of an array of problems—light-headedness, nausea, dyspareunia, irregular menses, shortnes of breath, heartburn—in a dramatic but rather vague manner. Physical examination and laboratory tests are within normal limits.

49.30. The most likely diagnosis is
   A. Munchausen's syndrome
   B. factitious disorder
   C. malingering
   D. hypochondriasis
   E. somatization disorder

Answers and Comments

49.1. (A) In this context, the adjective "basic" is meant to convey the idea that the trust blends into the total personality and forms a base for later development. Erikson's concept of "psychosocial stages" should be differentiated from Freud's stages of "psychosexual development" (oral—anal—phallic Oedipal—latency). The student should also note the difference in spelling between the last names of Erik Erikson and Milton Erickson, an influential medical hypnotist (Ref. 1, p. 244).

49.2. (B) Reaction—formation, isolation, intellectualization, rationalization, and undoing are common defense mechanisms used by people who have an obsessive—compulsive disorder (Ref. 1, p. 401).

49.3. (A) People with borderline and psychotic conditions use primitive defense mechanisms such as denial, projection, and splitting. Splitting refers to experiencing the self or others as "all good" or "all bad," rather than as whole people with both good and bad aspects. It is considered the defense, par excellence, of people who manifest a "borderline personality organization" (Kernberg) (Ref. 3, p. 1083).

49.4. (E) The ego is most easily defined by listing its functions, of which there are at least 30: reality testing (ability to distinguish fantasy from reality); sense of reality (ability to tell whether one is awake or dreaming); synthetic function (ability to integrate other functions); ability to tolerate stress, anxiety, and frustration; the autonomous functions of mobility, perception, and memory; self- and object representations; defense mechanisms; and interpersonal relationships (Ref. 1, p. 747).

49.5. (D) A large body of research supports the idea that social support systems are a major factor in maintaining our health and in protecting us from the effects of external stressors. Normal individuals have a large number of people and more nonkin than kin in their social networks. Schizophrenics, in contrast, have smaller networks—typically only one relative, a doctor, and caseworker (Ref. 4, pp. 1278—1279).

49.6. **(E)** The WAIS is a testing of intelligence, but it is influenced by culture and achievement. It includes both verbal and performance subtests. Various patterns among the subtests may be of value in differentiating different types of pathology (Ref. 9, p. 205).

49.7. **(A)** The TAT is a projective test. However, it should be noted that skilled psychologists can use almost any test for a variety of purposes. For this reason, the physician is wise to specify the information he wishes to know, not to specify the test (Ref. 4, p. 968).

49.8. **(E)** Many patients have trouble falling asleep. This is not, however, a symptom of melancholia. This distinction is important because the symptoms of melancholia respond to antidepressant medication. In very low doses, tricyclics have a hypnotic effect. This should not be confused with their antidepressant effect. Because of the dangerous side effects, antidepressants should not be used as "sleeping pills" but reserved for the treatment of melancholia (Ref. 5, p. 215).

49.9. **(C)** The 6-month criterion is important in distinguishing schizophrenic disorder from schizophreniform disorder. A similar condition that lasts more than a few hours but less than 2 weeks may be an atypical psychosis or a brief reactive psychosis (if a stressor is present) (Ref. 5, p. 188).

49.10. **(E)** Many drugs can produce a secondary depression. Incubus, however, is a stage-four sleep disorder: the victim awakens in panic (Ref. 2, p. 463).

49.11. **(D)** A fluctuating level of consciousness, defects in recent memory and orientation, as well as visual hallucination are characteristic of organic pathology. A fluctuating level of consciousness is typical of delirium. Auditory hallucinations, in contrast, are more typical of schizophrenic disorders (Ref. 2, pp. 333–336).

49.12. **(E)** Competency is a legal concept and is judged by a court; it is not a medical concept. This is a process separate from commitment. Testamentary capacity refers to competence to make a will. The term is derived from the fact that during the middle ages, men made their wills while holding their testicles (Ref. 9, pp. 859–860).

49.13. (B)
49.14. (A)
49.15. (C)
49.16. (D)
49.17. (E) This section tests your knowledge of defense mechanisms. Defenses work automatically, out of a person's awareness, to protect him from anxiety and intrapsychic conflict. In reaction— formation, an unacceptable urge or characteristic is replaced, in consciousness, by its opposite. Repression is the exclusion of an idea from consciousness; it is a form of forgetting. In regression, the personality may regress as a whole or only certain aspects of it may regress. Rationalization refers to making good reasons for one's behavior. Splitting, discussed earlier, refers to the experiencing of one's self and others as either "all good" or "all bad" (Ref. 9, pp. 91–111).

49.18. (C)
49.19. (C)
49.20. (D) This section tests your knowledge of the biogenic hypothesis of depression. Low levels of 3, 4 MHPG in the urine are believed to reflect low levels of norepinephrine in brain synapses. Such a state suggests the utility of prescribing a drug such as imipramine, which is believed to block the reuptake of norepinephrine. Levels of 5 HIAA in the CSF are believed to reflect levels of serotonin in the brain. Consequently, a patient with low levels might well be given a drug such as amitryptyline, which blocks the reuptake of serotonin. It should be noted, however, that recent research has raised doubts about the validity of this hypothesis (Ref. 6, p. 2309).

49.21. (A) Overidealization is characteristic of narcissistic personality disorders and sometimes of the histrionic and borderline personality disorders (Ref. 5, p. 320).

49.22. (E) Attention-deficit disorder, with or without hyperactivity, is frequently associated with a developmental reading disability. It is most important that the child is not labeled retarded by parents and school (Ref. 5, p. 93).

49.23. (E) There are several families of antipsychotic medications. They all seem to share one effect: they block dopamine receptors.

Although no longer much used, Rauwolfia alkaloids, which deplete biogenic amines (and cause depression), may occasionally work as well when newer antipsychotics do not (Ref. 6, p. 2274).

49.24. **(B)** Drugs which cause this extrapyramidal side effect, may also be able to inhibit its symptomatic manifestation. Thus, the patient may be "treated" with haloperidol. The resulting muscle tone may make the movement disorder less noticeable. This is like putting powder on a pimple. Although the abnormal movements, which disappear when the patient is asleep and which usually do not bother him, are most commonly seen in the mouth area, they can spread to other parts of the body. At this point, there is no good treatment for the condition (Ref. 7, p. 661).

49.25. **(E)** Anticholinergic side-effects include: dry mouth, blurred vision, palpitations, tachycardia, constipation, urinary retention, paralytic ileus, and a central anticholinergic syndrome (Ref. 6, p. 2298).

49.26. **(A)** Not all auditory hallucinations meet the diagnostic criteria for schizophrenic disorder as delineated in DSM-III (Ref. 2, p. 415).

49.27. **(E)** It is important to pick up this man's feeling tone and the fact that he may be suicidal. Every depressed patient should be asked about suicide. Later, there will be time for the investigation and treatment of his premature ejaculation, alcoholism, and marital conflicts—but not if the patient is already dead. All answers but E change the feeling tone (Ref. 7, pp. 144–171).

49.28. **(B)** This man has not a single symptom of schizophrenic disorder. He does have several symptoms of melancholia (Ref. 5, p. 307).

49.29. **(E)** Mourning is not a sign of melancholia. This is important in terms of pharmacotherapy, because the symptoms of melancholia are likely to respond to antidepressants (Ref. 5, p. 215).

49.30. **(E)** Somatization disorder usually begins in the 20s and runs a fluctuating course. The patient is rarely free of symptoms but lacks the characteristic signs and symptoms of depression. Hypochondriasis is characterized by the obsessive fear that one may have an illness and an unrealistic interpretation of symptoms as abnormal. Munchausen's syndrome, or chronic factitious illness with physical symptoms, is the diagnosis of people who feign a serious illness and make hospitalization a way of life. These patients differ from malingerers in that their only gain is hospitalization, to which they seem addicted (Refs. 4, p. 2002; 5, p. 247).

References

1. Arieti, S. (ed.): *American Handbook of Psychiatry*, 2nd Ed., Vol. 1, Basic Books, New York, 1975.

2. Allen, J.R. and Allen, B.A. *Psychiatry: A Guide*, Medical Examination Publishing, New Hyde Park, 1984.

3. Kaplan, H. I., Freedman, A.M., and Sadock, B.J.: *Comprehensive Textbook of Psychiatry*, 3rd Ed., Vol. 1, Williams and Wilkins, Baltimore,1980.

4. Kaplan, H.I., Freedman, A.M., and Sadock, B.J.: *Comprehensive Textbook of Psychiatry*, 3rd Ed., Vol. 2, Williams and Wilkins, Baltimore, 1980.

5. American Psychiatric Association. *Diagnostic and Statistical Manual of Mental Disorders*, 3rd Ed., American Psychiatric Association, Washington, D.C., 1980.

6. Kaplan, H.I., Freedman, A.M., and Sadock, B.J.: *Comprehensive Textbook of Psychiatry*, 3rd Ed., Vol. 3, Williams and Wilkins, Baltimore, 1980.

7. Arieti, S. (ed.): *Ibid*, Vol. 3, 1975.

8. Froelich, R. and Bishop, F.M.: *Clinical Interviewing Skills*, 3rd Ed., C.V. Mosby, St. Louis, MO, 1977.

9. Kolb, L. and Brodie, K.: *Modern Clinical Psychiatry*, 10th Ed., W.B. Saunders, Philadelphia, 1982.

PUBLIC HEALTH
AND COMMUNITY
MEDICINE

50

Public Health and Community Medicine
Raymond O. West, M.D., M.P.H.

DIRECTIONS: Each of the questions or incomplete statements below is followed by five suggested answers or completions. Select the **one** that is best in each case.

50.1. An adequate screening program for the persistent hyper-phenylalinemias, including PKU (phenylketonuria), and for congenital hypothyroidism (CH) should assure all of the following EXCEPT

    A. at least two-thirds participation of the eligible population

    B. notification of parents about newborn screening and their participation therein

    C. reliable and prompt performance of the screening test

    D. prompt follow-up of subjects with positive tests

    E. appropriate diagnosis of subjects with confirmed positive tests

50.2. Cases of toxic shock syndrome can be divided into two categories, namely, those which are associated with menstruation and those unassociated with menstruation. Nonmenstrual cases have been found in each of the following conditions EXCEPT
   A. subcutaneous lesions such as burns, abrasions, and insect bites
   B. septic surgical wounds
   C. therapeutic abortions
   D. vaginal delivery but not cesarean section
   E. furuncles and deep abscesses

50.3. Kawasaki syndrome has been called a "new multisystem disease of very young children." Because it is new, it has public health and community implications. There are six principal diagnostic criteria. Which of the following is NOT true?
   A. Fever for more than 5 days
   B. Changes in the mouth, such as strawberry tongue and diffuse oropharyngeal erythema
   C. Changes in the peripheral extremities, including induration of hands and feet and erythema of palms and soles
   D. A papular rash that rises to vesicles and pustules
   E. Enlarged lymph node mass, 1.5 cm in diameter

50.4. Statistics deal with material subject to inherent variability and it helps by providing a measure of doubt about theories. Which of the following is NOT true?
   A. Statistical theories can never be proved
   B. The null hypothesis states that the experimental results would not be due to chance variation
   C. The usual significant levels are 0.05 and 0.01
   D. If the null hypothesis is wrongly rejected, this is a type 1 error
   E. Failure to reject the null hypothesis when it is wrong is a type 2 error

50.5. Concerning cancer mortality in the United States:
- **A.** Lung cancer is still the leading cause of cancer death in men
- **B.** Cancer of the lung and cancer of the breast are equal causes of mortality in women
- **C.** Cancer of the colon and the rectum is the second cause of cancer death in men and third in women
- **D.** Cancer of the prostate is the third cause of cancer death in men
- **E.** The third cause of cancer death in women is uterine cancer

50.6. All of the following except one are significant pollutants of the air in the United States
- **A.** argon
- **B.** carbon monoxide
- **C.** sulphur oxides
- **D.** nitrogen oxides
- **E.** hydrocarbons

50.7. Regarding nutritional syndromes of public health importance, which of the following is NOT true?
- **A.** Xerophthalmia is a vitamin D deficiency
- **B.** Kwashiorkor results from a deficiency of protein relative to calories
- **C.** Marasmus occurs when both protein and calorie intake have been very limited to about the same degree
- **D.** Obesity is perhaps the most prevalent form of malnutrition in the United States and other industrialized countries
- **E.** Hemorrhagic disease of the newborn is a vitamin K deficiency

50.8. The prevention of dental caries is an important public health consideration. Which of the following statements is NOT true concerning fluoridation and prevention?
  A. The recommended daily dosage of fluoride for children above 3 years of age is less than 0.01 mg
  B. Adjusting the fluoride content of communal water supplies to approximately one part per million is the single most important method of dental caries prevention
  C. Children consuming a therapeutically optimum amount of fluoride in their drinking water experience 50—60% less dental decay than children using fluoride-deficient water
  D. Most large U.S. cities have fluoridated their water supply
  E. Worldwide, approximately 320 million people are consuming drinking water containing optimal levels of fluorides

50.9. Regarding suicide and parasuicide, which of the following is NOT true?
  A. Those who have never married and those who have divorced carry a higher risk of suicide than those who are married
  B. Women have higher rates than men in all age groups
  C. Suicide rates are traditionally highest in the middle- and old-age groups
  D. There is a higher than average frequency of suicide among alcoholics
  E. About 10% of those with a history of parasuicide will eventually kill themselves

50.10. Regarding preventable mental illnesses, which of the following is NOT true?
- **A.** The decline in cases of general paresis psychosis is not so much because of the decline in the annual incidence of syphilis as because of public health meaures to find cases and insure effective treatment in the early stages
- **B.** Pellagra psychosis is the best example of a documented mental disorder produced by nutritional deficiency
- **C.** The likelihood of a child being born with Down's syndrome declines steeply as the mother ages
- **D.** Gregg, the Australian ophthalmologist, observed in 1941 an epidemic of congenital cataracts following an epidemic of German measles and associated the two
- **E.** The number of cases of brain damage following an attack of measles far exceeds the number with clinically obvious encephalitis

50.11. All of the following are metabolic disorders that can cause chronic, disabling conditions of public health importance EXCEPT
- **A.** Tay-Sachs disease
- **B.** galactosemia
- **C.** maple syrup urine disease
- **D.** senile dementia, Alzheimer's type
- **E.** homocystinuria

50.12. Data derived from the Framingham study illustrate the risk factor status of hypertension for all of the following EXCEPT
- **A.** CHD (coronary heart disease)
- **B.** Intermittent claudication
- **C.** Atherothrombotic brain infarction
- **D.** Congestive heart failure
- **E.** Pulmonary infarct

50.13. Which of the following is not a valid reason why, in a food-borne outbreak, not everyone who eats the implicated food becomes ill?
  A. Food histories may be faulty because of uncertain recall, lying, or errors in recording
  B. Incubation period so short that the association between eating and becoming ill is ignored
  C. The implicated food may not be contaminated throughout
  D. Dosage (the quantity consumed) varies
  E. Host susceptibility varies

DIRECTIONS: The group of questions below consists of five lettered headings followed by a list of numbered words or statements. For each numbered word or statement, select the **one** lettered heading that is most closely associated with it. Each lettered heading may be selected once, more than once, or not at all.

  A. Arithmetic mean
  B. Median
  C. Gaussian distribution
  D. Skewed
  E. Mode

50.14. One-half the observations fall below and one-half above the value

50.15. Most frequently encountered measurement

50.16. Mean, median, and mode are located at different points on a curve

50.17. Mean, median, and mode all fall in the same location on a curve

50.18. Average

DIRECTIONS: The set of lettered headings below is followed by a list of numbered words or phrases. For each numbered word or phrase select

    (A)   if the item is associated with A only
    (B)   if the item is associated with B only
    (C)   if the item is associated with both A and B
    (D)   if the item is associated with neither A nor B

  A. The ability of a test to single out subjects who have a disease that the test should be able to identify
  B. The ability of a test to classify subjects who do not have a specific illness as negative
  C. Both
  D. Neither

50.19. Sensitivity

50.20. Specificity

50.21. Predictive value

DIRECTIONS: For each of the questions or incomplete statements below, **one or more** of the answers or completions given is correct. Select

    (A)   if only 1, 2, and 3 are correct
    (B)   if only 1 and 3 are correct
    (C)   if only 2 and 4 are correct
    (D)   if only 4 is correct
    (E)   if all are correct

50.22. Descriptive epidemiology is concerned with the study of the distribution of disease in population groups. The objectives are

  1. to permit evaluation of trends in health and comparisons among subgroups within (and between) countries
  2. to provide a basis for planning, provision and evaluation of health services
  3. to identify problems to be studied by analytic methods
  4. to suggest areas that may be fruitful for investigation

50.23. Which of the following statements refer to gonorrhea as it occurs currently in the United States?
1. Gonorrhea is the most frequently reported communicable disease in the United States
2. A sharp increase of reported cases in the late 1960s and early 1970s probably represents a real increase in the occurrence of this disease
3. The same increase also is felt to represent improved case detection procedures
4. Reported cases number approximately one million per year

50.24. A strain of gonococci resistant to all forms of penicillin has emerged—penicillinase-producing *Neisseria gonorrhoea* (PPNG). A significant proportion of PPNG cases are related to importation of infection from
1. Southeast Asia
2. Canada
3. the west coast of Africa
4. Mexico

50.25. The extent to which injury saps the resources of the nation is not commonly recognized. Which of the following is true?
1. Unintentional injury is the fourth leading cause of death in the United States
2. Unintentional injuries are the leading cause of death under age 40
3. Among the young, unintentional injuries contribute more deaths than all other causes combined
4. In contrast, homicides and suicides contribute less than 10,000 deaths/year in the United States

50.26. In general, demography, the study of human population, deals with fertility, mortality, and migration. Which of the following is true?
1. Demographers define fertility as the production of live births
2. Fecundity is the ability to produce live births
3. Pregnancy rates refer to the number of conceptions
4. Fertility rates include only live births and do not count fetal deaths or abortions

DIRECTIONS: This section of the test consists of situations, each followed by a series of questions. Study each situation and select the **one** best answer to each question following it.

Questions 50.27–50.28: A 27-year-old man developed mild rhinorrhea and shortly thereafter experienced pain in his left leg, fever, and headache. He was hospitalized and found to have marked weakness of muscle groups in the left leg, including footdrop. A cerebrospinal fluid examination was abnormal in that it contained an increased amount of white blood cells and the protein was 38 mg/dl.

50.27. The most likely diagnosis that should be considered by his physician is
   A. botulism
   B. chemical food poisoning
   C. poliomyelitis
   D. Reye's syndrome
   E. Guillain-Barré syndrome

50.28. Regarding polio vaccine and vaccinations, which of the following is NOT true?
   A. Two kinds of polio vaccine are used. They are inactivated polio vaccine (IPV) and oral polio vaccine (OPV)
   B. OPV is the vaccine of choice for primary vaccination of children in the United States
   C. Few adults in the United States possess immunity to the three types of polio virus
   D. Poliomyelitis among contacts of vaccinees could be prevented if all persons were immune to all three polio virus types before having contact with a vaccinee
   E. Responsible adults should be informed of the small risk of vaccine-associated poliomyelitis when OPV is administered to a child who may have household contact with adults

Questions 50.29–50.30: A 14-year-old girl is seen in the emergency room of a local hospital with gradually increasing muscular weakness, difficulty in swallowing, bilateral ptosis, and diplopia. She is afebrile and has no meningeal signs. No muscle twitching is noted. She is hospitalized and within 2 days two other members of the family present similar signs and symptoms. At this time the 14-year-old girl expires. All members of the family live on a farm and have not left the community for 18 months. No others in the community have been found to have similar complaints.

50.29. The most likely diagnosis is
A. acute encephalitis
B. tetanus
C. botulism
D. poliomyelitis
E. rabies

50.30. A check shows that four members of the family who were not taken ill did not consume canned string beans, whereas those who were taken ill had eaten them. The most likely diagnosis now is
A. *Salmonella* food poisoning
B. botulism
C. typhoid fever
D. rabies
E. trichinosis

Question 50.31: Refer to Figure 111.

50.31. Figure 111, which concerns tuberculosis, leads to which of the following possible conclusions?
A. Tuberculosis is increasing in the United States
B. Tuberculosis is decreasing in the United States
C. The data presented is in the form of rates and does not provide a *total number* of cases
D. This is point prevalence data
E. This data means nothing without first adjusting for sex, race, and socioeconomic status

TUBERCULOSIS

TUBERCULOSIS — Reported cases and cases per 100,000 population by age group,
United States, 1980

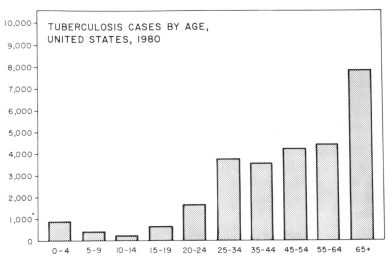

Figure 111

Answers and Comments

50.1. (A) Two-thirds participation is not enough. Participation must be by the entire eligible population. All of the other points are correct and, in addition to these, appropriate counseling and treatment of patients must be included. In the United States, a reliable screening test is a blood sample taken from every infant before he or she leaves the nursery regardless of age. Heel blood is used for PKU and either heel or cord blood for CH. The sample should be taken as close as possible to the time of discharge from the nursery (Ref. 1, p. 186).

50.2. (D) Indeed, menstrual cases of TSS have been associated with both childbirth by vaginal delivery and cesarean section. Cases associated with menstruation are far more common than the 15% or so that are considered to be nonmenstrual. Women can reduce the risk of TSS by not using tampons and women who choose to wear them can reduce the risk by wearing them intermittently during the menstrual period (Ref. 2, pp. 202–204).

50.3. (D) The rash of Kawasaki syndrome is erythematous. Diagnosis must be made by strict adherence to the six criteria, which include lymph node enlargement. This latter is seen in only half of the cases. Many other illnesses, such as measles, leptospirosis, streptococcal scarlet fever, exanthematous diseases such as Rocky Mountain spotted fever, enteroviral illnesses, and many others, must be excluded. About 2% of Kawasaki syndrome patients die, usually of massive myocardial infarction that results from acute thrombosis of aneurysmally dilated coronary arteries (Ref. 3, pp. 99–106).

50.4. (B) The null hypothesis, in fact, states that the experimental results are due only to chance variation. It is accepted as true until sufficient evidence is collected to reject it. The value of significance testing is that the tests give us a measure for our doubts about the reality of observed differences (Ref. 4, p. 140).

50.5. (E) All of the statements are true except E. Cancer of the uterus is now only 5% in women; a fortuitous drop in the past several years, no doubt because of the improvements in diagnosis and treatment. Percentages for cancer deaths in men are, lung 35%, colon and rectum 12%, prostate, 10%, and leukemia and lymphomas 8%. For women they are, breast 18%, lung 18%, colon and rectum 15%. Ovary and uterus are 5% each (Ref. 5, p. 19).

50.6. (A) Argon, although a constituent of air is not a pollutant. It is a normal constituent of air, polluted or otherwise. All of the others are correct. More than two hundred million tons of toxic materials are released into the atmosphere above the United States yearly. This is about one ton per person. About 60% comes from approximately 100 million internal combustion engines and the other 40% from factories fired by incinerators. In the United States more than 6000 communities are considered affected in varying degrees by air pollution (Ref. 11, p. 330).

50.7. (A) Xerophthalmia is a vitamin A deficiency. Vitamin A is a component of the visual purple of the retina and is essential to normal vision. In vitamin A deficiency, secreting epithelium tends to keratinize and cease functioning, resulting in a wide variety of symptoms. One of the common symptoms is nyctalopia, sometimes called "night blindness." This is defective vision in dim light, related to interference with formation of the visual purple of the rods of the retina (Ref. 6, pp. 1474–1477).

50.8. (A) The recommended daily dosage of fluoride for children above 3 years of age is 1 mg. This can be obtained by drinking 1 L of water with a concentratrion of one part per million fluoridation. In the United States, of the 57 cities with populations of one quarter of a million or more, only 13 do not have optimal fluoride levels and of the 6 largest cities, only Los Angeles is not fluoridated. The Republic of Ireland is the only country to adopt legislation requiring nationwide fluoridation (Ref. 6, pp. 1429–1433).

50.9. (B) Men have higher rates than women at all age groups. However, the gap between men and women is decreasing because of increased suicide rates for all female age groups. Suicide is an important factor at both extremes of socioeconomic status. Alcohol is often used when suicide is being committed. Suicide shows seasonal variations, with the highest rate being in the spring (Ref. 6, pp. 1364–1365).

50.10. (C) The likelihood of a child being born with Down's Syndrome rises steeply after his mother reaches age 35. Indeed, amniocentesis in the 40 and over age group is clearly justified because the risk in this age group is 1 in 50 compared with 1 in 1000 in the youngest maternal age group (Ref. 6, pp. 1324–1325).

50.11. (D) One can hardly call Alzheimer's syndrome metabolic because the cause or causes are totally unknown. Tay-Sachs disease is caused by the defective metabolism of gangliosides. Maple syrup urine disease is a disorder of branched-chain amino acids. Galactosemia results from a deficiency of the enzyme galactokinase. Homocystinuria is caused by the diminished activity of cystachioline synthetase, an enzyme important in the pathway that converts methionine to cystine. So these are all metabolic except SDAT (Ref. 6, pp. 1260–1261).

50.12. (E) The risk of these cardiovascular diseases increases from normal tension to borderline to hypertensive. We know of no data to indicate that pulmonary infarct is related to hypertension, whether borderline or severe (Ref. 6, p. 1207).

50.13. (B) Short incubation period poses no epidemiologic problem. Contrariwise, it's the long incubation illnesses (such as hepatitis A) that are hard (often impossible) to relate to a specific food item eaten at a specific time—maybe as long ago as 30 days (Ref. 6, pp. 308–309).

50.14. (B)
50.15. (E)
50.16. (D)
50.17. (C)
50.18. (A) The arithmetic mean is usually called the average, whereas the median is defined as one-half the observations falling below and one-half above the value. The mode is the most frequently encountered measurement. The Gaussian distribution is another name for the "normal curve," a curve in which the mean, median, and mode are located all at the same location on a curve. And if the curve is skewed, then the mean, median, and mode are located at different points on the curve (Ref. 7, p. 122).

50.19. (A) Sensitivity is a test power to find an illness if it is present. For example, high serum glucose is a relatively sensitive study to diagnose diabetes mellitus (Ref. 7, pp. 157–158).

50.20. (B) Specificity is the ability of a test to reject the diagnosis of an illness if it is not present. For example, a negative x-ray of the chest is fairly specific to rule out lobar pneumonia (Ref. 7, pp. 157–158).

50.21. (D) Predictive value of a "diagnostic endeavor" gives the frequency with which a positive test actually signifies disease (Ref. 7, pp. 157–158).

50.22. (E) All four of these answers are correct. Descriptive epidemiology describes populations of persons who have health conditions in common. Common descriptive variables are person, place, and time (Ref. 8, p. 150).

50.23. (E) The graph shown in Figure 112 indicates reported civilian case rates by year in the United States from 1941 to 1980. Since 1973, federally assisted state and local programs have been implemented to control gonorrhea and the reported number of cases has plateaued at about a million cases a year (Ref. 9, pp. 34–35).

GONORRHEA

Gonorrhea — Reported civilian case rates by year, United States, 1941-1980

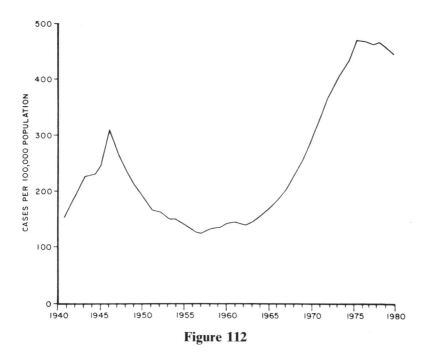

Figure 112

50.24. (B) Canada and Mexico are not thought to be significant in the importation of PPNG. Indeed, data from 1980 suggests an increasing occurrence of PPNG cases within the United States. Control efforts include intensive surveillance, case detection, treatment, and contact tracing. These efforts have been able to contain all outbreaks and most cases continue to be imported or linked to imported cases (Ref. 9, pp. 34–35).

50.25. (A) Homicide constitutes about 20,000 and suicides close to 30,000 deaths/year. The financial costs of injury are considerable— an estimate of 47 billion dollars in 1977 (Ref. 6, pp. 1554–1555).

50.26. (E) Fecundity is difficult to measure because it refers to the theoretical ability of a woman to conceive and carry a fetus to term.

For this reason, most demographic studies relate to fertility rather than fecundity. One should note that the words fertility and fecundity in French and Spanish are reversed. For example, the English "fertility" translates as "fecundite" in French (Ref. 6, pp. 1504–1505).

50.27. **(C)** This is most likely poliomyelitis, at least on the basis of information provided. Neither botulism or Guillain-Barré syndrome are likely to result in weakness of specific muscle groups. The cerebrospinal fluid in Guillain-Barré syndrome would almost certainly show increased protein of 100 mg/100 ml. Chemical food poisoning almost certainly would result in an acute illness characterized by nausea, vomiting, and abdominal pain. Reye's syndrome is much more likely to attack a younger individual and result in coma if untreated. This, indeed, was a case of poliomyelitis. The man had spent a day with relatives, including an 8-week-old infant who had received her first oral polio virus vaccine 8 days before the visit (Ref. 10, pp. 97–98).

50.28. **(C)** Most adults in the United States do possess immunity even with no record of ever being vaccinated. It is recommended that responsible adults be informed of the risk, etc. and that OPV be administered to a child regardless of the vaccination status of adult household contacts. Both OPV and IPV are effective in preventing polio but the Immunization Practices Advisory Committee of the Public Health Service has considered the benefits and risks of each vaccine to the entire population and have recommended OPV as the vaccine of choice for primary vaccination of children in the United States. Fortunately, OPV-associated polio is rare. Between 1969 and 1980, close to 300 million doses of OPV were distributed in the United States and only 93 cases of vaccine-associated poliomyelitis were reported. Of the 93 cases, 36 occurred among vaccine recipients and 57 among household or community contacts of vaccinees. Vaccine-related poliomyelitis is most frequently associated with polio virus types II and III (Ref. 10, pp. 97–98).

50.29. **(C)** Botulism is an intoxication characterized by frequent ptosis, blurred or double vision, and dry, sore throat. Progressive, descending paralysis, usually but not always symmetrical, may develop. Conspicuously absent are objective sensory abnormalities, altered mental status, and fever. The case/fatality rate for classical food-borne botulism was formerly about 60% but in the last decade less than 30% of cases expired. Respiratory paralysis is generally the immediate cause of death (Ref. 6, pp. 314–315).

50.30. (B) Most cases of classic botulism are caused by foods that received some preliminary heat treatment such as canning or smoking. About 90% of all outbreaks in recent years were due to improper home canning, rather than commercial canning. The string beans involved in this outbreak had been canned at home. Home canning at temperatures insufficient to destroy spores is the usual problem. Resistance of spores to heat sterilization is reduced at a low pH and this is why highly acid fruits are rarely implicated in outbreaks and why acidification of home canned vegetables (with vinegar or lemon juice) is recommended before pressure cooking as an extra measure of protection (Ref. 6, pp. 314–315).

50.31. (C) These are rates, specific for age; without denominators they tell nothing of total number of new cases. This is incidence data. There is no need for adjusting (or standardizing) because no comparison with other years or other nations is made. Increase or decrease (secular change) is not discernible from this data (Ref. 9, p. 88).

References

1. Morbidity and Mortality Weekly Report, Vol. 31, No. 15, April 23, 1982.

2. Morbidity and Mortality Weekly Report, Vol. 31, No. 16, April 30, 1982.

3. Melish, M.E., et al.: Kawasaki syndrome: An update. Hosp. Pract. March, 1982.

4. Castle, W.M.: *Statistics in Small Doses*, 2nd Ed., Churchill Livingstone, Edinburgh, 1977.

5. CA—A Cancer Journal for Clinicians, Vol 35, No. 1, February 1985.

6. Last, J.M.: *Public Health and Preventive Medicine*, 11th Ed., Appleton-Century-Crofts, New York, 1980.

7. Gehlbach, S.H.: *Interpreting the Medical Literature—A Clinician's Guide*, Collamore Press, D.C. Health and Co., Lexington, MA, 1982.

8. Mausner, J.S. and Bahn, A.K.: *Epidemiology, Introductory Text*, W.B. Saunders, Philadelphia, 1985.

9. Morbidity and Mortality Weekly Report Annual Summary, 1980, Vol. 29, No. 54, September, 1981.

10. Morbidity and Mortality Weekly Report, Vol. 31, No. 8, March 5, 1982.

11. Hanlon, J.J. and Pickett, G.E.: *Public Health Administration and Practice*, 8th Ed., Times Mirror/Mosby, St. Louis, 1985.